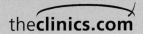

NEUROIMAGING CLINICS

Molecular Neuroimaging

Guest Editor
DAWID SCHELLINGERHOUT, MD

Consulting Editors
MAURICIO CASTILLO, MD, FACR
SURESH K. MUKHERJI, MD

November 2006 • Volume 16 • Number 4

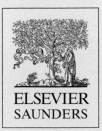

ELSEVIER
SAUNDERS

An imprint of Elsevier, Inc
PHILADELPHIA LONDON TORONTO MONTREAL SYDNEY TOKYO

W.B. SAUNDERS COMPANY

A Division of Elsevier Inc.

1600 John F. Kennedy Boulevard • Suite 1800 • Philadelphia, Pennsylvania 19103-2899

http://www.theclinics.com

NEUROIMAGING CLINICS Volume 16, Number 4
November 2006 ISSN 1052-5149, ISBN 1-4160-3893-0

Editor: Barton Dudlick

The ideas and opinions expressed in *Neuroimaging Clinics* do not necessarily reflect those of the Publisher. The Publisher does not assume any responsibility for any injury and/or damage to persons or property arising out of or related to any use of the material contained in this periodical. The reader is advised to check the appropriate medical literature and the product information currently provided by the manufacturer of each drug to be administered to verify the dosage, the method and duration of administration, or contraindications. It is the responsibility of the treating physician or other health care professional, relying on independent experience and knowledge of the patient, to determine drug dosages and the best treatment for the patient. Mention of any product in this issue should not be construed as endorsement by the contributors, editors, or the Publisher of the product or manufacturers' claims.

Neuroimaging Clinics (ISSN 1052-5149) is published quarterly by Elsevier Inc., 360 Park Avenue South, New York, NY 10010-1710. Months of issue are February, May, August, and November. Business and editorial offices: 1600 John F. Kennedy Blvd., Suite 1800, Philadelphia, PA 19103-2899. Business and editorial offices: 6277 Sea Harbor Drive, Orlando, FL 32887-4800. Periodicals postage paid at New York, NY, and additional mailing offices. Subscription prices are USD 218 per year for US individuals, USD 336 per year for US institutions, USD 112 per year for US students and residents, USD 252 per year for Canadian individuals, USD 413 per year for Canadian institutions, USD 302 per year for international individuals, USD 413 per year for international institutions and USD 151 per year for Canadian and foreign students and residents. To receive student/resident rate, orders must be accompanied by name of affiliated institution, date of term, and the *signature* of program/residency coordinator on institution letterhead. Orders will be billed at individual rate until proof of status is received. Foreign air speed delivery is included in all *Clinics* subscription prices. All prices are subject to change without notice. POSTMASTER: Send address changes to *Neuroimaging Clinics*, Elsevier Periodicals Customer Service, 6277 Sea Harbor Drive, Orlando, FL 32887-4800. **Customer Service: 1-800-654-2452 (US). From outside of the US, call (+1) 407-345-4000. E-mail: hhspcs@harcourt.com**.

Reprints. For copies of 100 or more, of articles in this publication, please contact the Commercial Reprints Department, Elsevier Inc., 360 Park Avenue South, New York, New York 10010-1710. Tel.: (+1) 212-633-3813; Fax: (+1) 212-462-1935; E-mail: reprints@elsevier.com.

Neuroimaging Clinics is covered by *Excerpta Medica/EMBASE*, the RSNA Index of Imaging Literature, Index Medicus, MEDLINE/MEDLARS, SciSearch, Research Alert, and Neuroscience Citation Index.

Printed in the United States of America.

GOAL STATEMENT

The goal of *Neuroimaging Clinics of North America* is to keep practicing radiologists and radiology residents up to date with current clinical practice in radiology by providing timely articles reviewing the state of the art in patient care.

ACCREDITATION

The *Neuroimaging Clinics of North America* is planned and implemented in accordance with the Essential Areas and Policies of the Accreditation Council for Continuing Medical Education (ACCME) through the joint sponsorship of the University of Virginia School of Medicine and Elsevier. The University of Virginia School of Medicine is accredited by the ACCME to provide continuing medical education for physicians.

The University of Virginia School of Medicine designates this educational activity for a maximum of 60 *AMA PRA Category 1 Credits*™. Physicians should only claim credit commensurate with the extent of their participation in the activity.

The American Medical Association has determined that physicians not licensed in the US who participate in this CME activity are eligible for *AMA PRA Category 1 Credits*™.

Category 1 credit can be earned by reading the text material, taking the CME examination online at http://www.theclinics.com/home/cme, and completing the evaluation. After taking the test, you will be required to review any and all incorrect answers. Following completion of the test and evaluation, your credit will be awarded and you may print your certificate.

FACULTY DISCLOSURE/CONFLICT OF INTEREST

The University of Virginia School of Medicine, as an ACCME accredited provider, endorses and strives to comply with the Accreditation Council for Continuing Medical Education (ACCME) Standards of Commercial Support, Commonwealth of Virginia statutes, University of Virginia policies and procedures, and associated federal and private regulations and guidelines on the need for disclosure and monitoring of proprietary and financial interests that may affect the scientific integrity and balance of content delivered in continuing medical education activities under our auspices.

The University of Virginia School of Medicine requires that all CME activities accredited through this institution be developed independently and be scientifically rigorous, balanced and objective in the presentation/discussion of its content, theories and practices.

All authors/editors participating in an accredited CME activity are expected to disclose to the readers relevant financial relationships with commercial entities occurring within the past 12 months (such as grants or research support, employee, consultant, stock holder, member of speakers bureau, etc.). The University of Virginia School of Medicine will employ appropriate mechanisms to resolve potential conflicts of interest to maintain the standards of fair and balanced education to the reader. Questions about specific strategies can be directed to the Office of Continuing Medical Education, University of Virginia School of Medicine, Charlottesville, Virginia.

The authors/editors listed below have identified no professional/financial affiliations for themselves or their spouse/partner:
Barton Dudlick (Acquisitions Editor); S. John Gatley, PhD; Juri Gelovani, MD, PhD; Alexander Hammers, PhD; Aparna H. Kesarwala, AB; Kimberly P. Lindsey, PhD; Anne Lingford-Hughes, PhD; Mark E. Mullins, MD, PhD; Andrea Pichler, PhD; Julie L. Prior, BA; Dawid Schellingerhout, MD, MBChB; Vijay Sharma, PhD; and, Pia C. Sundgren, MD, PhD.

The authors listed below have identified the following professional/financial affiliations for themselves or their spouse/partner:
Thomas L. Chenevert, PhD is on the speaker's bureau for Philips Medical Systems and is a patent holder at the University of Michigan.
Christopher H. Contag is a consultant for Xenogen Corp./Caliper Life Science.
Homer A. Macapinlac, MD is on the speaker's bureau for GE Healthcare, Siemens, and Radiology Corp of America; and, is on the advisory committee/board for GE Healthcare and Radiology Corp of America.
David Piwnica-Worms, MD, PhD is a consultant for Bristol Meyers Squibb.
Brian D. Ross, PhD has part ownership in the company Imbio; the technology of Diffusion MRI, which has been licensed to Imbio, is being commercialized by Cedera Software through an agreement with Imbio.

Disclosure of Discussion of non-FDA approved uses for pharmaceutical products and/or medical devices.
The University of Virginia School of Medicine, as an ACCME provider, requires that all authors/editors identify and disclose any "off label" uses for pharmaceutical products and/or for medical devices. The University of Virginia School of Medicine recommends that each reader fully review all the available data on new products or procedures prior to instituting them with patients.

TO ENROLL

To enroll in the Neuroimaging Clinics of North America Continuing Medical Education program, call customer service at 1-800-654-2452 or sign up online at *http://www.theclinics.com/home/cme*. The CME program is available to subscribers for an additional annual fee of USD 175.

MOLECULAR NEUROIMAGING

MARK E. MULLINS, MD, PhD
Assistant Professor of Radiology, Assistant
Professor of Neurology and Neurological Surgery,
Director of Medical Student Radiology Education,
Associate Director of Radiology Residency
Training Program, Director of Stroke Imaging,
Radiology, Emory University Hospital, Atlanta,
Georgia

ANDREA PICHLER, PhD
Molecular Imaging Center, Washington
University Medical School, St. Louis,
Missouri

DAVID PIWNICA-WORMS, MD, PhD
Molecular Imaging Center, Mallinckrodt
Institute of Radiology and Department
of Molecular Biology and Pharmacology,
Washington University Medical School, St. Louis,
Missouri

JULIE L. PRIOR, BA
Molecular Imaging Center, Washington University
Medical School, St. Louis, Missouri

BRIAN D. ROSS, PhD
Department of Radiology, University of Michigan
Health Systems, Ann Arbor, Michigan

DAWID SCHELLINGERHOUT, MD
Assistant Professor, Neuroradiology Section,
Department of Radiology and Experimental
Diagnostic Imaging, Division of Diagnostic
Imaging, M D Anderson Cancer Center, Houston,
Texas

VIJAY SHARMA, PhD
Molecular Imaging Center, Washington University
Medical School, St. Louis, Missouri

PIA C. SUNDGREN, MD, PhD
Department of Radiology, University of Michigan
Health Systems, Ann Arbor, Michigan

MOLECULAR NEUROIMAGING

Volume 16 • Number 4 • November 2006

Contents

Many breakthrough scientific discoveries have been made using opioid imaging, particularly in the fields of pain, addiction and epilepsy research. Recent developments include the application of ever higher resolution whole-brain positron emission tomography (PET) scanners, the availability of several radioligands, the combination of PET with advanced structural imaging, advances in modeling macroparameters of PET ligand binding, and large-scale statistical analysis of imaging datasets. Suitable single-photon emission computed tomography (SPECT) tracers are lacking, but with the increase in the number of available PET (or PET/CT) cameras and cyclotrons thanks to the clinical successes of PET in oncology, PET may become widespread enough to overcome this limitation. In the coming decade, we hope to see a more widespread application of the techniques developed in healthy volunteers to patients and more clinical impact of opioid imaging.

Recent technologic advances make it increasingly possible to image neurotransmitter systems in living human brain. The dopamine system has been most intensively studied owing to its involvement in several brain disorders, including motor disorders such as Parkinson's disease and Huntington's disease, as well as psychiatric disorders such as schizophrenia, depression, and compulsive behavioral disorders of multiple types. A variety of aspects of dopamine receptor density, function, and dopaminergic terminal status can now be assessed using the minimally invasive neuroimaging techniques of positron emission tomography and single-photon emission computed tomography. Although these techniques are currently used most often in the context of research, clinical applications are rapidly emerging.

David Piwnica-Worms, Aparna H. Kesarwala, Andrea Pichler, Julie L. Prior, and Vijay Sharma

Overexpression of multi-drug resistant P-glycoprotein (Pgp) remains an important barrier to successful chemotherapy in cancer patients and impacts the pharmacokinetics of many important drugs. Pgp is also expressed on the luminal surface of brain capillary endothelial cells wherein Pgp functionally comprises a major component of the blood–brain barrier by limiting central nervous system penetration of various therapeutic agents. In addition, Pgp in brain capillary endothelial cells removes amyloid-beta from the brain. Several single photon emission computed tomography and positron emission tomography radiopharmaceuticals have been shown to be transported by Pgp, thereby enabling the noninvasive interrogation of Pgp-mediated transport activity in vivo. Therefore, molecular imaging of Pgp activity may enable noninvasive dynamic monitoring of multi-drug resistance in cancer, guide therapeutic choices in cancer chemotherapy, and identify transporter deficiencies of the blood–brain barrier in Alzheimer's disease.

Homer A. Macapinlac

Positron emission tomography (PET) is a technique that allows imaging of the temporal and spatial distribution of positron-emitting radionuclides. The purpose of this article is to outline the current clinical use for PET imaging in the brain and other radiopharmaceuticals used for assessing various physiologic parameters pertaining to tumor metabolism.

Mark E. Mullins

MR spectroscopy involves the examination of molecules in a much more transparent manner than does routine, clinical, conventional MR imaging. Its performance and interpretation goes back to the origins of MR imaging in nuclear magnetic resonance and also points to a future in which functional-type techniques such as molecular imaging tell more than simple anatomy, but also the physiology of what is seen when looking at a patient's radiological images. A brief discussion of the past, present, and possible future of MR spectroscopy is examined herein to provide a framework for appreciation of MR spectroscopy as a molecular imaging modality. Several techniques, applications, and controversies also are discussed in this article.

Thomas L. Chenevert, Pia C. Sundgren, and Brian D. Ross

Diffusion MR imaging techniques are based on the molecular mobility of water, which is sensitive to interaction with intracellular elements, macromolecules, cell membranes, the density of cells, and microstructural organization. Disease processes that alter cell-water homeostasis, cell density, and cytoarchitecture affect water mobility and are quantifiable by diffusion MR imaging methodologies. Similarly, therapeutic intervention that alters these properties may be monitored for efficacy via diffusion MR imaging. This article outlines basic technical concepts and applications of diffusion imaging with an emphasis on oncology.

Molecular Imaging Using Visible Light to Reveal Biological Changes in the Brain 633

Christopher H. Contag

Advances in imaging have enabled the study of cellular and molecular processes in the context of the living body that include cell migration patterns, location and extent of gene expression, degree of protein–protein interaction, and levels of enzyme activity. These tools, which operate over a range of scales, resolutions, and sensitivities, have opened up broad new areas of investigation where the influence of organ systems and functional circulation is intact. There are a myriad of imaging modalities available, each with its own advantages and disadvantages, depending on the specific application. Among these modalities, optical imaging techniques, including in vivo bioluminescence imaging and fluorescence imaging, use visible light to interrogate biology in the living body. Optimal imaging with these modalities requires that the appropriate marker be used to tag the process of interest to make it uniquely visible using a particular imaging technology. For each optical modality, there are various labels to choose from that range from dyes that permit tissue contrast and dyes that can be activated by enzymatic activity, to gene-encoding proteins with optical signatures that can be engineered into specific biological processes. This article provides an overview of optical imaging technologies and commonly used labels, focusing on bioluminescence and fluorescence, and describes several examples of how these tools are applied to biological questions relating to the central nervous system.

Molecular Imaging of Novel Cell- and Viral-Based Therapies 655

Dawid Schellingerhout

Drugs, surgery, and radiation are the traditional modalities of therapy in medicine. To these are being added new therapies based on cells and viruses or their derivatives. In these novel therapies, a cell or viral vector acts as a drug in its own right, altering the host or a disease process to bring about healing. Most of these advances originate from the significant recent advances in molecular medicine, but some have been around for some time. Blood transfusions and cowpox vaccinations are part of the history of medicine… but nevertheless are examples of cell- and viral-based therapies. This article focuses on the modern molecular incarnations of these therapies, and specifically on how imaging is used to track and guide these novel agents. We survey the literature dealing with imaging these new cell and viral particle therapies and provide a framework for understanding publications in this area. Leading technology of gene modifications are the fundamental modifications applied to make these new therapies amenable to imaging.

Clinical Trials in a Molecular World 681

Dawid Schellingerhout and Juri Gelovani

New therapies aimed at molecular abnormalities are often more efficacious and less toxic than nontargeted therapies; however, with current technology, major treatment decisions are being made with inadequate data. This problem needs to be fixed by molecular imaging technology, enabling the noninvasive establishment of the presence of a molecular target, its spatial distribution and heterogeneity, and how this changes over time. This article discusses the status of molecular imaging in clinical trails today, and looks forward to what physicians would like it to become.

Index 695

NEUROIMAGING CLINICS OF NORTH AMERICA

Neuroimag Clin N Am 16 (2006) xi–xii

Foreword

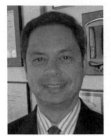 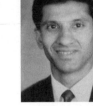

Mauricio Castillo, MD   Suresh K. Mukherji, MD
Guest Editors

Mauricio Castillo, MD
Professor and Chief
Division of Neuroradiology
Department of Radiology
University of North Carolina School of Medicine
Campus Box 7510
Chapel Hill, NC 27599-7510, USA

E-mail address:
castillo@med.unc.edu

Suresh K. Mukherji, MD
Professor and Chief
Neuroradiology and Head & Neck Radiology
Professor
Radiology and Otolaryngology Head & Neck Surgery
Associate Fellowship Program Director
Department of Radiology, B2 A209-0030
University of Michigan Health System
1500 East Medical Center Drive
Ann Arbor, MI 48109-0030, USA

E-mail address:
mukherji@umich.edu

The natural progression of the imaging sciences is clearly evident by the topic chosen for this issue of *Neuroimaging Clinics*. Radiology started as only an anatomic specialty, often using contrast agents to indirectly identify aberrations in this anatomy. This era of imaging lasted until the advent of nuclear medicine, which allowed us to indirectly probe and visualize some physiological and biological changes in the human body. The introduction of magnetic resonance imaging provided investigators with greater spatial resolution and the possibility of evaluating many physiological processes. Thus, although radiology debuted as an anatomic specialty, it then progressed to gross physiology,

microscopical physiology, chemistry, and now molecular imaging!

In this extremely interesting issue, Dr. Schellingerhout, colleagues, and guest authors offer us, clinical neuroradiologists, a view into the future of imaging. Certainly molecular neuroimaging is not something that most of us are familiar with. It does, however, behoove us to become familiar with at least some aspects of it because it clearly is the way of the future. Although molecular neuroimaging as a whole is still something that is not routinely used in clinical practice, some aspects of it—such as MR spectroscopy—have become very popular and widely used as of late. PET is another technique that

doi:10.1016/j.nic.2006.11.003

has been smoothly incorporated into our neuro-imaging armamentarium. Of the newer techniques, perhaps the one that neuroradiologists are most familiar with is diffusion imaging. These topics are well discussed in this issue, yet this issue goes further, providing the reader with more than a glimpse into topics such as opioid receptor and dopamine imaging. Cellular and viral-based therapies are also addressed, and the issue comes to a close with an overview of clinical trials in a molecular world. We thank Dr. Schellingerhout and his collaborators for providing us with a brief, but powerful and informative, view into the exciting future of not only neuroimaging but radiology as a whole.

NEUROIMAGING
CLINICS
OF NORTH AMERICA

Neuroimag Clin N Am 16 (2006) xiii–xiv

Preface

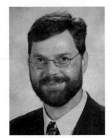

Dawid Schellingerhout, MD
*Neuroradiology Section, Department of Radiology
and Experimental Diagnostic Imaging, Division
of Diagnostic Imaging, University of Texas, M D
Anderson Cancer Center, 1515 Holcombe Blvd.,
Houston, TX 77030, USA*

E-mail address:
dawid.schellingerhout@di.mdacc.tmc.edu

Dawid Schellingerhout, MD
Guest Editor

*It is the glory of God to conceal a matter; to search out
a matter is the glory of kings. Proverbs 25:2*

Molecular imaging is the study of molecular and cellular events in living organisms by means of imaging. This relatively new field is becoming increasingly important as our understanding of the molecular basis of disease increases. It is adding great scope and depth to the imaging armamentarium we offer to patients and is opening up new vistas of research in both the laboratory and the clinic.

In this issue of *Neuroimaging Clinics*, we hope to take the reader on a tour through this exciting field, pointing out various interesting areas and giving a sense of how wide the territory stretches. We have to cover quite a bit of ground, because molecular imaging is quite expansive. It is also complicated in the sense that multiple and diverse disciplines are involved. In fact, one way to view molecular imaging is as a chain of disciplines, starting with basic science research into molecular targets and disease processes, handing of these targets to chemists who design probes and ligands to interact with them, passing these ligands to radiochemists or labeling chemists of various persuasions to create imaging probes—which then get tested by biologists in cell- and animal-based models of disease—only to be handed off yet again to imagers who are able to image these models on machines designed and maintained by physicists and engineers... and this is all just the preclinical part and is by no means comprehensive.

It is clear therefore that there are multiple players in molecular imaging, each with a vital contribution. In striving to provide the reader with a reasonable view of the field, we had to incorporate three viewpoints in this issue: targets, imaging, and therapy.

Biological targets are the bread and butter of a large part of the molecular imaging community. These individuals discover new biological pathways and signaling cascades. They identify and isolate key proteins and cellular events, make model systems, and synthesize inhibitors and imaging probes to interact with these models. Among their number are molecular biologists, biochemists, synthetic chemists, radiochemists, and many others who look at the world of molecular imaging from the perspective of biological targets.

Imagers live for imaging. These professionals use sophisticated equipment to create images of various biological processes, often using the imaging

doi:10.1016/j.nic.2006.10.001

probes and model systems to do research on these processes, but also often in the clinic to obtain information needed to treat patients. Their numbers include radiologists, physicists, nuclear medicine physicians, and many others. They see molecular imaging from the perspective of imaging.

Therapists care about disease and interventions to change outcomes. They are often the end users of the data produced by a molecular imaging modality, and their primary interest is in the impact of imaging on therapy.

A full understanding of molecular imaging requires comprehending, or at least appreciating, all of these perspectives. In this issue, we have outstanding articles dealing with targets (the first three articles), imaging (the following four articles), and therapy (the final two articles), all of which are written by experts in the field, each showing their view of the world. We invite the reader to step into the shoes of these authors, particularly if the author's viewpoint is not already familiar to the reader.

It is our hope that this work will contribute to a greater understanding of molecular imaging and, thus, ultimately contribute to the restoration of health for our patients.

ELSEVIER SAUNDERS

NEUROIMAGING
CLINICS
OF NORTH AMERICA

Neuroimag Clin N Am 16 (2006) xv

Dedication

To God, who delights in mysteries for us to unravel.

To my teachers in science, Juri Gelovani and Ralph Weissleder. To Jack Wittenberg and James H. Thrall, for giving me a chance. To the many other teachers, colleagues, and patients I've had the privilege to encounter and learn from.

To my wife, my parents, and, especially, to my children.

Dawid Schellingerhout, MD

1052-5149/06/$ – see front matter © 2006 Elsevier Inc. All rights reserved.
neuroimaging.theclinics.com

doi:10.1016/j.nic.2006.11.001

NEUROIMAGING
CLINICS
OF NORTH AMERICA

Neuroimag Clin N Am 16 (2006) 529–552

Opioid Imaging

Alexander Hammers, PhD[a,b,c],*, Anne Lingford-Hughes, PhD[d,e]

Opioids derive their name from the Greek όπιου for poppy sap. Various preparations of the opium poppy *Papaver somniferum* have been used for pain relief for centuries. Structure and stereochemistry are essential for the analgesic actions of morphine and other opiates, leading to the hypothesis of the existence of specific receptors. Receptors were identified simultaneously by three laboratories in 1973 [1–3]. The different pharmacologic activity of

agonists provided evidence for the existence of multiple receptors [4]. In the early 1980s, there was evidence for the existence of at least three types of opiate receptors: μ, κ, and δ [5,6]. A fourth "orphan" receptor (ORL1 or NOP1) displays a high degree of structural homology with conventional opioid receptors and was identified through homology with the δ receptor [7], but the endogenous ligand, orphanin FQ/nociceptin, does not interact directly

Dr. Hammers was funded by an MRC Clinician Scientist Fellowship (G108/585).

[a] Department of Clinical Neuroscience, Division of Neuroscience and Mental Health, Imperial College London, Hammersmith Hospital, DuCane Rd., London W12 0NN, UK

[b] Epilepsy Group, MRC Clinical Sciences Centre, Room 243, Cyclotron Building, Hammersmith Hospital, DuCane Rd., London W12 0NN, UK

[c] Department of Clinical and Experimental Epilepsy, Institute of Neurology, University College London, Queen Square, London WC1N 3BG, UK

[d] Academic Unit of Psychiatry, University of Bristol, Cotham House, Cotham Hill, Bristol BS6 6JL, UK

[e] Imaging Department, Division of Clinical Sciences, Faculty of Medicine, Hammersmith Hospital, Imperial College London, DuCane Rd., London W12 0NN, UK

* Corresponding author. Epilepsy Group, MRC Clinical Sciences Centre, Room 243, Cyclotron Building, Hammersmith Hospital, DuCane Rd., London W12 0NN, UK.

E-mail address: alexander.hammers@imperial.ac.uk (A. Hammers).

doi:10.1016/j.nic.2006.06.004

with classical opioid receptors [8] and is not discussed further herein. Endogenous opioids have been identified [9]. These substances were originally distinguished from exogenous opiates, but the term *opioids* is now generally used for all ligands.

Besides their role as endogenous and exogenous pain killers, opioids and their receptors are implicated in reward, addiction, mood regulation and mood disorders, epilepsy, movement disorders, and dementia.

Derivation, release, peptide action, and metabolism

All opioid peptides are derived from three different gene products: proopiomelanocortin, proenkephalin, and prodynorphin. Proopiomelanocortin gives rise to β-endorphin (μ- and δ- preferring) and nonopioid peptides. Proenkephalin contains four copies of different enkephalins (most δ-preferring). Prodynorphin gives rise to several dynorphin peptides and neoendorphin (all κ-preferring) (Table 1) [10]. Endogenous opioids consist of between four (endomorphin) and 31 amino acids (β-endorphin).

Similar to other neuropeptides, opioids are stored in large dense core vesicles [11], which are distinguishable electron microscopically from small clear vesicles containing the fast-acting transmitters such as GABA and glutamate. Opioid vesicle containing neurons also contain classical fast-acting transmitters; therefore, opioids act as co-transmitters to modulate the actions of the primary transmitter. Exocytosis of the dense core vesicles is calcium dependent [12] but, unlike small clear vesicles, exocytosis is not limited to restricted zones of the plasma membrane. Exocytosis requires high-frequency stimulation of the opioid-containing neurons [13,14].

In contrast to amino acid transmitters, opioid peptides can affect the excitability of neurons at the relatively large distance of 50 to 100 μm from the site of release [15] owing to their diffusion through the extracellular space and their high affinities for their receptors, with nanomolar concentrations of the peptides being effective [16]. After release from nerve terminals, opioid peptides are rapidly degraded by a variety of peptidases [9].

The time courses of changes of transmitter peptides and receptor protein are of great interest when interpreting positron emission tomography (PET) studies of opioid function in experiments designed to show the role of neurotransmitters, usually by employing two PET scans acquired at different delays from an experimental manipulation or spontaneously occurring event.

As is true for most G-protein coupled receptors, short-term exposure of opioid receptors to agonists leads to receptor desensitization, and long-term exposure to agonists leads to receptor downregulation [17]. Desensitization is achieved through phosphorylation of agonist-activated receptors and subsequent receptor endocytosis via clathrin-coated pits. The ubiquitin/proteasome pathway seems to be important in agonist-induced downregulation as well as basal turnover of opioid receptors. Monoubiquinated receptors are simply internalized, whereas ubiquitin chains of more than three units target the receptor to the proteasome. Further downstream, trafficking to lysosomes may have a role.

Triggered release of endogenous opioids (eg, in seizure models) leads to major changes [18]. In laboratory animals, transmitter peptide levels generally decrease to about 40% to 50% of baseline in the hours after release. Levels of transmitter peptide mRNA tend to increase temporarily. Depending on the model, increases can be relatively minor (approximately 150% of baseline) or major (300% to 1400%). Limited data are available on opioid receptor level changes following events like epileptic seizures. Acute release leads to decreased availability of receptors as measured by [^{3}H]diprenorphine binding [13] or [^{3}H]U69,593 binding [14]. Over slightly longer time courses, both decreases, particularly for δ-opioid receptors [19], and increases (of the μ receptor) [20] have been found. Receptor endocytosis may be irreversible for δ receptors, requiring de novo protein synthesis [17].

Opioid receptor function changes over the hours following neuronal events have received far less attention. After 4 hours of exposure to the μ-agonist DAMGO to induce desensitization, some functional resensitization of the μ receptor occurred after 10 minutes, with 100% of control responses reached after 60 minutes [21]. In another study, μ-receptor protein reached normal levels and function after 6 hours through recycling [22]. Basal levels can be achieved through recycling in 30 [23] to 60 minutes, with some agonists inducing receptor levels of 110% to 120% of control as measured with [^{3}H]diprenorphine [24].

Receptors and ligands

Receptors

There are three main types of opioid receptors, μ, δ, and κ. For all, the existence of subtypes has been proposed [10], and one subtype each has been cloned in several species including man. The receptor proteins consist of about 370 amino acids [17]. They belong to the G-protein coupled receptor family and have their characteristic structure with seven hydrophobic transmembrane domains, connected by relatively short intracellular and extracellular loops. The amino acid sequences are about 60%

Table 1: Opioid receptors and their ligands

Receptor	μ (MOR)	δ (DOR)	κ (KOR)
Endogenous ligand potency	β-endorphin > dynorphin A > met-enkephalin, leu-enkephalin	β-endorphin, leu-enkephalin, met-enkephalin > dynorphin A	Dynorphin A >> β-endorphin > leu-enkephalin > met-enkephalin
Agonists	DAMGO DAGO Dihydromorphine	DPDPE DSLET DADLE (δ, μ)	Enadoline (CI-977) U69,593
Selective antagonists	CTAP	Naltrindole	nor-BNI
Nonselective antagonists		Naloxone Naltrexone (orally active)	
PET ligands	[¹¹C]carfentanil (CFN) (agonist)	[¹¹C]methylnaltrindole (MeNTI) (antagonist)	[¹⁸F]cyclofoxy (CFX) (κ, μ; antagonist) [¹¹C]GR103545 (κ; agonist)

[¹¹C]diprenorphine/[¹⁸F]fluorodiprenorphine (DPN) (partial agonist at δ and κ, antagonist at μ)

[¹¹C]buprenorphine (partial agonist at μ, antagonist at δ, κ)

Abbreviations: DAMGO, [D-Ala², N-Me-Phe⁴,Gly-ol⁵]-enkephalin; DAGO, D-Ala2-MePhe4-Gly(ol)5 enkephalin: DPDPE, [D-Pen2,5]-enkephalin; DSLET, [D-Ser2, Leu5] enkephalin-Thr6; DADLE, D-Ala2-D-Leu5 enkephalin; CTAP, D-Phe-Cys-Tyr-D-Trp-Arg-Thr-Pen-Thr-NH2; nor-BNI, nor-binaltorphimine.

identical between opioid receptor types and about 90% identical between the same receptor types cloned from different species. There are marked differences in the degree of sequence conservation between domains. Most transmembrane segments and the three intracellular loops are highly conserved [17], the latter probably because they mediate the G-protein coupling. Extracellular loops are more variable and are responsible for receptor selectivity and affinity. The determinants of the opioid receptor binding pocket differ from ligand to ligand for a given receptor. This difference means that there is not a single receptor binding site, as is true for ionotropic receptors; rather, opioid receptors are capable of considerable plasticity regarding engagement of ligands and subsequent events leading to receptor activation.

Species differences

There are well-known species differences. In general, there is relatively less δ binding in the human compared with the rat brain and relatively more κ binding [25]. The latter finding has been corroborated by quantitative autoradiography [26,27] and by the detection of a more widespread κ-opioid receptor mRNA expression in humans compared with rodents [28]. Other examples include κ-opioid receptors found in deep cortical layers in human but not in rat brain and the lack in humans of the typical patchy distribution of μ receptors seen in rodents [29]. It is prudent to be careful in extrapolating results from rodent studies to humans.

Regional and layer-specific subtype distributions

The receptor subtypes are unevenly distributed between regions. Outside the medial occipital lobe, human neocortical binding consists of 40% to 50% κ, 20% to 40% δ, and 15% to 40% μ [25,29]. In the thalamus, μ binding predominates at approximately two-thirds, whereas in mesial temporal structures, approximately 60% of binding is attributed to κ receptors. Absolute levels are about 120 to 145 fmol receptors/mg protein in most of the neocortex, compared with about 72 to 74 fmol receptors/mg protein in the lateral and medial occipitotemporal gyri [26].

Importantly for PET studies, there is evidence of μ-receptor binding and, at a lower level, κ-receptor binding in the human cerebellum [30], indicating that, in contrast to many other transmitter systems, it cannot be used as a classical reference region for μ- or κ-receptor PET tracers; however, the medial occipital lobe is a potential reference region for μ-receptor PET tracers.

Mu receptors are found abundantly in the human thalamus, amygdala, striatum, and neocortex (except medial occipital), as well as some midbrain and deeper nuclei [31]. μ-opioid receptor binding is present in all of these areas but is most dense in layers I, IIIa, and IV [26,28,29], suggesting a somatodentritic expression. Functional coupling of μ receptors to intracellular signal transduction mechanisms, measured as DAMGO-stimulated [^{35}S]GTPγS-binding, was around 200% above basal levels and evenly distributed throughout human frontal gray matter [32,33]. In comparison, mRNA, receptor protein, and functional coupling are all much lower in the human hippocampus, whereas μ receptors contribute considerably to the high density of opioid receptors in the amygdala.

Delta receptors are generally less prominent in the human brain than in rodent brains. They are most numerous in the striatum and throughout the neocortex, and occur notably in medial occipital cortex [25,29]. δ-opioid receptor binding is present in all layers and shows peak densities in layers I to IIIa [26,29]. Functional coupling of δ receptors, assessed as DPDPE-stimulated [^{35}S]GTPγS-binding, was evenly distributed throughout human frontal gray matter [32]. There is comparatively little δ-opioid receptor binding in hippocampus and amygdala, very little in the thalamus (approximately 9% of total [25]), and none in the cerebellum, making the cerebellum a possible reference region for δ-opioid receptor ligands.

Kappa receptors are most numerous in the neocortex, amygdala, and hippocampus and notably sparse in the striatum [29]. κ-opioid receptor binding is present in all layers but concentrated in layers V and VI, matching the distribution of mRNA expression [26,29]. Enadoline-stimulated [^{35}S]GTPγS-binding, indicating functional coupling of κ receptors to intracellular signal transduction mechanisms, was present throughout human frontal gray matter but twice as strong in lamina V-VI when compared with lamina I-IV [32]. κ-opioid receptor binding in the human hippocampus is higher than μ- or δ-receptor binding [25] and restricted to the pyramidal cell layer [26]. About 60% of the high level of opioid receptor binding in the amygdala represents κ-opioid receptor binding [25,29]. In contrast to the rat, mRNA and κ-binding sites are present in the human cerebellum [30].

At least for the μ receptor, in some regions a substantial influence of age and sex on the binding potential of the μ-selective ligand [^{11}C]carfentanil as measured by PET has been found [34] in a total of 36 men and 30 women spanning several decades and scanned in two different scanners.

Ligands

Selective agonists and antagonists are now available (Table 1). Selectivity is never complete, but the affinity for the subtype or subtypes indicated is usually more than an order of magnitude higher than for the other subtypes. PET ligands are discussed in detail in the following sections.

Positron emission tomography imaging of opioid receptors

Introduction PET imaging

PET enables tomographic imaging of local concentrations of injected biologically active substances that have been radioactively labeled (radioligands or tracers) [35–37]. Subjects can be investigated in the resting state or in relationship to an event such as the injection of a substance, the induction of pain, or the occurrence of a seizure. Positron-emitting isotopes used for opioid receptor imaging have half-lives of approximately 20 minutes (^{11}C) and 110 minutes (^{18}F); therefore, the use of PET is limited by the need for an on-site cyclotron to produce ^{11}C, whereas ^{18}F-labeled substances can be transported off site. Only minimal or "tracer doses" of neuroreceptor radiotracers (in the microgram range) need to be injected to estimate receptor parameters; importantly for potent substances like opioid agonists, such small doses are usually without clinical effect. Radiotracers for receptor imaging need to have certain physical properties (ie, a suitable lipophilicity [measured as logP octanol-water] for penetrating the blood brain barrier), and biologic properties (ie, they should not be substrates for multidrug transporters). The radiation dose depends on the tracer used and the activity injected but is typically in the range of 2.5 to 5 mSv using contemporary tomographs and three-dimensional scanning, which should always be used for brain imaging. The raw data collected by the PET scanner is mathematically reconstructed to produce tomographic images of tissue radioactivity concentration. Requirements for absolute quantification are normalization for the current efficiency of detector blocks, correction for nonuniform efficiency along the longitudinal (z) axis, and scatter and attenuation correction.

Quantification of images

The distribution of the radioligand changes over time, and scanning is subdivided into time frames. Shortly after injection, radioactivity distribution reflects blood flow and radioligand delivery. Later, radioactivity levels and their changes will gradually reflect the ligand-receptor interaction more than blood flow and delivery.

Radiotracer availability in the brain depends on the blood concentration of the parent radioligand, its partitioning between blood cells and plasma, its binding to plasma proteins, and its metabolism.

A measure of the brain availability of the parent radiotracer is desirable. This measurement can be achieved with arterial blood sampling in which total radioactivity and radiolabeled metabolites in plasma are assayed in blood samples throughout the scanning period. These data can be used to produce an "input function" for the available unmetabolized ligand in arterial plasma. Mathematical modeling techniques are then used to derive parameters of interest from the data. These models make the assumption that the time-activity curve in each region or voxel of interest represents the convolution of the input function and the tissue response function. Compartmental models are typically used, usually with two tissue compartments, of which one represents free and nonspecific binding and the other specific binding. Outcome parameters are the volume-of-distribution (VD) or sometimes individual rate constants of radioligand exchange between different compartments. When a brain region devoid or nearly devoid of specific binding is available, for example, in the medial occipital lobe for μ receptors and the cerebellum for δ receptors, an image-based input function can be derived by measuring the tissue kinetics in this "reference region" [38]. A simpler method is to use late summed images, subtract a reference region's integrated radioactivity concentration from that of the target region, and divide by the reference region's integrated radioactivity concentration (ratio images). Radioligand properties, the radiation dose to patients and particularly healthy volunteers, accuracy, bias, reproducibility, reliability, and the sensitivity to clinically meaningful changes should always be considered before choosing a particular method of analysis. In addition, in more clinically orientated settings, it may not be possible to implement more complex acquisition techniques, such as those involving arterial cannulation and metabolite analysis. Simpler methods may often be less sensitive to changes and require the scanning of larger numbers of subjects, with additional cost and radiation protection implications [39–41].

Spectral analysis [42] is an alternative modeling technique to compartmental modeling that has the advantage of not requiring a predefined number of compartments to produce estimates of VD and has been widely used in the analysis of opioid receptor PET data. Spectral analysis convolves a multiexponential function with the parent tracer arterial plasma input function to generate an optimum fit for the observed tissue data and can often be used at the voxel level for the generation of parametric maps. The number and components of the exponentials represent the spectral contributions of the impulse function. The integral of the impulse response function (IRF), extrapolated to infinity, corresponds to the total VD of the tracer; however, for tracers with slow kinetics, VD estimates may be noisy owing to poor extrapolation of the late time courses. In this situation, suitable restrictions of the expected range of slow exponential decays can be used but will lead to underestimation of high binding regions. Alternatives or extensions currently under study include derivations of spectral analysis such as rank shaping [43], basis pursuit [44], bootstrapped techniques to derive error estimates simultaneously [45,46], or the use of a specific time point on the fitted time course of the unit IRF (eg, IRF_{60} at 60 minutes), which is less dependent on the extrapolation to infinity than VD.

Information derived from a reference region can be used to correct VD for nonspecific binding, yielding binding potentials (BP). VD and BP are proportional to the available receptor density (B_{max}) over receptor affinity (K_d). More complex experimental protocols usually requiring multiple injections may be used to derive B_{max} and K_d separately. Region- and voxel-based methods (the latter when tracer characteristics allow the generation of parametric maps) are used for the analysis of changes; both are complementary [47].

Quantitative or semi-quantitative evaluation of datasets, typically in comparison with healthy controls, is often more sensitive to abnormalities than the qualitative assessment of PET images [47–50]. Automatic methods for the co-registration of MR imaging and PET data are readily available and allow the interpretation of functional data compared with higher resolution structural data [51].

Partial volume effects arise owing to the restricted spatial resolution PET provides. When structural changes are present, that is, the anatomy differs between patients and controls, these effects are particularly important because they can lead to spurious differences. In these situations, they should be corrected for [52,53]. Region-based correction methods [54–56] and voxel-based methods [57] are used.

Even in the absence of partial volume effects differing between conditions or groups, interpretation of binding estimates tends not to be unequivocal. For example, reductions in binding estimates can be due to reduced receptor concentration, reduced receptor affinity, increased occupancy by endogenous ligands, or opposite changes in the control group or control condition. In the following sections, the interpretation thought to be most likely in the circumstances of the study has been indicated.

Available ligands and their quantification

Available ligands are tabulated in Table 1. Diprenorphine (DPN) binds with similar, approximately 1 nmol/L, affinities at all three major opioid receptor subtypes [58] and does not have a reference region because binding in all putative reference regions can be blocked with naloxone [59]. It is a partial agonist at δ and κ receptors and an antagonist at the μ receptor [60]. It has been labeled with ^{11}C [61,62] and ^{18}F [63], with the ^{18}F derivative having similar properties [63]. Ratio images derived from the use of an occipital reference region despite the presence of δ and κ receptors [25,28,29] have repeatedly been shown to have less sensitivity to detect changes in patients than images quantified with spectral analysis [40,41]. [^{11}C]buprenorphine is a partial agonist at μ receptors and an antagonist at κ and δ receptors but has not found widespread use compared with [^{11}C]DPN. In rats, the signal is smaller than that of [^{11}C]DPN, with more nonspecific binding.

The agonist [^{11}C]carfentanil (CFN) is used for imaging μ receptors. Its affinity for μ receptors (K_I at 37°C, 0.051 nM) is approximately 100-fold higher than for δ receptors and more than 200-fold higher than for κ receptors. Medial occipital cortex can be used as a reference region, and quantification has often been performed as the specific-nonspecific ratio on late summed images (eg, 35–70 minutes) as (region of interest − occipital)/occipital [64]. More recently, the use of graphic methods and the simplified reference tissue model [65] have been more accurate in quantifying [^{11}C]CFN binding [66]. Similar ^{18}F-labeled tracers are under development for use by centers without access to a cyclotron [67].

Delta receptors are visualized with the antagonist [^{11}C]methylnaltrindole (MeNTI). Its affinity for δ receptors of 0.02 nM is approximately 700-fold higher than for μ receptors and more than 3000-fold higher than for κ receptors [68]. Cerebellum has been used as a reference region, and quantification has been performed on late summed images (eg, 34–90 minutes [68] or 50–90 minutes [69]) as (region of interest − cerebellum)/cerebellum. [^{11}C]MeNTI binding is essentially irreversible over the time course of a 90-minute PET scan [68,70]. It is unclear how far flow effects will enter these binding estimates, and the ratio method was abandoned by the same researchers in a later systematic modeling study [70].

[^{18}F]cyclofoxy (CFX) is an antagonist at μ and κ receptors. Affinities were reported as a Ki of 2.6 nM for μ sites, 9.3 nM for κ sites, and 89 nM for δ sites [71]. The medial occipital cortex may contain some κ receptors [28] but has been successfully used as a reference region following estimation of total VD with an arterial input function and kinetic modeling with a one tissue compartment model [72–74].

[^{11}C]GR103545 is the active (−) enantiomer of the racemate GR89696 and a selective κ agonist, with subnanomolar to low nanomolar affinities

[75]. It has shown promise as the first κ-selective PET tracer in mice [76] and baboons [75] but will require radiochemistry improvements to increase specific activity and reduce co-injected unlabeled ligand to become useful in humans.

Opioid receptor imaging in healthy volunteers

The marked regional differences in overall opioid receptor concentrations and subtype distributions described previously are reproduced by in vivo imaging techniques. Regarding total opioid receptor binding, Jones and coworkers [77] commented on a marked difference, estimated from [¹¹C]DPN ratio images, between the "medial" or "affective" pain system (which comprises the medial thalamus, amygdala, caudate nucleus, insula, cingulate gyrus, and orbitofrontal cortex) (Fig. 1) with high opioid receptor binding and the "lateral" or "discriminating" pain system (projecting to the somatosensory cortex) with much lower binding. This difference is also obvious on parametric maps of [¹¹C]DPN VD (Fig. 2). Other areas now thought to be part of the lateral nociceptive system, such as parts of

the insula and the parietal operculum, have high [¹⁸F]DPN BPs [78]. Genotype has an important role in regional binding estimates [79]. There is a common co-dominant valine/methionine polymorphism in the gene encoding catechol-O-methyl-transferase (COMT), leading to higher activity of this enzyme that metabolizes catecholamines like dopamine, adrenaline, and noradrenaline in the order of val/val > val/met > met/met carrying individuals. The more met polymorphism, the less breakdown of catecholamines, presumably leading to more continuous stimulation of the dopaminergic system. In animal models, such chronic activation has been shown to lead to reduced enkephalin (Table 1) levels and compensatory increases in regional μ receptors. Although global [¹¹C]CFN BP, reflecting μ receptor concentration, was not influenced by the polymorphism in 18 subjects of whom 11 were heterozygous, marked differences in the expected direction were seen regionally in the thalamus [79]. Comparison of the various groups showed further effects of genotype on baseline [¹¹C]CFN BP in ventral pallidum and nucleus accumbens, in the order of about 30% (Fig. 3). The finding of higher μ-receptor binding in

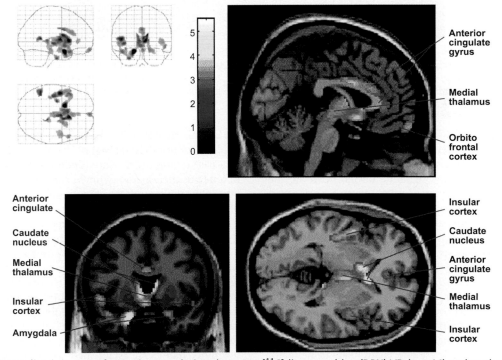

Fig. 1. Localized clusters of negative correlations between [¹¹C]diprenorphine (DPN) VD (n = 14) and restless legs syndrome severity, measured on the International Restless Legs Scale, analyzed with SPM99 and displayed at $P < .01$ uncorrected threshold, cluster extent of 50 voxels. All clusters throughout the whole brain are demonstrated (*top left*) in the maximum intensity projection "glass brain." The top right and bottom two panels show significant clusters overlain on a single subject brain [133]. Color bar represents Z-values. Many structures of the medial pain system show this negative correlation. (*From* von Spiczak S, et al. The role of opioids in restless legs syndrome: an [11C]diprenorphine PET study. Brain 2005;128(Pt 4):911; with permission.)

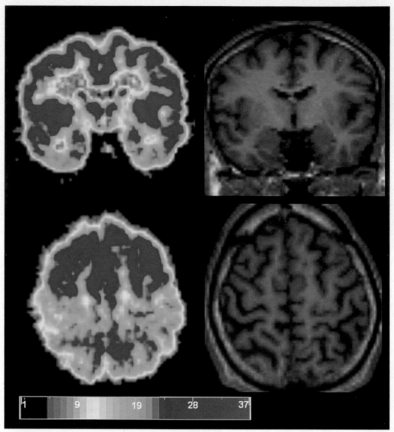

Fig. 2. Parametric maps of [¹¹C]diprenorphine (DPN) VD in a healthy male volunteer, acquired after injection of approximately 185 MBq of [¹¹C]DPN on a Siemens/CTI HR++ scanner displayed alongside co-registered MR imaging slices. (*Top*) Coronal slices at the level of the amygdala. (*Bottom*) Superior transverse slices. Note the heterogeneity of binding in the coronal slices and the relative lack of binding centered on the postcentral gyrus in the transverse slices. Color bar represents the VD.

individuals with the met/met phenotype was confirmed by a different group in postmortem autoradiographic studies in the caudate and accumbens nucleus and some thalamic nuclei; however, that study showed increased mRNA levels for pre-proenkephalin, contrary to predictions [80].

Other factors affect receptor concentrations. Age may regionally increase or decrease receptor concentrations as seen in postmortem studies and using [¹¹C]CFN BP via a ratio method in subjects aged between 19 and 79 years [34]. Women had generally higher μ receptor BP, thought to relate at least partly to hormonal status [34]. A high estradiol state induced with patches led to higher μ-receptor availability in eight women ranging between 15% and 32% [81]. These effects are likely to be region specific, and some regions may show interactions between age and sex, adding to difficulties in interpretation. In the thalamus, μ receptor BP was higher in premenopausal women when compared with their male contemporaries, whereas the opposite relationship was seen in postmenopausal women

[34]. Similarly, total VD and specific VD (regional total VD minus occipital VD) of [¹⁸F]CFX, reflecting μ- as well as κ-opioid receptor binding, were reduced in nine postmenopausal women compared with 15 men in the thalamus but not in several other regions of interest, including caudate and putamen [74].

The opioid system is involved in mood regulation. μ agonists tend to be rewarding, whereas κ agonists induce dysphoria. In 14 healthy women scanned with a bolus-infusion paradigm [82], neutral and sad mood states were induced in a counterbalanced order between 5 and 45 and 45 and 100 minutes, respectively, after the start of the radiotracer infusion. Sadness was induced by instructing subjects to concentrate on an autobiographical event that, before scanning, had been established to be associated with profound sadness. Logan plot derived VD ratios (over occipital lobe) for the periods of 10 to 45 and 50 to 100 minutes were compared using statistical parametric mapping. Increased availability of μ receptors (ie, a "deactivation" of the opioid system) was seen in the perigenual anterior cingulate gyrus,

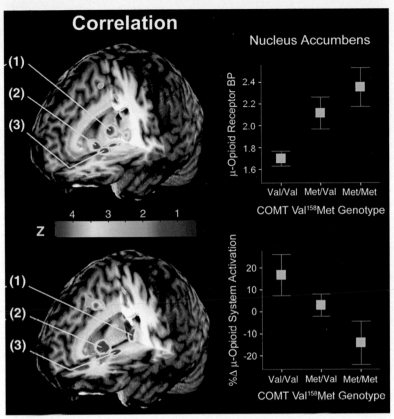

Fig. 3. Catechol-*O*-methyl-transferase (COMT) polymorphism with substitution of valine (val) by methionine (met) at codon 158 (*val^158^met*). Effect of genotypes and associated COMT activity on [^{11}C]carfentanil (CFN) volume-of-distribution ratio (DVR) binding potential (BP), reflecting μ-opioid receptor binding and μ-opioid receptor system activation in response to sustained pain. (*Upper left*) Correlations between COMT *val^158^met* polymorphisms and baseline μ opioid receptor BP. Significant correlations were obtained in the anterior thalamus (1), the nucleus accumbens (2), and adjacent ventral pallidum (3) ipsilateral to pain. (*Upper right*) Mean ± standard deviation of nucleus accumbens (ipsilateral) BP values. (*Lower left*) Correlations between COMT activity and μ-opioid system activation in the ipsilateral posterior thalamus (1), nucleus accumbens (2), and ventral pallidum (3), bilaterally, and the contralateral amygdala and adjacent temporal cortex. (*Lower right*) Mean ± standard deviation values for the percent change in the magnitude of μ-opioid receptor system activation in the nucleus accumbens. Color bar represents the Z-scores. Threshold for display of results was set at $P < .01$ for all analyses. (*From* Zubieta JK, Heitzeg MM, Smith YR, et al. COMT *val^158^met* genotype affects μ-opioid neurotransmitter responses to a pain stressor. Science 2003;299(5610):1241; with permission. Copyright 2003 AAAS.)

left inferior temporal cortex, and amygdala and ventral pallidum bilaterally. Most of these changes were more clearly seen after global normalization of VD ratios. The magnitude of deactivations correlated with the increase in negative affect ratings or the decrease in positive affect ratings in the perigenual cingulate gyrus, ventral pallidum bilaterally, and on the left in the amygdala, insula, and hypothalamus. The study provides direct in vivo evidence for a role of the μ-opioid receptor system in affect regulation in humans. In another study in 12 healthy men, higher baseline Logan plot VD ratios were weakly associated with smaller blood flow responses to aversive visual stimuli in the left anterior middle temporal gyrus [83].

Opioid imaging in the wider sense also includes indirect measures of opioid neurotransmission, that is, studies investigating cerebral blood flow in relation to opioid receptor agonists. Although these studies are not discussed herein, a recent detailed review is available elsewhere [84].

Opioid imaging in pain-related studies

Changes in receptor availability in pain and discomfort: between-group comparisons

Four patients with central neuropathic pain (mainly resulting from strokes) when compared with an undisclosed number of healthy controls had reduced [^{11}C]DPN VD centered on medial pain system structures (cingulate gyrus, insula, and thalamus), with some reductions in the lateral pain system (inferior parietal cortex) [85]. The effect sizes were around 15% to 30%. In this particular study, it was thought to be unlikely that the reductions were due to occupancy of receptors by endogenous opioids, and the interpretation of a disease-related loss of binding sites with subsequent failure of the opioid system to suppress pain was favored, partly supported by the lack of clinical change after prolonged infusions of naloxone in two patients. A different group reported a similar finding of regionally reduced [^{11}C]DPN ratios in medial (contralateral thalamus, insula, cingulate gyrus, midbrain) and lateral (parietal, somatosensory, and lateral frontal cortices) pain system structures in five patients with poststroke pain compared with 12 controls using the occipital lobe as a reference region [86], expanding on an earlier case report [87]. In contrast to the previous study [85], all images had been preprocessed to show the anatomic lesion on the same side, and decreases showed lateralization to the side contralateral to the perceived pain.

When compared with healthy controls, 15 patients with meticulously evaluated primary restless legs syndrome had no global or regional differences in [^{11}C]DPN VD [40]; however, the more severe the restless legs syndrome, the less [^{11}C]DPN VD in much of the medial pain system (**Fig. 1**), suggesting enhanced release of endogenous opioids. Similarly, ratings on the McGill Pain Questionnaire correlated inversely with [^{11}C]DPN VD in the orbitofrontal cortex and anterior cingulate gyrus.

Overall, these studies are remarkable for delineating the medial pain system irrespectively of the type of pain or anatomic localization of lesions. They offer no explanation of how such systematic changes could be mediated.

Six men with left-sided cluster headache when compared with eight healthy controls had decreased signal of [^{11}C]DPN (quantified as IRF_{60}) in the pineal gland, and binding in hypothalamus and cingulate gyrus correlated negatively with disease duration [88]. The validity of quantifying [^{11}C]DPN with IRF_{60} for the pineal gland, which is situated outside the blood-brain barrier, was not explicitly examined. Although the changes are in brain regions previously implicated in the pathophysiology of cluster headache [89], this makes them harder to interpret.

Ultimately, patients should be the beneficiaries and subjects in imaging research; however, experimental paradigms offer the possibility of tightly controlling several variables that would be impossible to standardize in real patients. In one such experiment [90], pain was induced in eight healthy volunteers by applying a heat stimulus (approximately 44°C) from 60 to 70 minutes after injection of [^{18}F]DPN. A VD from data 80 to 120 minutes post injection was calculated using an invasive Logan plot and compared with the findings in another eight healthy volunteers of similar age and sex distribution scanned with the same protocol but without pain induction. In the group with pain stimulation, there were decreases in [^{18}F]DPN VD in the ipsilateral nucleus accumbens and amygdala and bilaterally in the middle frontal gyri, the anterior insulae, the thalami, and the perigenual anterior cingulate gyrus.

Direct intrasubject comparisons of periods with pain and pain-free states

Such studies are more complex to perform, because paired studies need to be obtained for patients in two different states and ideally compared with paired control scans. Nevertheless, they allow the attribution of changes in a neurotransmitter system to changes in clinical or experimental stage and provide more powerful evidence than studies comparing groups of patients and controls.

Four patients with rheumatoid arthritis were examined twice with [^{11}C]DPN [91]. Global increases in opioid receptor availability and additional regional increases in the frontal and temporal lobe and cingulate gyrus were seen in the reduced pain state, consistent with the idea that occupancy by endogenous ligands, triggered by pain, may lead to reduced availability. The same group obtained similar results in six patients undergoing thermocoagulation for refractory trigeminal neuralgia. Regional increases of [^{11}C]DPN VD after surgical pain relief were seen in frontal, insular, perigenual, midcingulate, and inferior parietal cortices, basal ganglia, and thalamus bilaterally [92]. Although the preceding studies suffer from the lack of a control group scanned twice, they have the merit of being the only ones attempting intrasubject comparisons in patients so far.

More work has been done in healthy controls in experimental paradigms. When pain was induced through capsaicin application to the hand, eight healthy volunteers showed reductions in contralateral thalamic [^{11}C]CFN 34- to 82-minute tissue ratios over the occipital lobe when compared with baseline; in addition, the magnitude of the decrease of μ-receptor binding correlated directly with pain intensity [93].

All studies discussed hereafter used healthy controls in a paradigm whereby sustained deep tissue pain was induced by infusion of 5% hypertonic saline into the masseter muscle, with nonpainful infusion of 0.9% (isotonic) saline in the control condition into the other masseter muscle. By controlling the rate of infusion, a similar level of pain was maintained, around 50 or slightly below on a visual analogue scale where 0 denotes no pain and 100 the most intense pain imaginable. Both scans were acquired on the same day, separated by at least six isotope half-lives. Intramasseter infusions were administered from 20 to 40 minutes after radiotracer administration [79,81,94,95] or from 40 to 60 minutes [96]. A bolus-infusion radiotracer administration protocol was used. Modified Logan graphical analysis with occipital cortex as a reference region on data from 20 to 70 [79,81,94,95] or 40 to 90 minutes [96] post radiotracer injection was used to quantify μ-receptor binding as DVR, a VD ratio (ie, the slopes of the Logan plot for voxels of interest divided by the reference region slope).

Using this paradigm, the Ann Arbor group has initially shown in 20 healthy volunteers that sustained pain can induce a release of endogenous opioids, measurable as a decrease in [¹¹C]CFN DVR, indicating interaction of endogenous opioids with μ opioid receptors in specific brain regions. μ-opioid receptor mediated activation is associated with reductions in pain ratings in the sensory domain (ipsilateral nucleus accumbens, thalamus, and amygdala) and affective domain (bilaterally in the cingulate gyrus and thalamus, and ipsilaterally in the nucleus accumbens) [94]. Having established this principle, the researchers went on to demonstrate sex differences in 14 men and 14 women aged between 20 and 30 years, with the women scanned during the low-estrogen, low-progesterone early follicular menstrual cycle phase [95]. The intensity-controlled paradigm did not show any differences in subjective positive and negative affect scores or pain questionnaire ratings. Nevertheless, men activated the μ-opioid receptor system contralaterally to pain infliction in the anterior thalamus, ventral pallidum/substantia innominata, and anterior insula, as well as ipsilaterally in the amygdala and ventral basal ganglia, whereas the latter was the only area with significant DVR decreases in women who, in addition, showed DVR increases following pain in the ipsilateral nucleus accumbens. Across all subjects, greater activation of μ-opioid receptors in ipsilateral nucleus accumbens and amygdala was correlated with less pain perception, a correlation in the expected direction.

Baseline [¹¹C]CFN DVR indicated higher binding in women only in one amygdala, in contrast to the group's earlier study showing more widespread and impressive increases in women compared with men [34]. Characteristics of this earlier study which might explain some of these differences include a wider age range, a ratio method of quantification, no correction for multiple comparisons, and a less objective method of region definition. Sex

differences in the same direction were replicated later for the nucleus accumbens and hypothalamus (but not the amygdala) [81].

To further characterize the role estradiol has in women's μ-opioid transmission in relation to pain, eight women were subjected to two paired studies—one pair in the low-estrogen, low-progesterone early follicular menstrual cycle phase and one pair after transdermal delivery of estradiol for 7 to 9 days, which increased estradiol plasma levels about fivefold [81]. In the high estradiol state, baseline DVRs of [¹¹C]CFN increased an average of 15% to 32% in the thalamus, amygdala, nucleus accumbens, and hypothalamus. These increases were correlated with estradiol plasma levels in the latter two. The high estradiol state also led to 12% to 19% decreases of pain-induced [¹¹C]CFN DVRs (ie, activation of μ receptors through endogenous opioid receptors) in the hypothalamus/nucleus accumbens and the amygdala ipsilateral to pain. Even more strikingly than in the earlier study [95], women in the low estradiol state did not show any activation of μ receptors but, on the contrary, "deactivations" in these same regions and the medial thalamus; these effects ranged from 11% to 16%.

Such increases are difficult to interpret, because opioid release generally requires high frequency firing [97], and the system overall does not seem tonically active, however, the authors discuss [81,95] some evidence that there may be a tonic release of endogenous opioids at baseline, particularly in the nucleus accumbens, but possibly also in the brainstem, amygdala, and other regions.

The group went on to demonstrate an effect of genotype on μ-receptor neurotransmission and used the common COMT val/met polymorphism described above in the section on opioid imaging in healthy volunteers. In addition to the substantial influence on baseline μ-receptor binding, with individuals with the met/met phenotype showing higher levels of μ-opioid receptors in the thalamus, ventral pallidum, and nucleus accumbens, these individuals also had substantially smaller activations of the μ-receptor system (with a gene "dose" effect and met/val heterozygotes intermediate between homozygotes) and, in parallel, higher negative ratings on affect scores and pain questionnaires.

Interestingly, the same group provided evidence that the placebo response is mediated via μ-opioid receptors. Fourteen healthy male volunteers underwent a three-scan paradigm consisting of a baseline scan and two scans with pain induction. During one of these, a placebo was administered with the expectation of pain relief. Placebo did relieve pain and also led to release of endogenous opioids in the middle frontal gyrus and nucleus accumbens ipsilateral to the pain and in the perigenual anterior cingulate gyrus and insula contralaterally when compared with the pain only condition [96].

In summary, work performed thus far has firmly established that activation of the endogenous opioid transmitter system in response to chronic or acute and prolonged pain can reliably be imaged using [11C]CFN and [11C]DPN in groups of healthy volunteers and patients. In addition, reductions of opioid receptor binding are seen as group effects when comparing pain patients with healthy controls using [11C]DPN or [18F]DPN, with a remarkably similar spatial pattern corresponding largely to the medial pain system despite different etiologies and localizations of the primary pathology. In paired studies, many of the effects could be seen in individual subjects. Having established some major determinants of baseline binding and opioid release, the next steps for the field will be to start investigating single patients—the ultimate beneficiaries of medical research—and establish clinical links that help in management and prognosis.

Opioid imaging in epilepsy

Epilepsy is the most common serious neurologic disorder, affecting 0.5% to 0.8% of the population. Epileptic seizures can arise from one part of the brain (focal epilepsies) or can appear generalized from the outset (generalized epilepsies). Among the focal epilepsies, temporal lobe epilepsy is the most common, and hippocampal sclerosis is the most frequent underlying cause. There is considerable interest in opioidergic mechanisms in epilepsy. Two recent reviews covering opioid imaging in epilepsy are available [98,99].

Focal epilepsies

Interictal studies

Overall opioid receptor binding has been studied with [11C]DPN in two studies. Using [11C]DPN ratios (region − occipital/occipital) for four regions (amygdala, anterior temporal/midtemporal/posterior temporal, ie, not hippocampus) derived from standard-sized rectangular regions of interest in a single PET plane in 11 patients with a video electroencephalogram confirmed temporal lobe epilepsy, no differences between the focus and nonfocus sides were seen [100]. Eleven controls were scanned but no results reported. A later study confirmed the absence of asymmetries of [11C]DPN binding in two patients [101]. In contrast, work in progress has shown abnormalities of [11C]DPN binding in 80% of patients with focal epilepsies due to malformations of cortical development [102].

[11C]CFN was used in the same 11 patients studied with [11C]DPN [100] and quantified in the same way in the same regions. In contrast to opioid receptors overall, increases of μ-receptor binding ratios were seen on the side of the epileptogenic focus in lateral midtemporal and posterior temporal neocortex, whereas binding in the amygdala was decreased. The latter finding might be due to partial volume effects that could be corrected for in contemporary studies [103]; however, the finding of lateral neocortical increases confirms an earlier study [104]. These increases of [11C]CFN binding coincided with areas of hypometabolism seen on [18F]FDG PET in the earlier [104] but not the later study [103]. Temporal neocortical binding increases were also seen in ten patients using the δ-receptor subtype selective antagonist [11C]MeNTI. Region definition was similar to that in the earlier study [100] but performed on three slices, and binding was quantified via ratios on 50- to 90-minute concentration images as (region − cerebellum)/cerebellum [69]. Because of [11C]MeNTI's essentially irreversible binding, this quantification method is likely suboptimal and was later abandoned [70]. Ratio increases for δ receptors were seen over all of the temporal neocortex ipsilateral to the seizure focus and included the amygdala. Significance was reached for the superior temporal pole, reaching more posteriorly in the most inferior of three PET slices available [69]. The increases in the inferior most slice coincided with increases of [11C]CFN ratios derived from the same patients. In contrast to the earlier study, no increases were seen in temporal neocortex at the level of the amygdala, although the amygdala [11C]CFN ratio decrease was replicated.

One speculative explanation is that an increase in μ receptors may be a manifestation of a tonic antiepileptic system in the temporal neocortex to limit the spread of epileptic activity, while the amygdalar decrease of [11C]CFN ratios could be related to mesial temporal hyperexcitability. Opposite changes of [11C]CFN and [11C]MeNTI ratios in the amygdala, implying increases of μ receptors but decreases of δ receptors, may explain why no asymmetries were detected with the nonselective tracer [11C]DPN.

Using [18F]CFX, the μ and κ antagonist, quantified with a kinetic model as a VD, there was no overall asymmetry in a group of 14 patients with temporal lobe epilepsy, but, in some individual patients, binding was increased in the ipsilateral temporal lobe [72]. Taken together with the temporal neocortical increases of μ receptors described previously, this finding would be consistent with a decrease in the affinity or number of κ receptors, or decreased availability of κ receptors through occupation by an endogenous ligand.

Ictal studies

Ictal studies have been performed in five patients with reading epilepsy compared with six controls with [^{11}C]DPN and a two-scan (rest-activation) paradigm [105]. Quantification was performed using a metabolite-corrected arterial plasma input function and spectral analysis. This approach allowed the computation of parametric maps of the IRF$_{60}$ and use of statistical parametric mapping. Reading epilepsy provides a model for focal epilepsy and has the advantage that seizures can be provoked easily through reading yet do not lead to significant head movement. Comparison of the resting condition in patients with that in controls revealed no significant differences. Reading-induced seizures were associated with reduced [^{11}C]DPN IRF$_{60}$ in the left parietotemporo-occipital cortex and to a lesser extent in the left middle temporal gyrus and posterior parieto-occipital junction (Fig. 4), implying release of endogenous opioids at the time of seizures. These areas are known to be involved in reading, visual processing, and recognition of words, and the researchers have since provided fMR imaging measures of increased cerebral blood flow during reading overlapping with these regions (Fig. 4).

Further evidence for the release of endogenous opioids at the time of seizures comes from a fortuitous ictal [^{18}F]CFX PET scan from the National Institutes of Health laboratory reported as a personal communication [106]. Frequent intermittent right medial temporal discharges developed about 6 minutes after injection, and the time-activity curve for the right medial temporal lobe remained constantly below that of the contralateral side for the remaining 60 minutes.

Taken together, these findings suggest an involvement of the opioid system in several forms of focal epilepsy. Currently, PET opioid studies are confined to research in a few centers and are not used clinically.

Idiopathic generalized epilepsy

[^{11}C]DPN VD was used to image all opioid receptor subtypes in eight patients with childhood and juvenile absence epilepsy compared with eight controls [107]. No significant differences were found, suggesting no overall interictal abnormalities of the opioid system in idiopathic generalized epilepsy. Nevertheless, changes were seen in a dynamic [^{11}C]DPN study investigating eight patients with primary generalized epilepsy and eight controls. In patients, absence seizures were induced by hyperventilation 30 to 40 minutes after tracer injection, and hyperventilation maintained for 10 minutes led to generalized spike-wave discharges for 10% to 51% of this period. After this provocation of serial absence seizures, a faster elimination of [^{11}C]DPN from association cortices but not thalamus, basal ganglia, or cerebellum was seen, suggested by simulations and a two-compartment model to correspond to an estimated 15% to 41% decrease in the specific tracer uptake rate constant (k3) [108], compatible with the release of endogenous opioids in association cortices at the time of seizures.

Summary

Opioid receptor alterations seem to be involved in temporal lobe epilepsy and other epilepsy syndromes. Some of the earlier studies could be replicated to benefit from the rapid progress in the

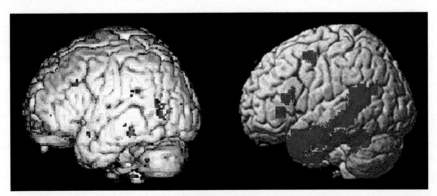

Fig. 4. Diprenorphine binding during reading-induced seizures compared with control conditions and cerebral blood flow during reading. (*Left*) Statistical parametric map on a normalized MR brain image. Areas with significantly decreased [^{11}C]diprenorphine (DPN) impulse response function at 60 minutes (IRF$_{60}$) during seizures are shown in yellow (Z = 5.22; $P < .05$ corrected) in the left parietotemporo-occipital cortex and red (uncorrected $P < .001$; not significant when corrected for multiple comparisons) in the right inferior parietal lobe (Z = 4.12), left superior temporal gyrus (Z = 4.02), left fusiform gyrus (Z = 4.00), left middle temporal gyrus (Z = 3.51), and left temporoparietal junction (Z = 3.37). (*From* Koepp MJ, Richardson MP, Brooks DJ, et al. Focal cortical release of endogenous opioids during reading-induced seizures. Lancet 1998;352:954; with permission.) (*Right*) fMR imaging results in healthy volunteers reading sentences versus pseudofont [134]. The activated areas overlap with those in which endogenous opioid release is seen.

fields of MR imaging and PET in the last decade. No detailed studies of extratemporal epilepsies and malformations of cortical development have been reported. In the absence of suitable κ-selective radioligands, the question of the interictal and ictal role of the κ-opioid system in the epilepsies remains open.

There is good evidence for ictal release of endogenous opioids in several syndromes. Because many of the opioid receptor ligands seem to be displaceable by endogenous transmitters, further systematic comparisons of the ictal state with the interictal state will be highly relevant. Future studies aiming to elucidate the pathophysiology of the epilepsies may benefit from the use of subtype-specific opioid ligands.

Opioid imaging in other specialties

Movement disorders

The high concentration of opioid peptides and receptors in the basal ganglia has prompted investigations in movement disorders. Parkinson's disease is the most common akinetic rigid movement disorder and is due to degeneration of nigral dopaminergic neurons projecting to the striatum; consequently, major differences have been shown in the dopaminergic system [109]. Several atypical parkinsonian syndromes, including multiple system atrophy and Steele-Richardson-Olszewski syndrome (SRO) (supranuclear palsy), typically do not respond to levodopa replacement therapy.

There were no differences in standard-sized putaminal and caudate region of interest [11C]DPN ratios over occipital cortex in eight normal controls and eight patients with a clinical diagnosis of Parkinson's disease [110]. In contrast, the same study showed that mean putaminal ratios were reduced in seven patients with multiple system atrophy (striatonigral degeneration subtype), with three of seven patients showing significant abnormalities defined as binding greater than 2.5 standard deviations below the control mean. Six patients with SRO syndrome (supranuclear palsy) showed decreased ratios in caudate and putamen as a group, with abnormal caudate binding in four of six patients and abnormal putaminal binding in all six. In the SRO group, mean binding was also significantly decreased when compared with that in Parkinson's disease patients.

Another study by the same group investigated six Parkinson's disease patients with dyskinesias (involuntary movements that are a complication of long-term treatment with levodopa therapy) compared with seven Parkinson's disease patients without dyskinesias and ten controls [111]. They used a region of interest approach on ratio images of [11C]DPN radioactivity concentration between 30 and 90 minutes postinjection, dividing caudate, putamen, and thalamus standard-sized region of interest values by occipital values, and in addition used spectral analysis to generate parametric images of IRF_{60} values. Again, no differences between non-dyskinetic Parkinson's disease patients and controls were seen. Dyskinetic patients showed reduced uptake ratios when compared with controls and their non-dyskinetic counterparts in the putamen and thalamus. A smaller difference was found between dyskinetic patients and controls in the caudate nucleus; this finding did not differentiate the dyskinetic from the non-dyskinetic group. There was a nonsignificant ($P < .1$) but large (11 years on average) age difference between the patient groups; however, the same group had seen no age effect on striatal [11C]DPN ratios in the earlier study [110]. The findings have some support in a decreasing putaminal uptake ratio with increased dyskinesia severity, defined as the summed scores (1–4) of the Unified Parkinson's Disease Rating Scale (UPDRS) items 32 and 33 (duration and disability), which just reached significance using a Pearson correlation, and the (nonsignificant) greater reduction of contralateral uptake ratios in two patients with unilateral dyskinesias. This study was one of the first to harness the power of statistical parametric mapping, developed in the same institution originally for blood flow studies, for the investigation of receptor binding studies. The statistical parametric mapping investigation of IRF_{60} not only confirmed the differences between dyskinetic Parkinson's disease patients and controls but also showed additional decreases in the pallidum and anterior cingulate gyrus, as well as increases in the middle and superior frontal gyri. Based on experimental evidence, the authors favored the interpretation that the striatal and thalamic reductions in opioid receptor binding were due to increased occupancy due to increased endogenous opioid transmission.

In view of no differences in dopamine D1 or D2 receptors between dyskinetic and non-dyskinetic Parkinson's disease patients and increased blood flow in basal ganglia and frontal cortex during levodopa-induced dyskinesias, this study overall suggests that dyskinesias are instead associated with alterations of opioid transmission in the basal ganglia, with resulting overactivity of basal ganglia–frontal connections [112].

Another condition in which opioid neurotransmission has been investigated is Huntington's disease, an autosomal dominantly transmitted neurodegeneration predominantly affecting the caudate nucleus which leads to psychiatric abnormalities, involuntary movements, and, ultimately, death in early middle age. In five patients with

Huntington's disease compared with nine controls, decreases of [^{11}C]DPN binding measures were seen with a variety of approaches. Importantly, IRF$_{60}$ images outperformed ratio images (striatal regions over occipital lobe for 30- to 90-minute radioactivity images), and statistical parametric mapping outperformed regional approaches in the sense that peak changes were more marked, and additional nonhypothesized decreases were found in the mid-to-anterior cingulate gyrus as well as nonhypothesized increases in thalami and pregenual cingulate gyrus/superior frontal gyrus [41], arguing strongly for the use of kinetic modeling techniques. Huntington's disease is accompanied by major atrophy, particularly of the caudate nucleus. The study did not correct for partial volume effects, and it is likely that this factor accounts at least for some of the observed decreases but not for the thalamic and cortical increases.

The findings in dyskinetic patients with Parkinson's disease and patients with Huntington's disease prompted investigation of carriers of a mutation in the DYT1 gene manifesting with primary torsion dystonia. There were no regional differences in [^{11}C]DPN VD in seven patients compared with 15 healthy controls and no correlation of opioid receptor binding with disease severity, arguing against a major role of opioid neurotransmission across all dyskinesias [113].

In the movement disorder restless legs syndrome, no differences between 15 patients and 12 age-matched healthy controls were seen using [^{11}C]DPN and either ratio methods or [^{11}C]DPN VD (n = 14 patients) [40]. [^{11}C]DPN VD was negatively correlated with the severity of restless legs syndrome in structures belonging to the medial pain system, and negatively correlated with the affect score of the McGill Pain Questionnaire in orbitofrontal cortex and anterior cingulate gyrus; both findings were interpreted as occupancy by endogenous opioids. Similar changes were seen using ratio images, but effect sizes and spatial extents were much smaller, underlining the value of quantitative kinetic analysis.

Tourette's syndrome is a tic disorder with motor and vocal tics starting before the age of 18 years. In five patients with this syndrome, basal ganglia total opioid receptor binding was not different from that in an undisclosed number of controls. Spectral analysis and statistical parametric mapping localized decreased binding in the cingulate gyrus, as well as increased binding in the insula bilaterally, the left premotor cortex and perigenual cingulate cortex [114]. These findings, although etiologically unclear, are interesting in the context of case reports of therapeutic utility of opioid neurotransmission modifying drugs (both antagonists and agonists).

Dementia

Opioid receptor alterations have been described in the most frequent dementia, Alzheimer's disease. A quantitative autoradiographic study investigated 11 brains of patients with Alzheimer's disease compared with 10 brains of age-matched controls who had had normal neurological status in life. There was decreased μ-receptor binding in the hippocampus (−48%) and subiculum (−46%), decreased δ-receptor binding in the amygdala (−51%) and ventral putamen (−30%), decreased κ-receptor binding in the hippocampus (−39%), and increased κ-receptor binding in the dorsal (+57%) and ventral (+93%) putamen and cerebellar cortex (+155%, but on the background of relatively low absolute binding) [27]. Quantifying receptor binding decreases in neurodegenerative diseases in vivo requires partial volume effect correction, which can be difficult. Nevertheless, the effect sizes shown in this postmortem study are remarkable, and the large increases in κ-receptor binding could potentially be useful for early diagnostic and therapeutic studies.

Early reports of μ-opioid receptor decrease in the amygdala in Alzheimer's disease measured by [^{11}C]CFN have not been pursued [115]. Work with [^{18}C]CFX in 12 patients with Alzheimer's disease and 12 age-matched controls using specific VD calculated as total VD minus medial occipital VD and standard-sized circular regions of interest in both groups revealed decreased specific VD in the Alzheimer patients in a global fashion but accentuated in parietal, frontal, and limbic areas [73]. It is unclear how partial volume effects affect kinetic modeling of time-activity curves derived from standard-sized regions of interest, and the global nature of changes as well as their smaller magnitude compared with cerebral blood flow changes make clinical usefulness of [^{18}C]CFX in Alzheimer's disease unlikely, particularly in view of the recent availability of in vivo markers of Alzheimer's pathology like [^{11}C]PIB or [^{18}F]FDDNP [116].

Cardiology

There are other areas in which opioid imaging could potentially be useful. For example, a recent preliminary study in five subjects showed BPs in myocardium of about 4 with [^{11}C]CFN and [^{11}C]MeNTI. High doses of naloxone, however, when given as a single pre-PET bolus without subsequent infusion, only reduced BPs by about 20% [117]. Nonetheless, this study shows the potential of opioid imaging techniques used outside the brain.

Opioid imaging in psychiatry: addiction

In contrast to the widespread use of PET/single-photon emission computed tomography (SPECT) imaging of dopaminergic systems in psychiatric disorders, opioid imaging has not been widely applied. The exception is in the addiction field. The opioid system is the target for opioid drugs of abuse and has a key role in modulating the dopaminergic system, mediating, for example, the pleasurable and reinforcing effects of alcohol [118].

The first study to explore the opioid system in addiction used [^{11}C]CFN to investigate the μ-opioid receptor in cocaine addiction. Increased levels of the μ-opioid receptor were found in ten cocaine addicts who were 1 to 4 days abstinent when compared with six controls [119]. Increased [^{11}C]CFN binding was seen throughout the brain in the anterior cingulate, frontal and temporal cortices, caudate, and thalamus. The increased levels in the amygdala, anterior cingulate, and frontal cortex positively correlated with the severity of cocaine craving reported. When rescanned at approximately 4 weeks of abstinence, in some but not all of the individuals, the increased levels of [^{11}C]CFN binding were reduced to levels comparable with those in healthy controls. A later study in 17 cocaine addicts compared with 16 controls also reported increased μ-opioid receptor levels as measured with [^{11}C]CFN in the anterior cingulate and frontal and lateral temporal cortices in cocaine addicts after 1 day of abstinence from cocaine [120]. Similar to the earlier study, the increased μ-opioid receptor levels correlated with self-reported craving in several brain regions (eg, the anterior cingulate, dorsolateral frontal cortex) but not ratings of depression or anxiety. Interestingly, the increased levels of [^{11}C]CFN binding in some frontal cortical regions (eg, dorsolateral frontal cortex) positively correlated with the amount of cocaine recently used. This finding suggests that the increased levels occur in response to cocaine use. Cocaine addicts were then scanned at 1 week and 12 weeks after monitored abstinence. The levels of [^{11}C]CFN binding and changes over time varied, depending on the brain region. For instance, μ-opioid receptors remained elevated in the anterior cingulate cortex after 1 week but in the dorsolateral cortex had reduced to control levels. Over the 12-week period, binding of [^{11}C]CFN decreased in all brain regions with the exception of the anterior cingulate cortex. Craving was still positively correlated with increased μ-opioid receptors at 1 week; however, after 12 weeks, craving was negligible, so correlational analysis was not performed.

The results of these two studies support a role for the opioid system in cocaine addiction. The level of μ-opioid receptor availability seems to be related to cocaine use and craving. [^{11}C]CFN is sensitive to endogenous opioid levels, and the reported increase in early abstinence from cocaine in dependent individuals could be due to an increase in receptor number or reduced endogenous opioid levels. The preclinical literature has reported that both may occur.

The opioid system has a key role in mediating the pleasurable effects of alcohol, and several lines of evidence suggest that altered function in the opioid system may be involved in vulnerability to alcohol dependence in humans [121]. In addition, the opioid antagonist naltrexone is an effective medication in treating alcohol misuse [122]. To test the hypothesis that increased opiate receptor levels may also mediate craving for alcohol, Heinz and coworkers [123] used [^{11}C]CFN PET to assess μ-opioid receptor levels in alcohol dependent individuals who had been abstinent for 1 to 3 weeks. Using regional analysis and statistical parametric mapping to compare [^{11}C]CFN levels in patients with that in controls, increased binding was seen in the ventral striatum, including the nucleus accumbens (**Fig. 5**). This area is involved in mediating reward-based learning, and its dopaminergic function is modulated by the opioid system. No differences were seen in other areas, including the cortex. Using statistical parametric mapping, a positive correlation between [^{11}C]CFN binding levels in the ventral striatum and self-reported craving was seen (**Fig. 5**). This finding is similar to observations in cocaine dependence. In addition, a positive correlation was seen between μ-opiate receptor levels in the frontal cortex and craving, as measured by the obsessive-compulsive drinking scale. This area of the cortex is involved in executive functioning; therefore, a dysfunctional μ-opioid system may contribute to the poor decision making often seen in dependent patients. Several other clinical variables were studied, including a family history of alcoholism, age, early versus late alcoholism (established dependency before and after the age of 25 years), and smoking, but none of these were significantly associated with μ-opioid receptor availability.

Some individuals maintained their sobriety and were rescanned 5 weeks later. Unlike in cocaine dependence, the higher [^{11}C]CFN binding levels persisted. It was not possible to determine whether the increased binding was due to reduced endogenous opioid levels or increased receptor levels; however, the researchers speculated that if receptor levels are increased, naltrexone may work through normalizing this increase and reducing the rewarding effects of alcohol.

In opiate addiction, a similar increase in opioid receptor availability in early abstinence has been reported. A preliminary study of three heroin dependent patients used [^{11}C]CFN PET to measure μ-opioid receptor availability during and after

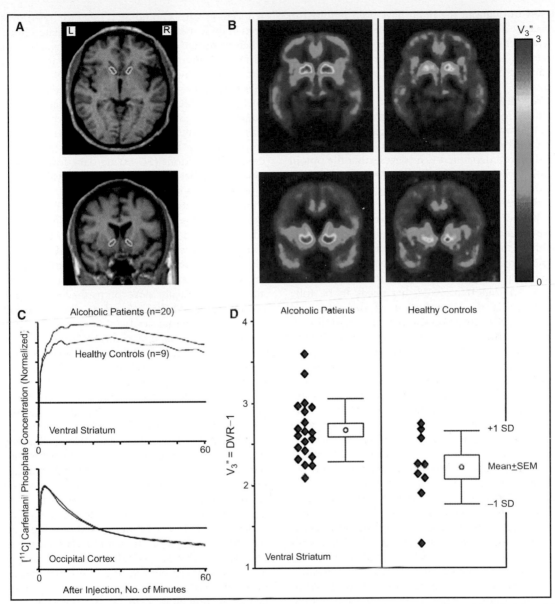

Fig. 5. Brain imaging of central μ-opiate receptor availability (V_3''). Region of interest analysis: (*A*) definition, (*C*) interindividually averaged time-activity curves, and (*D*) V_3'' of all participants, obtained from Logan plot. (*B*) Voxelwise averaged V_3'' parametric images of detoxified alcoholic patients, abstinent for 1 to 3 weeks (*top left*) compared with healthy volunteers (*top right*). The highest V_3'' in alcoholic patients and the largest difference between alcoholic patients and controls were found in the ventral striatum and the adjacent putamen. [11C]carfentanil indicates 11C-labeled carfentanil. In part (*D*), the open circles represent the mean; the box surrounding the circles, the standard error of the mean; and the bars, the standard deviation. (*From* Heinz A, Reimold M, Wrase J, et al. Correlation of stable elevations in striatal mu-opioid receptor availability in detoxified alcoholic patients with alcohol craving: a positron emission tomography study using carbon 11-labeled carfentanil. Arch Gen Psychiatry 2005;62(1):59; with permission.)

a brief 6-week ascending and descending regimen of the substitute drug, buprenorphine [124]. Buprenorphine is a partial agonist at the μ-opiate receptors and a κ antagonist. After withdrawal from buprenorphine, a significant increase in [11C]CFN binding was seen compared with that in controls in the inferofrontal and anterior cingulate cortices. The small number of patients studied likely contributed to the restricted areas showing a significant increase. Using [11C]DPN PET, higher binding levels throughout the brain have been reported in recently abstinent methadone-maintained heroin dependent patients compared with control subjects [125]. Unlike for cocaine or alcohol dependence, no significant correlation with craving was found.

Together these studies suggest that early abstinence from dependence is associated with increased availability of μ-opioid receptors. Because this increase has been shown for alcohol, cocaine, and opioid dependence, it suggests that the opioid system may have a fundamental role in addiction and that changes occur regardless of the substance of abuse. Although an increase in receptor availability is associated with craving in alcohol and cocaine dependence, this is not true in opioid dependence. Perhaps the direct action of the opioid abuse on the opioid receptors obscures any more subtle effects on the opiate system involved in reward and addiction. An important issue that needs to be fully explored is the contribution of the effects of substances of abuse on the opioid system, the effects of abstinence, or underlying vulnerability to the raised opioid receptor levels seen.

PET imaging has been widely used to explore the dose-occupancy relationship for a number of drugs in psychiatry, in particular D2 occupancy by the antipsychotic drugs [126]. In clinical practice, it became clear that high doses of these drugs were unnecessary because most D2 receptors were already blocked, and the risk of adverse side effects outweighed any small potential increase in antipsychotic efficacy. In the management of opioid addiction, patients are generally put on a substitute drug such as methadone or buprenorphine. In clinical practice, the dose of the substitute drug given is generally based on converting how much "street" opioid drugs such as heroin the patient is using, together with clinical observation of withdrawal or intoxication once on the substitute drug. There can be a wide variation in the dose of substitute drug, particularly methadone, that the patient eventually is maintained on (eg, tens of milligrams to over 100 mg). In addition, patients can request more substitute drug when it is not clear to the clinician that they are in withdrawal or need more. PET imaging can assess the dose-occupancy relationship for these two substitute drugs at the opioid receptor in an attempt to determine how much drug to give to a patient.

Methadone, a μ agonist, is the most widely prescribed substitute drug. A group of opioid dependent patients who had been maintained on methadone for many years (2–27 years) and were stable underwent a [^{18}C]CFX PET scan [127]. In regions of interest such as the anterior cingulate cortex, thalamus, caudate nucleus, and amygdala, reduced [^{18}C]CFX binding (19% to 32%) was seen in these methadone-maintained opiate addicts when compared with controls. The scans were performed 22 hours after the last dose of methadone, almost at a time when their next daily dose was due. Plasma levels of methadone only weakly correlated with [^{18}C]CFX binding in the caudate and putamen and not significantly in any other region. It was speculated that only a small number of opioid receptors were occupied by clinically efficacious doses of methadone (30–90 mg/day), leaving a significant number of opioid receptors available for other functions such as pain relief.

Another study using [^{11}C]DPN PET has also explored the dose-occupancy relationship for methadone [128]. In this study, no significant relationship between the dose of methadone and [^{11}C]DPN binding was evident, and complementary preclinical work revealed that [^{11}C]DPN binding was not altered by an acute dose of methadone despite having profound behavioral effects. The conclusion was that methadone needs to occupy a small percentage of receptors to be clinical efficacious and at a level that is undetectable using [^{11}C]DPN PET. These findings were slightly at odds with a previous study from the same group that had shown blockade of opioid agonist effects in a similar group of methadone-maintained patients [129], suggesting that few opioid receptors were available.

Although both studies suggest that methadone does not need to occupy a large percentage of opioid receptors for efficacy, neither can help with rational prescribing, that is, how much methadone to give to reach a maximal clinical effect. The studies suggest that the tolerance seen to opiates in such patients is due to altered opioid receptor function other than removal of the opioid receptor binding site, because this site is clearly still available for the radiotracers to bind to. It is likely that mechanisms involved in transmembrane signaling underlie this phenomenon. Evidence from preclinical or human postmortem studies is also not consistent as to what happens to the opioid receptor in opioid dependence, with increases, reductions, or no change reported [130,131]. It is notable that opioid withdrawal can be ameliorated with non-opioid drugs, suggesting that this system is not critical in mediating all of the effects of abused opioid drugs [132].

By contrast, a clear dose-occupancy relationship is apparent with buprenorphine, a partial agonist at the μ receptor and κ antagonist. In a preliminary study of three heroin dependent patients using [^{11}C]CFN PET, 2 mg of buprenorphine, a relatively low clinical dose, occupied 36% to 50% of opioid receptors [124]. A relatively large clinical dose, 16 mg, resulted in 79% to 95% occupancy; however, there was a large variation in the percentage occupancy seen. In a follow-up study using more patients, buprenorphine resulted in significant reduction of [^{11}C]CFN binding by 41% with 2 mg, 80% with 16 mg, and 84% with 32 mg [132]. This degree of occupancy was seen throughout the brain, including areas of interest such as the anterior cingulate gyrus, amygdala, and frontal cortical regions, and was correlated with plasma buprenorphine levels. In addition, blockade of opioid agonist effects correlated with buprenorphine occupancy. PET opioid receptor imaging has been informative, showing the amount of buprenorphine required to result in almost complete occupancy of opioid receptors.

Summary

The excitement of the 1970s, when opioid receptors and the various subtypes were described, has been matched in the 1990s and early years of this century by the application of ever higher resolution whole-brain PET scanners, the availability of several radioligands, the combination of PET with advanced structural imaging, advances in modeling of macroparameters of PET ligand binding, and efforts in large-scale statistical analysis of imaging datasets. Suitable SPECT tracers are lacking, but with the current increase in the number of available PET (or PET/CT) cameras and cyclotrons owing to the clinical success of PET in oncology, PET may become widespread enough to overcome this.

Many breakthrough scientific discoveries have been made using opioid imaging. It is to be hoped that, in the coming decade, there will be a more widespread application of the available techniques to patients and an impact in clinical medicine.

Acknowledgments

The authors would like to thank their colleagues at the MRC Clinical Sciences Centre, Hammersmith Hospital, and the Department of Clinical and Experimental Epilepsy, Institute of Neurology, particularly Dr. Matthias Koepp and Professor John Duncan for helpful discussions, Dr. Federico Turkheimer for proofreading parts of this review, and Dr. Matthias Glaser for the drawings of the chemical structures.

References

[1] Pert CB, Snyder SH. Properties of opiate-receptor binding in rat brain. Proc Natl Acad Sci USA 1973;70:2243–7.

[2] Simon EJ, Hiller JM, Edelman I. Stereospecific binding of the potent narcotic analgesic (3H) Etorphine to rat-brain homogenate. Proc Natl Acad Sci USA 1973;70:1947–9.

[3] Terenius L. Stereospecific interaction between narcotic analgesics and a synaptic plasma membrane fraction of rat cerebral cortex. Acta Pharmacol Toxicol (Copenh) 1973;32:317–20.

[4] Martin WR, Eades CG, Thompson JA, et al. The effects of morphine- and nalorphine-like drugs in the nondependent and morphine-dependent chronic spinal dog. J Pharmacol Exp Ther 1976; 197:517–32.

[5] Lord JA, Waterfield AA, Hughes J, et al. Endogenous opioid peptides: multiple agonists and receptors. Nature 1977;267:495–9.

[6] Kosterlitz HW, Paterson SJ, Robson LE. Characterization of the kappa-subtype of the opiate receptor in the guinea-pig brain. Br J Pharmacol 1981;73:939–49.

[7] Darland T, Heinricher MM, Grandy DK. Orphanin FQ/nococeptin: a role in pain and analgesia, but so much more. Trends Neurosci 1998; 21:215–21.

[8] Mogil JS, Pasternak GW. The molecular and behavioral pharmacology of the orphanin FQ/nociceptin peptide and receptor family. Pharmacol Rev 2001;53:381–415.

[9] Pleuvry BJ. Opioid receptors and their ligands: natural and unnatural. Br J Anaesth 1991;66: 370–80.

[10] Alexander S, Peters J, Mead A, et al. TiPS receptor and ion channel nomenclature supplement 1999. Trends Pharmacol Sci 1999;19(Suppl 1): 62–3.

[11] Simmons ML, Chavkin C. Endogenous opioid regulation of hippocampal function. Int Rev Neurobiol 1996;39:145–96.

[12] Bayon A, Rossier J, Mauss A, et al. In vitro release of [5-methionine] enkephalin and [5-leucine] enkephalin from the rat globus pallidus. Proc Natl Acad Sci USA 1978;75:3505–6.

[13] Neumaier JF, Chavkin C. Release of endogenous opioid peptides displaces [^{3}H] diprenorphine binding in rat hippocampal slices. Brain Res 1989;493:292–302.

[14] Wagner JJ, Evans CJ, Chavkin C. Focal stimulation of the mossy fibers releases endogenous dynorphins that bind kappa 1-opioid receptors in guinea pig hippocampus. J Neurochem 1991; 57(1):333–43.

[15] Drake CT, Terman GW, Simmons ML, et al. Dynorphin opioids present in dentate granule cells may function as retrograde inhibitory neurotransmitters. J Neurosci 1994;14:3736–50.

[16] Corbett A, Paterson S, McKnight A, et al. Dynorphin (1–8) and dynorphin (1–9) are ligands for the kappa-subtype of opiate receptor. Nature 1982;299:79–81.

[17] Chaturvedi K, Christoffers KH, Singh K, et al. Structure and regulation of opioid receptors. Biopolymers 2000;55:334–46.

[18] Simonato M, Romualdi P. Dynorphin and epilepsy. Prog Neurobiol 1996;50:557–83.

[19] Crain BJ, Chang KJ, McNamara JO. An in vitro autoradiographic analysis of mu and delta opioid binding in the hippocampal formation of kindled rats. Brain Res 1987;412:305–10.

[20] Perry DC, Grimes LM. Administration of kainic acid and colchicine alters mu and lambda opiate binding in rat hippocampus. Brain Res 1989;477:100–8.

[21] Pfeiffer M, Kirscht S, Stumm R, et al. Heterodimerization of substance P and mu-opioid receptors regulates receptor trafficking and resensitization. J Biol Chem 2003;278(51):51630–7.

[22] Minnis JG, Patierno S, Kohlmeier SE, et al. Ligand-induced mu opioid receptor endocytosis and recycling in enteric neurons. Neuroscience 2003;119(1):33–42.

[23] Lecoq I, Marie N, Jauzac P, et al. Different regulation of human delta-opioid receptors by SNC-80 [(+)-4-[(alphaR)-alpha-((2S,5R)-4-allyl-2,5-dimethyl-1-piperazinyl)-3-meth oxybenzyl]-N,N-diethylbenzamide] and endogenous enkephalins. J Pharmacol Exp Ther 2004;310(2):666–77.

[24] Chen LE, Gao C, Chen J, et al. Internalization and recycling of human mu opioid receptors expressed in Sf9 insect cells. Life Sci 2003;73(1):115–28.

[25] Pfeiffer A, Pasi A, Mehraein P, et al. Opiate receptor binding sites in human brain. Brain Res 1982;248:87–96.

[26] Hiller JM, Fan LQ. Laminar distribution of the multiple opioid receptors in the human cerebral cortex. Neurochem Res 1996;21:1333–45.

[27] Mathieu-Kia AM, Fan LQ, Kreek MJ, et al. Mu-, delta- and kappa-opioid receptor populations are differentially altered in distinct areas of postmortem brains of Alzheimer's disease patients. Brain Res 2001;893(1–2):121–34.

[28] Peckys D, Landwehrmeyer GB. Expression of mu, kappa, and delta opioid receptor messenger RNA in the human CNS: a ^{33}P in situ hybridization study. Neuroscience 1999;88:1093–135.

[29] Pilapil C, Welner S, Magnan J, et al. Autoradiographic distribution of multiple classes of opioid receptor binding sites in human forebrain. Brain Res Bull 1987;19:611–5.

[30] Schadrack J, Willoch F, Platzer S, et al. Opioid receptors in the human cerebellum: evidence from [11C]diprenorphine PET, mRNA expression and autoradiography. Neuroreport 1999;10(3):619–24.

[31] Kuhar MJ, Pert CB, Snyder SH. Regional distribution of opiate receptor binding in monkey and human brain. Nature 1973;245:447–50.

[32] Platzer S, Winkler A, Schadrack J, et al. Autoradiographic distribution of mu-, delta- and kappa 1-opioid stimulated [^{35}S]guanylyl-5'-O-(gamma-thio)-triphosphate binding in human frontal cortex and cerebellum. Neurosci Lett 2000;283:213–6.

[33] Rodríguez-Puertas R, González-Maeso J, Meana JJ, et al. Autoradiography of receptor-activated G-proteins in post mortem human brain. Neuroscience 2000;96:169–80.

[34] Zubieta J-K, Dannals RF, Frost JJ. Gender and age influences on human brain mu-opioid receptor binding measured by PET. Am J Psychiatry 1999;156:842–8.

[35] Cherry SR, Phelps ME. Imaging brain function with positron emission tomography. In: Toga AW, Mazziotta JC, editors. Brain mapping: the methods. San Diego: Academic Press; 1996. p. 191–221.

[36] Wienhard K, Wagner R, Heiss W-D. PET. Grundlagen und Anwendungen der Positronen-Emissions-Tomographie. Berlin, Heidelberg, New York: Springer-Verlag; 1989.

[37] Valk PE, Bailey DL, Townsend DW, et al, editors. Positron emission tomography: basic science and clinical practice. London, Berlin, Heidelberg: Springer-Verlag; 2003. p. 884.

[38] Gunn RN, Lammertsma AA, Hume SP, et al. Parametric imaging of ligand-receptor binding in PET using a simplified reference region model. NeuroImage 1997;6(4):279–87.

[39] Hammers A, Asselin MC, Osman S, et al. Towards improved test-retest reliability in quantitative ligand PET: [^{11}C]diprenorphine as an example. [abstract]. J Cereb Blood Flow Metab 2005;25:S665.

[40] von Spiczak S, Whone AL, Hammers A, et al. The role of opioids in restless legs syndrome: an [11C]diprenorphine PET study. Brain 2005;128(Pt 4):906–17.

[41] Weeks RA, Cunningham VJ, Piccini P, et al. ^{11}C-diprenorphine binding in Huntington's disease: a comparison of region of interest analysis with statistical parametric mapping. J Cereb Blood Flow Metab 1997;17:943–9.

[42] Tadokoro M, Jones AKP, Cunningham VJ, et al. Parametric images of ^{11}C-diprenorphine binding using spectral analysis of dynamic PET images acquired in 3D. In: Uemura K, et al, editors. Quantification of brain function: tracer kinetics and image analysis in brain PET. Amsterdam: Excerpta Medica; 1993. p. 289–94.

[43] Turkheimer FE, Hinz R, Gunn RN, et al. Rank-shaping regularization of exponential spectral analysis for application to functional parametric mapping. Phys Med Biol 2003;48(23):3819–41.

[44] Gunn RN, Gunn SR, Turkheimer FE, et al. Positron emission tomography compartmental models: a basis pursuit strategy for kinetic modeling. J Cereb Blood Flow Metab 2002;22(12):1425–39.

[45] Turkheimer F, Sokoloff L, Bertoldo A, et al. Estimation of component and parameter distributions in spectral analysis. J Cereb Blood Flow Metab 1998;18(11):1211–22.

[46] Kukreja SL, Gunn RN. Bootstrapped DEPICT for error estimation in PET functional imaging. Neuroimage 2004;21(3):1096–104.

[47] Hammers A, Koepp MJ, Labbé C, et al. Neocortical abnormalities of [11C]-flumazenil PET in mesial temporal lobe epilepsy. Neurology 2001; 56:897–906.

[48] Theodore WH, Sato S, Kufta C, et al. Temporal lobectomy for uncontrolled seizures: the role of positron emission tomography. Ann Neurol 1992;32:789–94.

[49] Hajek M, Antonini A, Leenders KL, et al. Mesiobasal versus lateral temporal lobe epilepsy: metabolic differences shown in the temporal lobe shown by interictal 18F-FDG positron emission tomography. Neurology 1993;43: 79–86.

[50] Henry TR, Mazziotta JC, Engel JJ, et al. Quantifying interictal metabolic activity in human temporal lobe epilepsy. J Cereb Blood Flow Metab 1990;10:748–57.

[51] Kiebel SJ, Ashburner J, Poline JB, et al. MRI and PET coregistration: a cross validation of statistical parametric mapping and automated image registration. Neuroimage 1997;5:271–9.

[52] Koepp MJ, Richardson MP, Labbé C, et al. 11C-flumazenil PET, volumetric MRI, and quantitative pathology in mesial temporal lobe epilepsy. Neurology 1997;49(3):764–73.

[53] Knowlton RC, Laxer KD, Klein G, et al. In vivo hippocampal glucose metabolism in mesial temporal lobe epilepsy. Neurology 2001;57: 1184–90.

[54] Labbé C, Koepp MJ, Ashburner J, et al. Absolute PET quantification with correction for partial volume effects within cerebral structures. In: Carson C, Daube-Witherspoon M, Herscovitch P, editors. Quantitative functional brain imaging with positron emission tomography. San Diego: Academic Press; 1998. p. 59–66.

[55] Rousset OG, Ma Y, Evans AC. Correction for partial volume effects in PET: principle and validation. J Nucl Med 1998;39:904–11.

[56] Aston JAD, Cunningham VJ, Asselin MC, et al. Positron emission tomography partial volume correction: estimation and algorithms. J Cereb Blood Flow Metab 2002;22:1019–34.

[57] Richardson MP, Friston KJ, Sisodiya SM, et al. Cortical grey matter and benzodiazepine receptors in malformations of cortical development: a voxel-based comparison of structural and functional imaging data. Brain 1997;120(Pt 11): 1961–73.

[58] Richards ML, Sadee W. In vivo opiate receptor binding of oripavines to mu, delta and kappa sites in rat brain as determined by an ex vivo labeling method. Eur J Pharmacol 1985;114(3): 343–53.

[59] Asselin M-C, Hammers A, Sethi FN, et al. Definition of a reference region for PET/ [11C]diprenorphine studies [abstract]. J Cereb Blood Flow Metab 2003;23(Suppl):679.

[60] Lee KO, Akil H, Woods JH, et al. Differential binding properties of oripavines at cloned mu- and delta-opioid receptors. Eur J Pharmacol 1999;378(3):323–30.

[61] Frost JJ, Wagner HN Jr, Dannals RF, et al. Imaging opiate receptors in the human brain by positron tomography. J Comput Assist Tomogr 1985;9:231–6.

[62] Jones AKP, Luthra SK, Maziere B, et al. Regional cerebral opioid receptor studies with [11C]diprenorphine in normal volunteers. J Neurosci Methods 1988;23:121–9.

[63] Wester HJ, Willoch F, Tolle TR, et al. 6-O-(2-[18F]fluoroethyl)-6-O-desmethyldiprenorphine ([18F]DPN): synthesis, biologic evaluation, and comparison with [11C]DPN in humans. J Nucl Med 2000;41(7):1279–86.

[64] Frost JJ, Douglass KH, Mayberg HS, et al. Multicompartmental analysis of [11C]-carfentanil binding to opiate receptors in humans measured by positron emission tomography. J Cereb Blood Flow Metab 1989;9(3): 398–409.

[65] Lammertsma AA, Hume SP. Simplified reference tissue model for PET receptor studies. Neuroimage 1996;4:153–8.

[66] Endres CJ, Bencherif B, Hilton J, et al. Quantification of brain mu-opioid receptors with [11C]carfentanil: reference-tissue methods. Nucl Med Biol 2003;30(2):177–86.

[67] Henriksen G, Platzer S, Marton J, et al. Syntheses, biological evaluation, and molecular modeling of 18F-labeled 4-anilidopiperidines as mu-opioid receptor imaging agents. J Med Chem 2005;48(24):7720–32.

[68] Madar I, Lever JR, Kinter CM, et al. Imaging of delta opioid receptors in human brain by N1'-([11C]methyl)naltrindole and PET. Synapse 1996;24(1):19–28.

[69] Madar I, Lesser RP, Krauss G, et al. Imaging of δ- and μ-opioid receptors in temporal lobe epilepsy by positron emission tomography. Ann Neurol 1997;41:358–67.

[70] Smith JS, Zubieta JK, Price JC, et al. Quantification of delta-opioid receptors in human brain with N1'-([11C]methyl) naltrindole and positron emission tomography. J Cereb Blood Flow Metab 1999;19(9):956–66.

[71] Rothman RB, Bykov V, Reid A, et al. A brief study of the selectivity of norbinaltorphimine, (-)-cyclofoxy, and (+)-cyclofoxy among opioid receptor subtypes in vitro. Neuropeptides 1988;12(3):181–7.

[72] Theodore WH, Carson RE, Andreasen P, et al. PET imaging of opiate receptor binding in human epilepsy using [18F]cyclofoxy. Epilepsy Res 1992;13:129–39.

[73] Cohen RM, Andreason PJ, Doudet DJ, et al. Opiate receptor avidity and cerebral blood

flow in Alzheimer's disease. J Neurol Sci 1997;
148(2):171–80.

[74] Cohen RM, Carson RE, Sunderland T. Opiate receptor avidity in the thalamus is sexually dimorphic in the elderly. Synapse 2000;38(2):226–9.

[75] Talbot PS, Narendran R, Butelman ER, et al. ¹¹C–GR103545, a radiotracer for imaging kappa-opioid receptors in vivo with PET: synthesis and evaluation in baboons. J Nucl Med 2005;46(3):484–94.

[76] Ravert HT, Scheffel U, Mathews WB, et al. [(11)C]-GR89696, a potent kappa opiate receptor radioligand; in vivo binding of the R and S enantiomers. Nucl Med Biol 2002;29(1): 47–53.

[77] Jones AK, Qi LY, Fujirawa T, et al. In vivo distribution of opioid receptors in man in relation to the cortical projections of the medial and lateral pain systems measured with positron emission tomography. Neurosci Lett 1991;126(1):25–8.

[78] Baumgartner U, Buchholz HG, Bellosevich A, et al. High opiate receptor binding potential in the human lateral pain system. Neuroimage 2006;30(3):692–9.

[79] Zubieta JK, Heitzeg MM, Smith YR, et al. COMT val158met genotype affects mu-opioid neurotransmitter responses to a pain stressor. Science 2003;299(5610):1240–3.

[80] Berthele A, Platzer S, Jochim B, et al. COMT Val108/158Met genotype affects the mu-opioid receptor system in the human brain: evidence from ligand-binding, G-protein activation and preproenkephalin mRNA expression. Neuroimage 2005;28(1):185–93.

[81] Smith YR, Stohler CS, Nichols TE, et al. Pronociceptive and antinociceptive effects of estradiol through endogenous opioid neurotransmission in women. J Neurosci 2006;26(21):5777–85.

[82] Zubieta JK, Ketter TA, Bueller JA, et al. Regulation of human affective responses by anterior cingulate and limbic mu-opioid neurotransmission. Arch Gen Psychiatry 2003;60(11):1145–53.

[83] Liberzon I, Zubieta JK, Fig LM, et al. mu-Opioid receptors and limbic responses to aversive emotional stimuli. Proc Natl Acad Sci USA 2002; 99(10):7084–9.

[84] Apkarian AV, Bushnell MC, Treede RD, et al. Human brain mechanisms of pain perception and regulation in health and disease. Eur J Pain 2005;9(4):463–84.

[85] Jones AK, Watabe H, Cunningham VJ, et al. Cerebral decreases in opioid receptor binding in patients with central neuropathic pain measured by [¹¹C]diprenorphine binding and PET. Eur J Pain 2004;8(5):479–85.

[86] Willoch F, Tolle TR, Wester HJ, et al. Central poststroke pain and reduced opioid receptor binding within pain processing circuitries: a [¹¹C]diprenorphine PET study. Pain 2004; 108(3):213–20.

[87] Willoch F, Schindler F, Wester HJ, et al. Central pain after pontine infarction is associated with changes in opioid receptor binding: a PET study with ¹¹C-diprenorphine. AJNR Am J Neuroradiol 1999;20(4):686–90.

[88] Sprenger T, Willoch F, Miederer M, et al. Opioidergic changes in the pineal gland and hypothalamus in cluster headache: a ligand PET study. Neurology 2006;66(7):1108–10.

[89] May A, Ashburner J, Buchel C, et al. Correlation between structural and functional changes in brain in an idiopathic headache syndrome. Nat Med 1999;5:836–8.

[90] Sprenger T, Valet M, Boecker H, et al. Opioidergic activation in the medial pain system after heat pain. Pain 2006;122(1–2):63–7.

[91] Jones AK, Cunningham VJ, Ha-Kawa S, et al. Changes in central opioid receptor binding in relation to inflammation and pain in patients with rheumatoid arthritis. Br J Rheumatol 1994;33(10):909–16.

[92] Jones AK, Kitchen ND, Watabe H, et al. Measurement of changes in opioid receptor binding in vivo during trigeminal neuralgic pain using [¹¹C] diprenorphine and positron emission tomography. J Cereb Blood Flow Metab 1999; 19(7):803–8.

[93] Bencherif B, Fuchs PN, Sheth R, et al. Pain activation of human supraspinal opioid pathways as demonstrated by [¹¹C]-carfentanil and positron emission tomography (PET). Pain 2002; 99(3):589–98.

[94] Zubieta JK, Smith YR, Bueller JA, et al. Regional mu opioid receptor regulation of sensory and affective dimensions of pain. Science 2001; 293(5528):311–5.

[95] Zubieta JK, Smith YR, Bueller JA, et al. μ-opioid receptor-mediated antinociceptive responses differ in men and women. J Neurosci 2002; 22(12):5100–7.

[96] Zubieta JK, Bueller JA, Jackson LR, et al. Placebo effects mediated by endogenous opioid activity on mu-opioid receptors. J Neurosci 2005; 25(34):7754–62.

[97] Tortella FC. Endogenous opioid peptides and epilepsy: quieting the seizing brain? Trends Pharmacol Sci 1988;9:366–72.

[98] Koepp MJ, Duncan JS. PET: opiate neuroreceptor mapping. Adv Neurol 2000;83:145–56.

[99] Hammers A. Flumazenil PET and other ligands for functional imaging. Neuroimaging Clin N Am 2004;14(3):537–51.

[100] Mayberg HS, Sadzot B, Meltzer CC, et al. Quantification of mu and non-mu receptors in temporal lobe epilepsy using positron emission tomography. Ann Neurol 1991;30:3–11.

[101] Bartenstein PA, Prevett MC, Duncan JS, et al. Quantification of opiate receptors in two patients with mesiobasal temporal lobe epilepsy, before and after selective amygdalohippocampectomy, using positron emission tomography. Epilepsy Res 1994;18(2):119–25.

[102] Hammers A, Koepp MJ, Richardson MP, et al. [¹¹C]-diprenorphine PET in malformations of

cortical development (MCD) [abstract]. Epilepsia 2001;42(S7):100.

[103] Meltzer CC, Zubieta JK, Links JM, et al. MR-based correction for brain PET measurements for heterogeneous gray matter radioactivity distribution. J Cereb Blood Flow Metab 1996;16:650–8.

[104] Frost JJ, Mayberg HS, Fisher RS, et al. Mu-opiate receptors measured by positron emission tomography are increased in temporal lobe epilepsy. Ann Neurol 1988;23:231–7.

[105] Koepp MJ, Richardson MP, Brooks DJ, et al. Focal cortical release of endogenous opioids during reading-induced seizures. Lancet 1998;352:952–5.

[106] Koepp MJ, Duncan JS. PET: opiate neuroreceptor mapping. In: Henry TR, Duncan JS, Berkovic SF, editors. Functional imaging in the epilepsies. Philadelphia: Lippincott Williams & Wilkins; 2000. p. 145–55.

[107] Prevett MC, Cunningham VJ, Brooks DJ, et al. Opiate receptors in idiopathic generalised epilepsy measured with ^{11}C-diprenorphine and PET. Epilepsy Res 1994;19:71–7.

[108] Bartenstein PA, Duncan JS, Prevett MC, et al. Investigation of the opioid system in absence seizures with positron emission tomography. J Neurol Neurosurg Psychiatry 1993;56:1295–302.

[109] Brooks DJ. Neuroimaging in Parkinson's disease. NeuroRx 2004;1(2):243–54.

[110] Burn DJ, Rinne JO, Quinn NP, et al. Striatal opioid receptor binding in Parkinson's disease, striatonigral degeneration and Steele-Richardson-Olszewski syndrome, a [^{11}C]diprenorphine PET study. Brain 1995;118(Pt 4):951–8.

[111] Piccini P, Weeks RA, Brooks DJ. Alterations in opioid receptor binding in Parkinson's disease patients with levodopa-induced dyskinesias. Ann Neurol 1997;42(5):720–6.

[112] Brooks DJ, Piccini P, Turjanski N, et al. Neuroimaging of dyskinesia. Ann Neurol 2000;47(4, Suppl 1):S154–8 [discussion: S158–9].

[113] Whone AL, Von Spiczak S, Edwards M, et al. Opioid binding in DYT1 primary torsion dystonia: an ^{11}C-diprenorphine PET study. Mov Disord 2004;19(12):1498–503.

[114] Weeks RA, Turjanski N, Brooks DJ. Tourette's syndrome: a disorder of cingulate and orbitofrontal function? QJM 1996;89(6):401–8.

[115] Mueller-Gaertner HW, Mayberg HS, Ravert HT, et al. Mu opiate receptor binding in amygdala in Alzheimer's disease: in vivo quantification by ^{11}C carfentanil and PET [abstract]. J Cereb Blood Flow Metab 1991;11(Suppl 2):S20.

[116] Nordberg A. PET imaging of amyloid in Alzheimer's disease. Lancet Neurol 2004;3(9):519–27.

[117] Villemagne PS, Dannals RF, Ravert HT, et al. PET imaging of human cardiac opioid receptors. Eur J Nucl Med Mol Imaging 2002;29(10):1385–8.

[118] Kreek MJ, LaForge KS, Butelman E. Pharmacotherapy of addictions. Nat Rev Drug Discov 2002;1(9):710–26.

[119] Zubieta JK, Gorelick DA, Stauffer R, et al. Increased mu opioid receptor binding detected by PET in cocaine-dependent men is associated with cocaine craving. Nat Med 1996;2(11):1225–9.

[120] Gorelick DA, Kim YK, Bencherif B, et al. Imaging brain mu-opioid receptors in abstinent cocaine users: time course and relation to cocaine craving. Biol Psychiatry 2005;57(12):1573–82.

[121] Lingford-Hughes A, Nutt D. Neurobiology of addiction and implications for treatment. Br J Psychiatry 2003;182:97–100.

[122] Lingford-Hughes AR, Welch S, Nutt DJ. Evidence-based guidelines for the pharmacological management of substance misuse, addiction and comorbidity: recommendations from the British Association for Psychopharmacology. J Psychopharmacol 2004;18(3):293–335.

[123] Heinz A, Reimold M, Wrase J, et al. Correlation of stable elevations in striatal mu-opioid receptor availability in detoxified alcoholic patients with alcohol craving: a positron emission tomography study using carbon 11-labeled carfentanil. Arch Gen Psychiatry 2005;62(1):57–64.

[124] Zubieta J, Greenwald MK, Lombardi U, et al. Buprenorphine-induced changes in mu-opioid receptor availability in male heroin-dependent volunteers: a preliminary study. Neuropsychopharmacology 2000;23(3):326–34.

[125] Williams TM, Daglish MRC, Lingford-Hughes AR, et al. Increased availability of opioid receptors in early abstinence from opioid dependence: an [^{11}C]diprenorphine PET study. Submitted.

[126] Pilowsky LS. Probing targets for antipsychotic drug action with PET and SPET receptor imaging. Nucl Med Commun 2001;22(7):829–33.

[127] Kling MA, Carson RE, Borg L, et al. Opioid receptor imaging with positron emission tomography and [(18)F]cyclofoxy in long-term, methadone-treated former heroin addicts. J Pharmacol Exp Ther 2000;295(3):1070–6.

[128] Melichar JK, Hume SP, Williams TM, et al. Using [^{11}C]diprenorphine to image opioid receptor occupancy by methadone in opioid addiction: clinical and preclinical studies. J Pharmacol Exp Ther 2005;312(1):309–15.

[129] Melichar JK, Myles JS, Eap CB, et al. Using saccadic eye movements as objective measures of tolerance in methadone dependent individuals during the hydromorphone challenge test. Addict Biol 2003;8(1):59–66.

[130] Goodman CB, Emilien B, Becketts K, et al. Downregulation of mu-opioid binding sites

following chronic administration of neuropeptide FF (NPFF) and morphine. Peptides 1996; 17(3):389–97.

[131] Zadina JE, Kastin AJ, Harrison LM, et al. Opiate receptor changes after chronic exposure to agonists and antagonists. Ann N Y Acad Sci 1995; 757:353–61.

[132] Greenwald MK, Johanson CE, Moody DE, et al. Effects of buprenorphine maintenance dose on mu-opioid receptor availability, plasma concentrations, and antagonist blockade in heroin-dependent volunteers. Neuropsychopharmacology 2003;28(11):2000–9.

[133] Holmes CJ, Hoge R, Collins L, et al. Enhancement of MR images using registration for signal averaging. J Comput Assist Tomogr 1998;18: 192–205.

[134] Noppeney U, Price CJ. An FMRI study of syntactic adaptation. J Cogn Neurosci 2004; 16(4):702–13.

NEUROIMAGING CLINICS OF NORTH AMERICA

Neuroimag Clin N Am 16 (2006) 553–573

Applications of Clinical Dopamine Imaging

Kimberly P. Lindsey, PhD[a,b], S. John Gatley, PhD[c,*]

- Dopamine
  Overview
  Dopamine circuitry: pathways
  Molecules and targets
- Dopamine imaging
  General overview
  Technique overview: PET and SPECT
    neuroimaging
  Radiotracers for PET and SPECT
- Transporter ligands
  Vesicular monoamine transporter 2
  Dopamine transporter
  (^{99m}Tc) TRODAT-1
  Nomifensine
  Methylphenidate
  WIN 35 428 (CFT)

- Dopamine receptor ligands
- Measuring dopaminergic function
  Pharmacologic manipulations
  F-DOPA
- Motor disorders
  Parkinson's disease
  Huntington's disease
  Transplanted tissue
- Psychiatric disorders
  Schizophrenia
  Major depression
  Attention deficit hyperactivity disorder
  Generalized social phobia
  Compulsive behavior
- Summary
- References

A variety of recent technologic advances make it increasingly possible to image neurotransmitter systems in living human brain. The dopamine system has been most intensively studied owing to its involvement in several brain disorders, including motor disorders such as Parkinson's disease and Huntington's disease, as well as psychiatric disorders such as schizophrenia, depression, and compulsive behavioral disorders of multiple types. A variety of aspects of dopamine receptor density, function, and dopaminergic terminal status can now be assessed using the minimally invasive neuroimaging techniques of positron emission tomography (PET) and single-photon emission computed tomography (SPECT). Although these techniques are currently used most often in the context of research, clinical applications are rapidly emerging.

Dopamine

Overview

The dopamine system is involved in the regulation of brain regions that subserve motor, cognitive, and motivational behaviors. Dopaminergic dysfunction has been implicated in some of the deficits associated with the aging of the human brain.

[a] Department of Psychiatry, Harvard University Medical School, 115 Mill Street, Belmont, MA 02478, USA
[b] Psychopharmacology Research Laboratory, McLean Hospital, 115 Mill Street, Belmont, MA 02478, USA
[c] Center for Drug Discovery, Northeastern University, 360 Huntington Avenue, Boston, MA 02115, USA
* Corresponding author. 116 Mugar Hall, 360 Huntington Avenue, Boston, MA 02115.
E-mail address: s.gatley@neu.edu (S.J. Gatley).

doi:10.1016/j.nic.2006.06.003

Additionally, neurologic and psychiatric illnesses including substance abuse have been associated with disruptions of dopaminergic function. The diverse roles of dopamine in health and disease have made the dopaminergic system an important topic of research in the neurosciences as well as an important set of molecular targets for drug discovery and development.

Dopamine circuitry: pathways

Dopaminergic cell bodies are located mostly in the midbrain, specifically in the substantia nigra and ventral tegmental area. From there, three major dopaminergic projections target the striatum and portions of the frontal lobes, as shown in Fig. 1A.

Nigrostriatal pathway—projects from cell bodies within the substantia nigra to the caudate and putamen (corpus striatum). These structures are components of the basal ganglia and are part of the extrapyramidal motor system within the brain. The nigrostriatal pathway has an important role in the coordination and maintenance of movement.

Mesolimbic pathway—Dopamine neurons located in the ventral tegmental area project to the nucleus accumbens and the amygdala. This pathway is thought to mediate social emotional behavior and motivation and reward. Drugs of abuse are thought to exert their reinforcing effects through this pathway.

Mesocortical pathway—The mesocortical pathway projects from the ventral tegmental area of the midbrain to the prefrontal cortex, especially the dorsolateral prefrontal cortex. The dorsolateral prefrontal cortex is highly involved in attention, initiative, motivation, planning, decision making, working memory, and other higher cognitive functions. Antipsychotic drugs are thought to work though this pathway.

Molecules and targets

Dopamine signaling is mediated primarily via G-protein coupled receptors of two major classes (Fig. 1B) termed *D1-like* and *D2-like*, whose activation increases and decreases, respectively, formation of the second messenger cyclic AMP. Both classes are localized mostly postsynaptically; however, D1-like and D2-like receptors are also found presynaptically where they are thought to modulate dopamine release. Dopamine signaling is terminated primarily by the action of the dopamine transporter (DAT), which acts to move dopamine from the synapse into the cytosol of the presynaptic neuron where it is either revesicularized by the vesicular monoamine transporter 2 (VMAT2) or

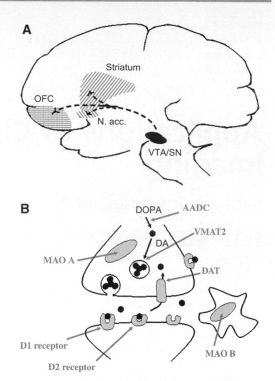

Fig. 1. (*A*) Cartoon representation of a sagittal section through the human brain showing the major projections of dopamine neurons from the cell bodies in the ventral tegmental area and substantia nigra (VTA/SN) to terminal field areas in the orbitofrontal cortex (OFC), nucleus accumbens (N. acc.), and dorsal striatum. (*B*) Cartoon representation of a typical dopaminergic synapse in the brain. In the presynaptic nerve terminal (*top*), dopamine (DA, ●) is made from its precursor L-dihydroxyphenyl alanine (DOPA) by aromatic amino acid decarboxylase (AADC) and concentrated in vesicles by the brain-type vesicular monoamine transporter (VMAT2). Dopamine released exocytotically into the synaptic cleft binds to postsynaptic dopamine receptors to elicit eventual physiologic responses. The extent to which D1 and D2 receptors are co-localized on individual neurons as shown is uncertain. The concentration of extracellular dopamine is controlled largely by its reuptake into nerve terminals, mediated by the dopamine transporter (DAT), the target of cocaine and other stimulant drugs. Most of this dopamine appears to be destroyed by monoamine oxidase A (MAO-A) located on mitochondria (*oval structure*), rather than being re-incorporated into vesicles. A portion of the extracellular dopamine is taken up by glial cells (*at right of figure*), where it is removed by monoamine oxidase B (MAO-B).

metabolized by intracellular monoamine oxidase. The action of the DAT regulates the concentration of extracellular dopamine, maintaining low (nanomolar) steady-state concentrations.

Radioligands for neuroimaging have been developed for the dopamine receptor types 1 and 2 and for the transporters (DAT and VMAT2). Additionally, a fluorine-labeled L-DOPA analogue, L-[18F]6-fluoro-DOPA (F-DOPA), has been used clinically since the mid-1980s [1,2]. This labeled dopamine precursor is taken up by dopaminergic neurons and converted to [18F]dopamine, which is stored in presynaptic vesicles. It gives a measure of the integrity of dopamine systems in parkinsonism. Table 1 provides a brief summary of selected radioligands and their uses.

Dopamine imaging

General overview

PET and SPECT neuroimaging are used to visualize the behavior of drug molecules in complex biologic systems. Although the physics of these techniques are somewhat different, they are used to answer the same types of questions. Most of the dopamine imaging that has been performed has used one or more of the following three strategies:

Studies of dopamine neuroreceptor density. This technique provides highly detailed information about regional patterns of specific patterns of radioligand binding within a receptor-rich tissue such as the brain. Alterations in neuroreceptor density can arise for a variety of reasons, including disease or chronic or acute exposure to drugs.

Studies of dopamine receptor or transporter occupancy. The ability of an abused or

Table 1: **Selected dopamine radioligands and their uses**

Target	Relevance	Radioligand	Mechanism and use
Aromatic amino acid decarboxylase (AADC)	Enzyme that produces dopamine from L-DOPA	[18F]fluoro-DOPA	Produces fluorodopamine that is stored in synaptic vesicles; indicates dopaminergic function
D1 receptor	Involved in addiction, movement disorders, parkinsonism, and schizophrenia	[11C]SCH23390	Receptor mapping
D2 receptor	Involved in movement disorders, parkinsonism, and schizophrenia—main target of neuroleptics	[11C]raclopride [18F]fallypride [123I]epidepride [123I]IBZM	Receptor mapping Receptor occupancy of neuroleptics Alterations in endogenous dopamine Receptor mapping Receptor mapping Similar to [11C]raclopride
D3 receptor	D2-like; restricted anatomically	None as yet	—
D4 receptor	D2-like; important in schizophrenia	None as yet	—
D5 receptor	D1-like	None as yet	—
Dopamine transporter (DAT)	Controls extracellular dopamine; target of cocaine and similar drugs	[11C]cocaine [11C]CFT [99mTc]TRODAT [123I]beta-CIT	Research, occupancy Transporter mapping Loss of dopamine terminals in parkinsonism
Vesicular monoamine transporter (VMAT2)	Concentrates dopamine (and other monoamine neurotransmitters) in vesicles; target of the drug reserpine	[11C] dihydrotetrabenazine	Loss of dopamine nerve terminals—may be superior to DAT radioligands
Monoamine oxidase A (MAOA)	Destroys dopamine after reuptake in nerve terminals	[11C]clorgyline	Enzyme mapping—selective suicide inhibitor
Monoamine oxidase B (MAOB)	Destroys monoamines after uptake into glial cells; marker of gliosis	[11C]L-deprenyl	Enzyme mapping—selective suicide inhibitor

therapeutic drug molecule to compete with or to displace a receptor-mapping radioligand for the same binding sites can be measured using imaging techniques. This information allows calculation of the amount of receptor occupancy provided by the given dose of drug. Measurement of the degree of receptor occupancy achieved by a drug potentially allows evaluation of the relationships between receptor occupancy and physiologic, behavioral, and subjective effects of the drug.

Studies of functional aspects of dopaminergic systems: drug effects on diverse neurotransmitter systems. Changes in extracellular dopamine at baseline and after pharmacologic or other challenges can be inferred from its competitive interaction with [^{11}C]raclopride at the D2 receptor. Additional information about dopaminergic function can be obtained using F-DOPA to assess DOPA uptake by dopaminergic cells.

Technique overview: PET and SPECT neuroimaging

PET is used to track the regional biodistribution and biokinetics of chemical compounds labeled with short-lived positron-emitting isotopes [3], enabling direct measurement of neurochemical systems in living human brain [4]. A great deal of progress has been made in the development of highly specific radiotracers that can be used to detect acute or chronic alterations in neurochemistry and physiology. The high sensitivity of PET scanners allows the detection of microgram quantities of radiolabeled molecules in vivo, that is, amounts so small that they do not exert measurable pharmacologic effects and occupy only a small fraction of drug-binding sites. Kinetic modeling approaches permit quantification and simple visualization of the distribution of receptor sites or enzymes within brain or other organs using suitable tracers.

SPECT can be used to measure some of the same components of the dopaminergic system as PET. SPECT scanners offer poorer resolution (6 mm rather than 3 to 4 mm), sensitivity, and quantification than PET scanners; however, SPECT is less expensive than PET, and SPECT scanners are more widely available because they are more often used for other clinical nuclear medicine procedures. Additionally, radiosynthesis of SPECT ligands is typically less involved, and the longer half-lived isotopes reduce the need for the tight coupling between radiotracer synthesis and imaging study required with PET. Table 2 provides a summary of nuclear decay properties of various radionuclides.

Table 2: Nuclear decay properties of common radionuclides

Nuclide	Half-life	Decay mode
^{11}C[a]	20 min	Positron (511 keV annihilation photon)
^{18}F[a]	110 min	Positron (511 keV annihilation photon)
^{99m}Tc[b]	6 h	Gamma, 140 keV
^{123}I[a]	13.2 h	Electron capture (gamma, 159 keV)

[a] Nuclides produced using cyclotrons.
[b] Nuclides produced using nuclear reactors. ^{99m}Tc is the metastable daughter of ^{99}Mo (half-life = 66 h). It is obtained inexpensively in the radiopharmacy from "generators" containing ^{99}Mo. ^{99m}Tc has favorable properties for clinical nuclear imaging.

Radiotracers for PET and SPECT

A major difference between PET and SPECT lies in the availability of radiopharmaceuticals. The PET nuclide ^{11}C can be used in principle to label any drug so that compounds of known pharmacology can be labeled; however, the half-life of only 20 minutes means that the imaging facility must be adjacent to a cyclotron and a chemistry laboratory staffed with appropriate professionals. If ^{123}I- or ^{99m}Tc-labeled compounds have been developed for an imaging target, these SPECT radiopharmaceuticals can readily be purchased from distant facilities or made in the radiopharmacy from kits; however, the initial development of labeled compounds containing inorganic elements, especially ^{99m}Tc, is more difficult. Currently, clinical PET relies heavily on the ^{18}F-labeled glucose analogue FDG, which can be made in house or purchased from regional positron radiopharmacies. It is likely that other ^{18}F radiopharmaceuticals, such as F-DOPA, will become available to institutions lacking cyclotrons in the near future.

By using appropriate radioligands that interact with specific constituents of dopaminergic circuitry, a variety of different types of information can be obtained (see Table 1). Studies can be designed to evaluate constitutive differences in neuroreceptor density, homeostatic or other changes in response to chronic drug, occupancy by pharmacologic doses of drug, or dopamine release in response to pharmacologic challenge. Some of the best-characterized radioligands are discussed in the next sections, but this is not meant to be an exhaustive listing. Figs. 2 and 3 list a variety of commonly used PET and SPECT radioligands along with their targets and structures.

Aromatic aminoacid decarboxylase (AADC)	[^{18}F]L-6-Fluoro-3,4-di-hydroxy-henylalanine (6FDOPA)	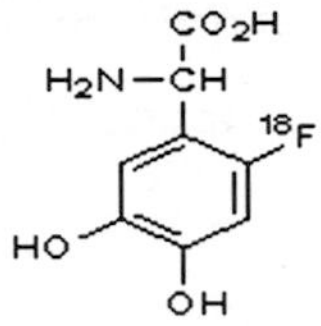
Brain vesicular monoamine transporter (VMAT2)	[^{11}C]Dihydrotetra-benazine	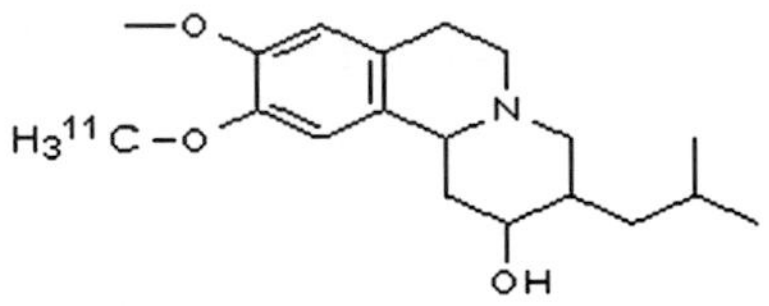
Neuronal dopamine transporter (DAT)	[^{11}C]CFT or[^{11}C]WIN 35428	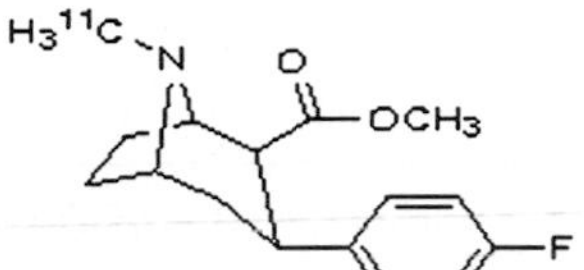
Dopamine D1 receptor	[^{11}C]SCH23390	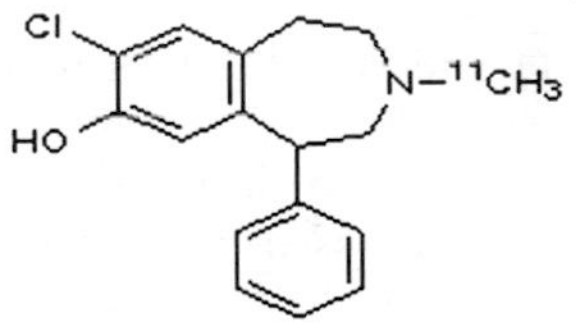
Dopamine D2 receptor	[^{11}C]Raclopride	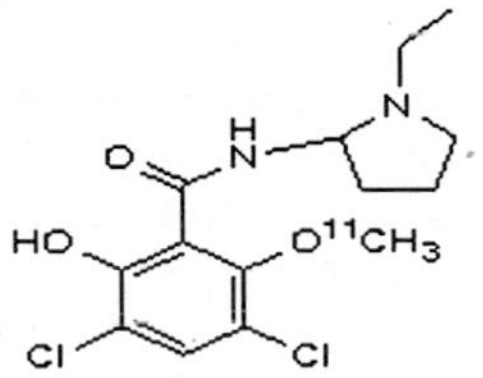
Monoamine oxidase A (MAO-A)	[^{11}C]Clorgyline	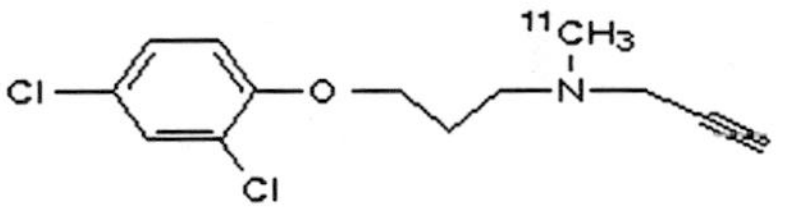
Monoamine oxidase B (MAO-B)	[^{11}C]L-Deprenyl or [^{11}C]Selegiline	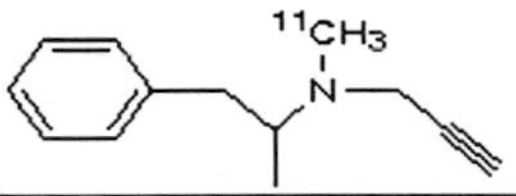

Fig. 2. Structures of representative PET radiopharmaceuticals for the dopamine system.

Transporter ligands

Vesicular monoamine transporter 2

[^{11}C]Dihydrotetrabenazine is a PET ligand that labels VMAT2, the intracellular dopamine transporter that functions to move dopamine from the cytosol into synaptic vesicles [5]. Based on animal studies, it is estimated that more than 95% of striatal VMAT2 is associated with dopaminergic nerve terminals [6]. Imaging with dihydrotetrabenazine or other VMAT2 ligand is an indicator of the integrity of dopamine vesicularization systems in dopamine nerve terminals. Decreases in the binding of VMAT2 have been interpreted to reflect dopamine neuronal death; however, it is possible that VMAT2 might be reduced in the absence of cell death or even in the absence of nerve terminal loss.

Dopamine transporter

Several DAT radioligands have been examined in reasonable detail in human subjects. These substances include [^{11}C]cocaine and three structurally related compounds containing the tropane moiety: WIN 35 428 (also known as CFT), RTI-55 (also

Neuronal dopamine transporter (DAT)	[^{123}I]β-CIT or [^{123}I]RTI-55 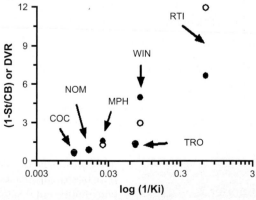
Dopamine D2 receptor	[^{123}I]Iodobenzamide or [^{123}I]IBZM

Fig. 3. Most common SPECT radiopharmaceuticals for the dopamine system.

known as β-CIT), and TRODAT-1. In vivo measures of binding are reasonably well correlated with radioligand affinity measured in vitro (Fig. 4). The structures of these radioligands are presented in Fig. 2.

The optimal choice of DAT radiopharmaceutical is still an open question in many situations but probably depends on the purpose. For verifying substantial loss of dopamine transporters in parkinsonism, a relatively high-affinity radioligand such as [^{11}C]CFT may be best, because this tracer gives high-quality images in circumstances where transporter concentration has decreased to low levels.

If the goal is to evaluate a moderate loss of transporters (eg, to detect incipient parkinsonism), a DAT radioligand of lower affinity such as [^{11}C]methylphenidate may be better. The reason is that a "ceiling effect" can exist where the concentration of binding sites is high enough to retain every molecule of radioligand extracted from the blood, such that a large loss of transporter or receptor is necessary before radiopharmaceutical uptake is appreciably diminished. A radioligand of moderate affinity can be best for detecting small decreases in receptor density.

Fig. 4. In vitro and in vivo behavior of DAT radioligands. The graph demonstrates the 100-fold range of affinities for DAT of radioligands that have proved useful in clinical or clinical research PET or SPECT studies, varying between the weak binding of cocaine and the much stronger binding of its analogue RTI-55 (β-CIT). It also indicates the general concordance between in vivo binding in rodents and human, which has facilitated translational research in this area. Overall, in vivo and in vitro binding is well correlated; this observation serves as an important validation of in vivo imaging of DAT. The x-axis represents the affinity (1/Ki) measure in vitro using rat striatal membranes. Open circles St/Cb represent the striatum-to-cerebellum radioactivity ratio in rodents. Closed circles DVR represent the distribution volume ratio in humans measured using PET or SPECT. RTI, [^{123}I]RTI-55 (β-CIT); WIN, [^{11}C]WIN 35,428 (CFT); TRO, TRODAT-1; MPH, [^{11}C]d-threomethylphenidate; NOM, [^{11}C]nomifensine; COC, [^{11}C]cocaine.

(⁹⁹ᵐTc) TRODAT-1

This compound, ([2-[[2-[[[3-(4-chlorophenyl)-8-methyl-8-azabicyclo[3,2,1]oct-2-yl]methyl] (2-mercaptoethyl)amino]ethyl]amino]-ethanethiolato(3-)-*N2,N2',S2,S2'*]oxo-[1*R*-(*exo-exo*)]), may be the most commonly used DAT ligand in SPECT. Prospects for widespread clinical imaging of dopamine nerve terminal loss were greatly enhanced in 1996 when Kung and coworkers [7] developed TRODAT-1, a cocaine derivative that incorporates a technetium atom. At about the same time, Madras and coworkers [8] introduced Technepine using a similar chelating strategy. Unlike TRODAT-1, Technepine has not been widely used in human subjects. An "improved" version of Technepine with better selectivity and biologic stability, called Fluoroatech, was later introduced by the Meltzer group, but information on its behavior in human subjects is lacking [9]. In contrast, at the time of this writing, at least 25 independent studies of TRODAT-1 in human subjects have been abstracted by MEDLINE. These studies and their topics are listed in **Box 1**. Structures of technetium-labeled radioligands for DAT are shown in **Fig. 5**.

The advantages of TRODAT-1 stem from the use of ⁹⁹ᵐTc-pertechnetate, available cheaply and conveniently from a generator system in the radiopharmacy at a much lower per millicurie cost than ¹²³I, which must be purchased from a commercial cyclotron facility. Nevertheless, the authors' impression is that β-CIT [10], the best studied ¹²³I-labeled SPECT radioligand for DAT, provides SPECT studies of superior quality to those obtained using TRODAT-1. Although no head-to-head comparisons of

TRODAT-1 with β-CIT in the same patients have been published, such a comparison has been made with the closely related [¹²³I]FP-β-CIT. It was concluded that the ¹²³I radiopharmaceutical had "superior accuracy for early differential diagnosis of idiopathic parkinsonism and non-degenerative extrapyramidal disorders, as well as better sensitivity for disease follow-up" [11].

To the authors' knowledge, DAT remains the only brain neuroreceptor for which a ⁹⁹ᵐTc radioligand is available. Attempts to develop ⁹⁹ᵐTc tracers for other targets have failed because the bulky labeling group required impedes brain penetration, receptor binding, or both [12,13]. Finding a way of introducing a relatively small ¹⁸F or ¹²³I atom into a biologically active molecule without destroying key properties is generally an easier proposition.

Nomifensine

This compound was the first PET radioligand specific for DAT and exhibits rapid and easily modeled uptake, with peak concentrations appearing in brain within about 20 minutes. Although nomifensine binds more tightly to the norepinephrine transporter than it does to DAT, this does not adversely affect its utility for imaging DAT, probably because DAT is present at much higher concentrations than the norepinephrine transporter.

Methylphenidate

This drug is commercially marketed as Ritalin, the most commonly prescribed psychotropic drug for children in the United States. Development of [¹¹C]d-threo-methylphenidate as a DAT radioligand was facilitated by the fact that Ritalin pharmacology in humans is fairly well characterized, and the drug is generally regarded as safe.

WIN 35 428 (CFT)

This tracer does not reach a binding peak in striatum within the time limits imposed by the half-life of ¹¹C. After 5+ half-lives have passed (110 minutes), the decay-corrected concentration in the striatum is still rising [14]. It is unclear what impact this failure to reach equilibrium has on the ability to detect small decreases in DAT using this tracer. Potentially under these conditions, a tissue with a threshold level of binding sites might bind every molecule of tracer delivered. If this happens, measures of binding can be robustly affected by alterations in tissue perfusion that cause changes in radioligand delivery. This phenomenon may account for the observation that studies with [¹¹C]WIN 35 428 (unlike those performed with other tracers) have failed to demonstrate a decline of DAT with age in human subjects [14]. The same

---

Box 1:   Conditions studied using TRODAT-1

Parkinson's disease [159–163]
Attention deficit hyperactivity disorder [112,117,164]
Alcohol hallucinosis [165]
Rubral tremor [161]
Vascular parkinsonism [166]
Machado-Joseph disease [167,168]
Tourette's syndrome [169]
Spinocerebellar ataxia [170,171]
DOPA-responsive dystonia [172]
Manganese intoxication [173]
Carbon disulfide toxicity [174,175]
Drug-naïve schizophrenia [176,177]
Major depression [106]
Wilson's disease [178]
Early corticobasal degeneration [179]
Multiple system atrophy [180,181]
Age and gender differences in DAT in relation to executive and motor functions [182,183]
Pharmacologic type studies [108,184,185]

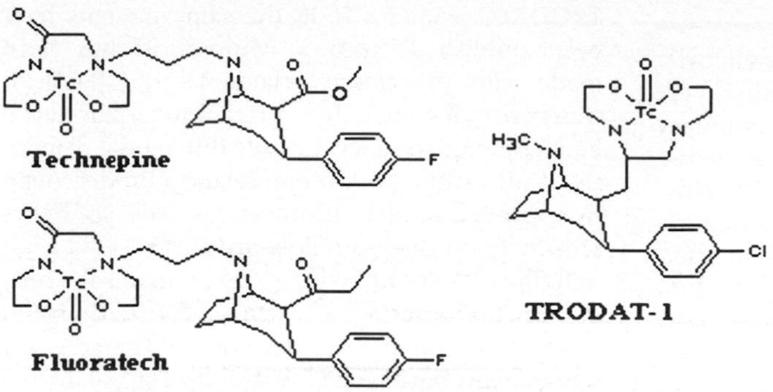

Fig. 5. Technetium radiopharmaceuticals for DAT.

is true to an even greater extent of [^{11}C]RTI-55 ([^{11}C]β-CIT). Although high-affinity PET radioligands such as WIN 35 428 may provide high-quality images and clearly visualize profound decreases in DAT in parkinsonism, they may not be sensitive to small changes in DAT levels.

Dopamine receptor ligands

Receptor ligands for D1- and D2-type receptors have been developed. D1 receptor ligands include SCH 23390 [15] and NNC 112 [16]. Although termed *D1 receptor ligands*, these substances fail to distinguish between the two D1-type receptors, D1 and D5; therefore, images acquired using these ligands reflect binding to both D1 and D5 receptors. The functional significance of these receptors remains unclear. Nevertheless, both of these radioligands have found application in schizophrenia [17,18], Huntington's disease [19–23], and Parkinson's disease [24].

Well-characterized D2-type receptor ligands include [^{11}C]raclopride for PET and [^{123}I]iodobenzamide for SPECT imaging. Neither of these radioligands discriminates between the D2 and D3 receptor. As for the D1-type ligands, neuroimaging measures the total binding to both of these receptor populations. Neuroanatomic differences in the distribution of these receptors make it possible to measure relatively pure D2 receptor binding in certain areas of the brain. The field awaits the development of radioligands that will distinguish all five dopamine receptor subtypes as well as further information about the functions of each.

Measuring dopaminergic function

Pharmacologic manipulations

Raclopride binding potential has been shown to be sensitive to changes in synaptic dopamine [25], making it suitable for evaluation of dopaminergic function in addition to evaluation of D2 receptor density. [^{123}I]iodobenzamide can be used in

SPECT, like the PET tracer raclopride, to assess changes in synaptic dopamine [25]. Agents that either release dopamine (eg, amphetamine) or deplete dopamine (eg, alpha-methyl-paratyrosine [AMPT], an inhibitor of tyrosine hydroxylase) can be used with these tracers to evaluate dopamine system function. The strategy for these studies with [^{11}C]raclopride involves a test-retest design wherein the patient is injected with radiotracer twice in the same scanning session, amphetamine being administered before the second scan. For [^{123}I]iodobenzamide, one radiotracer injection is made and the decrease in brain radioactivity measured after a subsequent injection of amphetamine or other dopamine-releasing drug.

F-DOPA

Dopamine and its analogues such as [^{18}F]6-fluoro-dopamine cannot enter the brain to an appreciable degree because they are polar molecules and the blood-brain barrier does not contain carriers for dopamine. The blood-brain barrier and brain cells do contain carrier systems for amino acids, and one of these (the so-called "large neutral amino acid transporter") is able to transport the dopamine precursor L-DOPA . Administration of L-DOPA is used therapeutically to boost brain dopamine levels in Parkinson's disease. The enzyme involved in the conversion of L-DOPA to dopamine is aromatic amino acid decarboxylase (AADC). Because the amino acid transporter and AADC also recognize 6-fluoro-L-DOPA, the latter compound in ^{18}F-labeled form can be used to monitor the brain's ability to produce and store dopamine. The decarboxylation of 6-[^{18}F]fluoro-DOPA by aromatic L-amino acid decarboxylase and retention of the product [^{18}F]fluorodopamine within vesicles of catecholamine fibers results in the labeling of dopamine-rich brain regions during F-DOPA/PET studies [26]. Fluoro-L-3,4,-dihydroxyphenylalanine (F-DOPA) was first used in 1983 to visualize the human basal ganglia [27]. Oral carbidopa is administered in the studies to reduce peripheral decarboxylation and enhance the fraction of injected radiotracer extracted by the brain.

In contrast to dopamine, the receptor-, transporter-, and enzyme-binding radiopharmaceuticals in Figs. 2 and 3 are lipophilic compounds that can readily pass through membranes without the aid of carrier systems. Empirically, it has been shown that compounds exhibiting logP (log n-octanol/water partition coefficients, a measure of lipophilicity/polarity) of between 1 and 3 can generally penetrate the blood-brain barrier with high efficiency and make suitable brain imaging radioligands. For compounds with higher logP values, brain penetration falls off, probably because of excessive binding to blood cell membranes and proteins.

Motor disorders

Dopamine imaging has found its widest clinical application in the study of motor disorders such as Parkinson's disease. Parkinson's disease is a common, age-related neurodegenerative disease characterized by akinesia, bradykinesia, and resting tremor that affects approximately 1% of all individuals over the age of 55 years. Given the role of dopamine in this disorder, dopamine neuroimaging has utility in assessing regional changes, determining differential diagnoses, and monitoring disease progression and treatment effects.

Parkinson's disease

The pathology of Parkinson's disease involves a relatively selective deterioration of dopaminergic neurons in substantia nigra pars compacta that project to the striatum and other basal ganglia nuclei. Several review articles focused entirely on imaging Parkinson's disease have recently appeared [28–33]. A principle finding is that dopamine transporters are reduced in Parkinson's disease patients in proportion to disease severity and range between 36% and 71% of control values [10,34,35]. Also, measurable reductions in DAT binding occur before the onset of clinical symptoms of Parkinson's disease [36,37]. Patients with Parkinson's disease have normal D2 receptor binding [38–43]. The etiology of these changes has not been elucidated. The findings may indicate that presynaptic terminals are intact in Parkinson's disease yet less able to take up dopamine from the synapse. In contrast, reduced D2 receptor binding potential has been shown in patients with multiple system atrophy or progressive supranuclear palsy using SPECT and [123I]iodobenzamide, [123I]iodolisuride, or [123I]epidepride [40–47], probably reflecting degeneration of medium spiny neurons [48]. Potentially, this difference could form the basis for an early distinction between these two diagnoses; however, large individual differences in baseline D2 receptor levels between subjects are likely to make this difficult [49].

Several studies confirm that the striatal uptake of F-DOPA is markedly reduced in Parkinson's patients when compared with controls, and this reduction is more pronounced in putamen than caudate [50–54]. These reductions are superimposed on a natural age-related decline in the number of dopamine neurons that occurs in healthy control subjects. Parkinson's disease seems to accelerate this decline. The annualized rate of reduction has been estimated to be approximately 0% to 2% in healthy controls compared with 6% to 13% in individuals with Parkinson's disease [55–57]. Furthermore, F-DOPA uptake in putamen has been shown to be inversely correlated with illness duration and motor disability [52,58–60]. Despite the measured reductions in F-DOPA uptake in the striatum, uptake in the globus pallidus interna increases by approximately 30% to 40% early in the course of Parkinson's disease, but these values fall later during disease progression [61]. Potentially, increasing the function of the dopaminergic projection in this region helps maintain normal pallidal output to the motor cortex and ventral thalamus [59]. The ability of this mechanism to compensate for striatal degeneration may be limited, and its loss may be a turning point in the acceleration of disease progression.

Functional studies of dopamine release using [11C]raclopride PET have also been conducted in Parkinson's disease patients. Piccini and colleagues reported in 2003 on differences in methamphetamine-induced dopamine release between Parkinson's disease patients and normal controls measured with [11C]raclopride PET. A 0.3 mg/kg dose of methamphetamine induced significant reductions in raclopride binding in caudate (17%) and putamen (25%) in control subjects. Reductions in the same regions in Parkinson's disease patients after methamphetamine challenge were also significant but much smaller in size (8% in caudate and 7% in putamen) [60]. Another recent study evaluated repetitive transcranial magnetic stimulation for its ability to release dopamine in patients with Parkinson's disease and unilateral motor symptoms [62]. Intriguingly, the researchers reported that, although the amount of dopamine release was smaller on the symptomatic side, as expected, the area of dopamine release was significantly greater (by approximately 60%). Findings such as these suggest additional mechanisms by which the brain can compensate for the loss of dopaminergic neurons.

Huntington's disease

Huntington's disease is a progressive, autosomal dominant neurodegenerative disorder characterized by involuntary choreiform movements, cognitive decline, and progressive neuronal degeneration primarily affecting the striatum. The gene responsible for the disorder has been identified and the abnormality characterized as an atypically large number of CAG repeats in the coding region of the huntingtin gene. Carriers of the gene have inevitable development of disease and a 50% chance of passing the gene to their children. No effective therapy for this disorder exists, and the function of huntingtin, the protein encoded by this gene, is not yet known. This mutation causes death of striatal medium spiny neurons via an unknown mechanism. Cholinergic interneurons are spared. Several excellent reviews have been published recently, including but not limited to articles by Brooks in 2004 [63], Anderson in 2005 [64], Rosas and coworkers in 2004 [65], and Rego and de Almeida in 2005 [66], which provide more information on this topic for the interested reader. Huntington's disease provides unique opportunities for research because at-risk carriers of the huntingtin mutation can be identified before symptoms of the disease are manifested. Neuroimaging techniques may be helpful in predicting disease onset and in the assessment of new medications for delaying or preventing the onset of symptoms.

Several studies of dopamine receptor density have been performed in Huntington's disease patients, and reductions in D1 and D2 receptor levels have been documented [21]. Functional correlates of dopamine receptor binding in Huntington's disease have also been investigated. Asymptomatic subjects at risk for Huntington's disease showed correlations between D1 receptor binding measured with [^{11}C]SCH 23390 PET and performance on tests of verbal fluency, memory, attention, and planning [67], with subjects approaching their calculated age of onset showing reduced D1 receptor binding and poorer performance on the cognitive tasks. In symptomatic Huntington's disease patients, larger reductions in D1 receptor binding of approximately 50% in caudate and putamen [20,68,69] or frontal cortex [22] have been shown. A recent study showed that asymptomatic carriers of the huntingtin mutation had 50% reduced D2 receptor binding when compared with normal controls [70]. Furthermore, reductions in D2 receptor binding were correlated with age and CAG repeat length. Dopamine D2 receptor levels have also been assessed with PET and [^{11}C]raclopride. The yearly decrease in D2 receptor binding potential as measured by [^{11}C]raclopride PET has been reported to be approximately 6.3% in gene-positive asymptomatic subjects [71]. Interestingly, follow-up studies in this group suggest that striatal glucose metabolism is reduced by only 2.3% per year, again confirming the nonlinearity of the relationship between numbers of neurons/receptors and regional neuronal function. These findings indicate that reductions in D2 receptor binding in asymptomatic subjects at risk for Huntington's disease may be more marked than striatal perfusion deficits and may be a better measure for early detection of this disease [72].

Few functional neuroimaging datasets have been collected in Huntington's disease patients. Mildly affected patients show approximately 30% reductions in striatal glucose metabolism. As discussed previously, impairment of regional glucose metabolism appears to lag behind loss of dopaminergic neuroreceptors [71]; however, given the large decreases in correlates of glucose metabolism and large decreases in receptor binding in Huntington's disease, dopamine imaging is likely to be a rich source of information about functional aspects of dopaminergic systems in Huntington's disease [59].

Transplanted tissue

A novel application of dopamine imaging has been found in experimental trials involving transplanted tissue or growth factors in patients who have Parkinson's disease and Huntington's disease. A variety of different transplantation methods have been tested for their ability to restore normal dopamine levels to the striatum. Several recent studies have documented viability, migration, or location of fetal nigral cells transplanted for this purpose in Parkinson's disease patients [73–76]. Other groups have attempted to replace GABAergic neurons in the striato-pallido-thalamo-cortical circuitry in Huntington's disease [63,77]. Most of the neuroimaging studies that have been performed to assess transplant viability and function have used PET with F-DOPA. In general, neuroimaging evidence suggests that robust increases in putamenal F-DOPA uptake can be produced with transplantation of fetal dopaminergic cells, but evidence for improvement in clinical endpoints is mixed [63].

Psychiatric disorders

Aside from motor disorders, the other most studied application of dopamine imaging has been in psychiatric disorders. Dopaminergic abnormalities have been documented in numerous psychiatric conditions, including schizophrenia, depression, attention deficit/hyperactivity disorder, phobia, and compulsive behavioral disorders such as drug or alcohol abuse and obesity. The discovery of D2 receptors was driven largely by findings that antipsychotic efficacy correlated with affinity for this site [78]. At the organismal level, PET and SPECT neuroimaging have an important role in quantifying the relationships between receptor occupancy, drug blood levels, oral dose, and therapeutic outcome for psychiatric drugs [79].

Schizophrenia

Based on the correlation between clinical doses of antipsychotic drugs and their potency to block D2 receptors as well as the psychotogenic effects of dopamine-enhancing drugs, schizophrenia has historically been thought to be the result of hyperactivity of dopaminergic systems [80]. Attempts to gain insight into the etiology of schizophrenia have been made through the use of dopaminergic imaging techniques. Densities of D1- and D2-type dopamine receptors have been measured in schizophrenics. Given the high affinity of antipsychotics for the D2 receptor, early investigators hypothesized that D2 receptor density might be altered in schizophrenia. Nevertheless, no differences in D2 receptor density or availability have been reported in drug-free schizophrenics when compared with normal controls. Furthermore, although D1 receptor function has been shown to be important for functionality in prefrontal brain regions in schizophrenia, results from imaging studies of D1 receptor levels have been mixed. Aside from two neuroimaging studies showing reduced D1 receptor binding in schizophrenics in the prefrontal cortex [17,81] and one showing increases in the dorsolateral prefrontal cortex [82], the preponderance of the evidence from neuroimaging studies and postmortem autoradiography suggests that no differences exist in D1 receptor binding between schizophrenics and control subjects [18,83–85]. Interpretation of these findings is complicated by several factors, including small sample sizes, subjects' exposure to medications, different timing of scans with respect to subjects' most recent neuroleptic dose, different radiotracers and modeling paradigms, and subject age. A twin study has yielded some evidence that increased striatal D2 receptor density may be a marker for schizophrenia risk [86]. It remains to be seen whether this finding will be useful clinically given the large amount of variability in normal D2 levels.

The mechanism of action of antipsychotic drugs has been linked to their actions at dopamine receptors since the mid-1970s [78,87,88]. This correlation is the backbone of the dopamine hyperactivity hypothesis of schizophrenia. PET neuroimaging has been used to investigate the occupancy of dopamine (and other receptors) by antipsychotic drugs. In general, it has been found that typical antipsychotics occupy about 70% of striatal D2 receptors [89]. Although all antipsychotics occupy D2 receptors to a significant degree, recent evidence suggests that downstream effects on other neurotransmitter systems such as glutamate

and serotonin may also be essential for antipsychotic efficacy [90,91]. These data, along with an increasing awareness of the importance of persistent negative and cognitive symptoms in schizophrenics medicated with typical antipsychotics, have led to a reformulation of the classical dopamine overactivity hypothesis of schizophrenia.

Dopamine neuroimaging has also contributed to understanding of the extrapyramidal side effects caused by antipsychotic drugs. The high levels of striatal D2 receptor occupancy produced by these drugs may be associated with their extrapyramidal adverse effects [89]. Second-generation antipsychotics such as clozapine and olanzapine have been introduced, which have better efficacy to relieve negative symptoms as well as reduced propensity for extrapyramidal side effects. Dopamine neuroimaging studies have yielded data that is beginning to shed some light on the mechanisms of action of these drugs compared with first-generation antipsychotics such as haloperidol. The D2 receptor occupancy of therapeutic doses of several different first- and second-generation antipsychotics has been assessed using [^{11}C]raclopride PET. Clozapine at therapeutically efficacious doses of 75 to 900 mg/day occupied a smaller proportion of D2 receptors (16%–68%) than therapeutic doses of risperidone, ranging from 2 to 12 mg/day (63%–89%), or olanzapine, ranging from 5 to 60 mg/day (43%–89%). Assessment of 5HT2 serotonin receptor occupancy in the same population showed that, as expected, atypical antipsychotics occupied a greater proportion of 5HT2 receptors than D2 receptors at all doses. In agreement with the clozapine imaging results are data from a similar PET study that found 44% mean whole-brain D2 occupancy produced by clinically used doses of clozapine in schizophrenics [92]. These researchers attributed clozapine's relatively low risk of extrapyramidal side effects to its approximately equivalent occupancy at D1 and D2 receptor sites. Another group has reported that olanzapine, another antipsychotic with a low risk of extrapyramidal side effects, binds D2/D3 receptors to an equivalent degree in most brain regions (including putamen ventral striatum, medial thalamus, amygdala, and temporal cortex). In that study, haloperidol and olanzapine produced occupancy in several brain regions that ranged from 68% to 78% in schizophrenic subjects chronically treated with either drug [93]. Interestingly, in the substantia nigra/ventral tegmental region, occupancy of D2 by olanzapine was significantly lower (40 ± 12%) than that of haloperidol (59 ± 9%). It was suggested that the sparing of this region explains the relative rarity of extrapyramidal symptoms in patients treated with olanzapine.

Increased amphetamine-induced release of endogenous dopamine in schizophrenia has been inferred using iodobenzamide SPECT [94,95] and [^{11}C]raclopride PET [96,97] measures of reduced D2 receptor availability. An additional study evaluated baseline D2 receptor occupancy by endogenous dopamine using an acute dopamine depletion procedure in schizophrenics [98]. This study found higher baseline D2 receptor occupancy at baseline in schizophrenics when compared with matched controls in the first episode of psychotic illness and in subsequent episodes of illness exacerbation.

To date, several studies probing neural metabolic correlates of schizophrenia have been published using F-DOPA or [^{11}C]DOPA PET. Of these, most describe elevated striatal DOPA uptake [99–103]; however, two studies failed to support these findings. No difference in F-DOPA uptake was detected by Dao-Castellana and colleagues [104] in schizophrenics when compared with controls, and Elkashef and colleagues [105] reported reduced striatal F-DOPA uptake. It is difficult to ascertain whether these discrepant findings result from methodologic differences, differences in diagnostic criteria and subject selection, a true heterogeneity in schizophrenic populations, or some combination of these factors.

Major depression

Several converging lines of evidence implicate dopamine abnormalities in depression. Increases in the number of DATs have been shown in 15 drug-free depressed patients compared with age-matched healthy controls using TRODAT-1 SPECT imaging [106]. Specifically, increases in TRODAT-1 uptake were reported in the right anterior putamen (23%), right posterior putamen (36%), left posterior putamen (18%), and left caudate nucleus (12%) over uptake measured in the same regions in the control subjects. Whether differences in DAT are a potential cause of depression or a consequence thereof remains uncertain.

Several reports describe decreased availability of the DAT occupancy after chronic treatment of depressed patients with bupropion [107–109], a DAT/norepinephrine transporter inhibitor; however, the bupropion was given for 3 to 4 weeks in all of these experiments and was also presumably present in the brain at the time of scanning. It is unclear whether the approximately 20% reduction in DAT binding that was measured reflects acute binding of bupropion to DAT, chronic bupropion-induced changes in DAT levels, or some combination.

PET and SPECT dopamine imaging have been used to demonstrate complex interactions between monoaminergic neurotransmitter systems in depressed patients treated with selective serotonin reuptake inhibitors. A 17% increase in DAT binding was associated with 8 days of treatment with 40 mg of citalopram in 17 depressed subjects compared with matched untreated normal control subjects (as assessed by [^{123}I]β-CIT SPECT) [110]. A similar increase in DAT binding was demonstrated in 10 depressed subjects treated with paroxetine [110]. In contrast, 16 days of treatment with bupropion at doses of 100 to 200 mg/day did not alter DAT binding in the same study using the same technique in depressed or normal subjects [110]. Although intriguing, these findings are difficult to interpret because of the confound between residual occupancy of the transporter at the time of scanning and its possible down-regulation due to chronic drug treatment, as discussed in the bupropion studies in the previous section.

Attention deficit hyperactivity disorder

Therapeutic agents for attention deficit hyperactivity disorder (ADHD), such as methylphenidate and amphetamine, target DAT. Several DAT imaging studies have been conducted in children and adults with ADHD using PET or SPECT with DAT ligands [111–115]. Most of these studies have found increased DAT binding in untreated adults and children with ADHD [111–113]; however, several articles report decreases in DAT binding compared with that in normal controls in methylphenidate-treated individuals with ADHD [112,113,116,117]. Interpretation of these results is complicated, because two of these reports give no information about the timing of the subjects' last therapeutic methylphenidate doses, and the third reports the results from scans performed only 90 minutes after the last methylphenidate dose [118]. It is possible that these findings reflect occupancy of the DAT by therapeutic methylphenidate rather than decreased numbers of DAT [119]. DAT occupancy by therapeutically relevant doses of methylphenidate, a selective DAT blocker clinically prescribed for ADHD, has been reported to be approximately 50% [120]. Additional work by this same group investigated whether variability in DAT blockade accounts for the large variability in therapeutic doses of methylphenidate in ADHD patients. DAT availability (using [^{11}C]cocaine PET) and functional dopamine release (using competitive [^{11}C]raclopride PET in the same subjects) were assessed in response to doses of oral methylphenidate. The findings suggest that the variability in dopamine release and not the variability in DAT blockade by methylphenidate accounts for the differences.

Generalized social phobia

Few neuroimaging studies have addressed this area. Decreased [^{123}I]iodobenzamide binding to D2 receptors has been documented in patients with social phobia, correlating with the Liebowitz Social Anxiety Scale Score [121]. DAT binding as measured with [123I]β-CIT was also significantly reduced in 11 patients with social phobia when compared with control subjects [122]. Coupland [123] has argued that data from three recent studies showing inverse relationships between social detachment (measured using the Karolinska Scales of Personality) and neuroimaging measures of dopamine D2 receptor [124,125] or transporter [126] density provide support for the idea that abnormalities in dopaminergic systems are involved in the etiology of this condition.

Compulsive behavior

Drug abuse

Aside from motor disorders and schizophrenia, the condition most often studied with dopamine imaging is drug dependence, because enhanced dopaminergic neurotransmission is thought to be responsible for the acutely reinforcing effects of abused drugs. Altered dopaminergic neuroreceptor levels may predispose individuals to addiction, and chronic use can result in compensatory adaptations in the levels and activity of these proteins. Chronic methamphetamine use has been associated with reduced DAT density as measured using [11C]WIN 35 428 PET. Significant differences in DAT radioligand binding were observed in the orbitofrontal cortex, dorsolateral prefrontal cortex, and amygdala [127]. Reductions in DAT in the orbitofrontal cortex and dorsolateral prefrontal cortex were correlated with psychiatric symptoms and the duration of methamphetamine use.

Methamphetamine abuse has also been associated with significantly lower levels of D2 receptor availability in the caudate and putamen using [11C]raclopride PET [128]. These reductions were associated with reductions in glucose metabolism in the orbitofrontal cortex in the same 15 methamphetamine users when compared with 20 normal controls [128]. [11C]d-threo-methylphenidate PET has been used to measure DAT density in methamphetamine abusers [129]. Methamphetamine-associated reductions in DAT binding were reported in the caudate (28% lower than normal controls) and putamen (21% lower than controls). Reductions in the whole striatum were associated with deficits in neuropsychologic tests including the Timed Gait, Grooved Pegboard, and Auditory Verbal Learning Task [129]; however, neither the methamphetamine dose nor the days since last methamphetamine use were correlated with DAT levels. Although reductions in DAT binding and D2 binding, along with reductions in measures of metabolic correlates, are consistent with neuronal death, protracted abstinence may partially reverse the methamphetamine-associated decrease in DAT density [130]. In a [11C]d-threo-methylphenidate PET study in five methamphetamine users, 9 to 15 months of protracted abstinence from methamphetamine was associated with a 19% DAT increase in the caudate and a 16% increase in the putamen (Fig. 6). A trend toward significant improvements in neuropsychologic test performance on Timed Gait and Delayed Recall was also noted [130]. This recovery of DAT binding may be associated with functional improvements in these individuals. Many researchers now believe that the loss of dopamine nerve terminal markers such as DAT and D2 receptors may not reflect neuronal death, and that dopaminergic cell bodies may remain

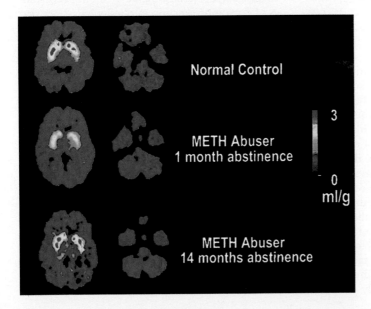

Fig. 6. Brain images of the distribution volume of [11C]d-threo-methylphenidate in a control subject and a methamphetamine (METH) abuser [129]. Images shown were obtained at the level of the striatum (*images to the left*) and the cerebellum (*images to the right*). Both subjects were evaluated twice, once during short-term abstinence (approximately 3 months) and once during protracted abstinence (approximately 14 months). Notice the significant increases in binding in striatum in the METH abuser with protracted abstinence. (*From* Volkow ND, Chang L, Wang G, et al. Loss of dopamine transporters in methamphetamine abusers recovers with protracted abstinence. J Neurosci 2001;21:9415. © Copyright 2001 by the Society for Neuroscience).

viable and re-form their connections with neighboring neurons with continued abstinence from methamphetamine.

Neuroreceptor imaging with PET can also be used to relate molecular events such as a drug occupying its target site to organismal events like behavior, clinical efficacy, or self-reported drug effects. The relationship between self-reported euphoria and cocaine occupancy of the DAT is fairly well documented [131–134]. Approximately 40% occupancy has been found to be required for cocaine to be perceivable to a user [133]. Doses commonly used by addicts result in DAT occupancy levels of about 60% to 77% [133]. Another elegant study has evaluated the impact of a drug's rate of onset on its reinforcing efficacy. Volkow and colleagues [135] related measured differences in the reinforcing efficacy of doses of cocaine by different routes of administration to DAT occupancy, finding that, even at equivalent occupancy, equivalent doses of drugs administered by routes with faster delivery to the brain were perceived as more reinforcing. The rate of change of synaptic dopamine concentration seems to be important as well as the absolute amount of increase from the baseline state [136]. Ongoing research in this area continues to identify other factors such as the pharmacokinetics of offset and drug half-life that are likely to have an important role in determining the reinforcing efficacy of drugs of abuse.

Alcoholism

Results from the relatively few dopamine imaging experiments investigating the density of dopaminergic neuroreceptors in alcoholics are mixed. One study reports no difference in DAT density between normal controls and alcoholics using [^{11}C]d-threo-methylphenidate PET [137], whereas two studies from a Finnish group reported reduced striatal DAT density in alcoholics as measured using [^{123}I]β-CIT SPECT. Radioligand binding was lower in 27 alcoholics at the time of their admission for detoxification than in 29 healthy controls [138]. The subjects who had alcohol in their blood at the time of the scan had the lowest binding. Furthermore, DAT binding returned to normal values within 4 weeks of cessation of alcohol consumption [138]. Differences in experimental design between the two studies may explain the seemingly discrepant findings. The studies performed by Laine and colleagues imaged alcoholics within days of cessation of heavy drinking, whereas the Volkow study imaged subjects later after cessation. The Finnish group also reported that a group of 10 nonviolent alcoholics had decreased DAT radioligand binding when compared with 19 healthy controls [139]. Binding was not significantly different

between 19 violent alcoholics and the same 10 controls [139].

At least four reports of decreased D2 receptor availability in alcoholic subjects have been published [137,140–142] using PET or SPECT. A follow-up study by Volkow and colleagues confirmed their original findings of no differences in DAT binding between alcoholics and controls and additionally reported that D2 receptor availability in alcoholics did not recover with alcohol detoxification (weeks of abstinence) or prolonged abstinence (months) [143]. To the authors' knowledge, no neuroimaging studies of dopamine D1 receptors or dopaminergic function have been performed in alcoholic subjects.

Obesity

In 10 severely obese men and women, [^{11}C]raclopride PET showed that D2 receptor binding was significantly reduced in obesity and, furthermore, was inversely proportional to body mass index [144]. Additionally, amygdalar D2 receptor binding in 16 normal individuals with various body mass indices was shown to correlate directly with body mass index and the personality trait "harm avoidance," as assessed with [^{11}C]FLB 457 PET and the Temperament and Character Inventory [145]. Other neuroimaging studies have implicated a role for the serotonin transporter in binge eating disorder in women. When compared with obese controls, patients with binge eating disorder were reported to have 27% increased serotonin transporter binding in midbrain regions [146]. Despite this finding, a role for dopamine is suggested by findings of reduced volume in dopaminergic brain regions in several recent morphometric MR imaging studies [147,148]. Although no neuroimaging studies of dopamine function in obesity have been performed, this is likely to be a fruitful avenue of clinical research in the near future.

Other behavioral disorders

Perhaps ironically, the prototypical compulsive behavior disorder, obsessive-compulsive disorder, has been little studied with dopamine neuroimaging techniques. To the authors' knowledge, only one such study has been conducted. In that study, [^{123}I]β-CIT SPECT was used to probe DAT density and found significantly reduced striatal DAT availability in 10 subjects with obsessive-compulsive disorder when compared with normal controls [149].

On the other hand, Tourette's syndrome, a neurologic disorder characterized by waxing and waning vocal and motor tics, has been studied extensively with dopamine neuroimaging. Abnormalities have been found in cortico-striatal-thalamic circuitry, and, based on the responsiveness of the disorder to dopaminergic medications, abnormalities in do-pamine neurotransmission are presumed to have a role. Increased DAT density as measured by [^{123}I]β-CIT SPECT has been reported in the basal ganglia of male and female neuroleptic-free Tourette's patients [150], in agreement with postmortem findings [151]. Tourette's patients have also been reported to exhibit increased amphetamine-induced dopamine release as assessed by [^{11}C]raclopride PET [152]. Other reported Tourette's-related dopaminergic abnormalities include increased D2 receptor binding [153]. These findings may be present only in a subset of patients [154]. Other studies have found no changes in D2 receptor binding [155–157], VMAT2 binding [158], or F-DOPA uptake [157]. Methodologic differences may help explain these discrepant findings.

Summary

Nearly a quarter of a century has passed since dopamine D2 receptors and dopamine metabolism were first visualized in living human brain using PET. Since those pioneering studies, the performance of PET and SPECT cameras has improved enormously, and radiotracers for both modalities have become available that can probe many aspects of the dopamine system and other neurotransmitter systems. Furthermore, the widening dissemination of PET technology for clinical [^{18}F]fluoroglucose studies as well as the growing use of SPECT in nuclear medicine should facilitate transfer of dopamine system imaging to the clinical arena. Future radiopharmaceutical development should enhance this process. One area where breakthroughs could come is in imaging aberrantly folded proteins such as a-synuclein and huntingtin for the evaluation of preclinical Parkinson's disease and Huntington's disease.

References

[1] Garnett ES, Nahmias C, Firnau G. Central dopaminergic pathways in hemiparkinsonism examined by positron emission tomography. Can J Neurol Sci 1984;11(1 Suppl):174–9.

[2] Nahmias C, Garnett ES, Firnau G, et al. Striatal dopamine distribution in parkinsonian patients during life. J Neurol Sci 1985;69(3):223–30.

[3] Wolf AP, Fowler JS. Positron emission tomography: biomedical research and clinical application. Neuroimaging Clin N Am 1995;5(1):87–101.

[4] Fowler JS, Wolf AP. The heritage of radiotracers for positron emission tomography. Acta Radiol Suppl 1990;374:13–6.

[5] Chan GL, Holden JE, Stoessl AJ, et al. Reproducibility studies with 11C-DTBZ, a monoamine vesicular transporter inhibitor in healthy human subjects. J Nucl Med 1999;40(2):283–9.

[6] Vander Borght TM, Sima AA, Kilbourn MR, et al. [3H]methoxytetrabenazine: a high specific activity ligand for estimating monoaminergic neuronal integrity. Neuroscience 1995;68(3):955–62.

[7] Kung HF, Kim HJ, Kung MP, et al. Imaging of dopamine transporters in humans with technetium-99m TRODAT-1. Eur J Nucl Med 1996;23(11):1527–30.

[8] Madras BK, Jones AG, Mahmood A, et al. Technepine: a high-affinity 99m-technetium probe to label the dopamine transporter in brain by SPECT imaging. Synapse 1996;22(3):239–46.

[9] Meltzer PC, Blundell P, Zona T, et al. A second-generation 99m-technetium single photon emission computed tomography agent that provides in vivo images of the dopamine transporter in primate brain. J Med Chem 2003;46(16):3483–96.

[10] Innis RB, Seibyl JP, Scanley BE, et al. Single photon emission computed tomographic imaging demonstrates loss of striatal dopamine transporters in Parkinson disease. Proc Natl Acad Sci USA 1993;90(24):11965–9.

[11] Van Laere K, De Ceuninck L, Dom R, et al. Dopamine transporter SPECT using fast kinetic ligands: 123I-FP-beta-CIT versus 99mTc-TRODAT-1. Eur J Nucl Med Mol Imaging 2004;31(8):1119–27.

[12] Johannsen B, Pietzsch HJ. Development of technetium-99m-based CNS receptor ligands: have there been any advances? Eur J Nucl Med Mol Imaging 2002;29(2):263–75.

[13] Kung HF, Kung MP, Choi SR. Radiopharmaceuticals for single-photon emission computed tomography brain imaging. Semin Nucl Med 2003;33(1):2–13.

[14] Wong DF, Yung B, Dannals RF, et al. In vivo imaging of baboon and human dopamine transporters by positron emission tomography using [11C]WIN 35,428. Synapse 1993;15(2):130–42.

[15] Farde L, Halldin C, Stone-Elander S, et al. PET analysis of human dopamine receptor subtypes using 11C-SCH 23390 and 11C-raclopride. Psychopharmacology (Berl) 1987;92(3):278–84.

[16] Abi-Dargham A, Martinez D, Mawlawi O, et al. Measurement of striatal and extrastriatal dopamine D1 receptor binding potential with [11C]NNC 112 in humans: validation and reproducibility. J Cereb Blood Flow Metab 2000;20(2):225–43.

[17] Okubo Y, Suhara T, Suzuki K, et al. Decreased prefrontal dopamine D1 receptors in schizophrenia revealed by PET. Nature 1997;385(6617):634–6.

[18] Karlsson P, Farde L, Halldin C, et al. PET study of D(1) dopamine receptor binding in neuroleptic-naive patients with schizophrenia. Am J Psychiatry 2002;159(5):761–7.

[19] Andrews TC, Weeks RA, Turjanski N, et al. Huntington's disease progression: PET and clinical observations. Brain 1999;122(Pt 12):2353–63.

[20] Ginovart N, Lundin A, Farde L, et al. PET study of the pre- and post-synaptic dopaminergic markers for the neurodegenerative process in Huntington's disease. Brain 1997;120(Pt 3): 503–14.

[21] Weeks RA, Piccini P, Harding AE, et al. Striatal D1 and D2 dopamine receptor loss in asymptomatic mutation carriers of Huntington's disease. Ann Neurol 1996;40(1):49–54.

[22] Sedvall G, Karlsson P, Lundin A, et al. Dopamine D1 receptor number—a sensitive PET marker for early brain degeneration in Huntington's disease. Eur Arch Psychiatry Clin Neurosci 1994;243(5):249–55.

[23] Guo N, Hwang DR, Lo ES, et al. Dopamine depletion and in vivo binding of PET D1 receptor radioligands: implications for imaging studies in schizophrenia. Neuropsychopharmacology 2003;28(9):1703–11.

[24] Ouchi Y, Kanno T, Okada H, et al. Presynaptic and postsynaptic dopaminergic binding densities in the nigrostriatal and mesocortical systems in early Parkinson's disease: a double-tracer positron emission tomography study. Ann Neurol 1999;46(5):723–31.

[25] Laruelle M. Imaging synaptic neurotransmission with in vivo binding competition techniques: a critical review. J Cereb Blood Flow Metab 2000;20(3):423–51.

[26] Sanchez-Pernaute R, Brownell AL, Isacson O. Functional imaging of the dopamine system: in vivo evaluation of dopamine deficiency and restoration. Neurotoxicology 2002;23(4–5): 469–78.

[27] Garnett ES, Firnau G, Nahmias C. Dopamine visualized in the basal ganglia of living man. Nature 1983;305(5930):137–8.

[28] Eckert T, Eidelberg D. Neuroimaging and therapeutics in movement disorders. NeuroRx 2005; 2(2):361–71.

[29] Au WL, Adams JR, Troiano AR, et al. Parkinson's disease: in vivo assessment of disease progression using positron emission tomography. Brain Res Mol Brain Res 2005;134(1):24–33.

[30] Kemp PM. Imaging the dopaminergic system in suspected parkinsonism, drug induced movement disorders, and Lewy body dementia. Nucl Med Commun 2005;26(2):87–96.

[31] Ravina B, Eidelberg D, Ahlskog JE, et al. The role of radiotracer imaging in Parkinson disease. Neurology 2005;64(2):208–15.

[32] Fischman AJ. Role of [18F]-dopa-PET imaging in assessing movement disorders. Radiol Clin North Am 2005;43(1):93–106.

[33] Fukuyama H. Functional brain imaging in Parkinson's disease—overview. J Neurol 2004; 251(Suppl 7):vII1–3.

[34] Asenbaum S, Brucke T, Pirker W, et al. Imaging of dopamine transporters with iodine-123-beta-CIT and SPECT in Parkinson's disease. J Nucl Med 1997;38(1):1–6.

[35] Frost JJ, Rosier AJ, Reich SG, et al. Positron emission tomographic imaging of the dopamine transporter with 11C-WIN 35,428 reveals marked declines in mild Parkinson's disease. Ann Neurol 1993;34(3):423–31.

[36] Tissingh G, Bergmans P, Booij J, et al. Drug-naive patients with Parkinson's disease in Hoehn and Yahr stages I and II show a bilateral decrease in striatal dopamine transporters as revealed by [123I]beta-CIT SPECT. J Neurol 1998; 245(1):14–20.

[37] Marek KL, Seibyl JP, Zoghbi SS, et al. [123I]beta-CIT/SPECT imaging demonstrates bilateral loss of dopamine transporters in hemi-Parkinson's disease. Neurology 1996;46(1): 231–7.

[38] Brucke T, Wenger S, Asenbaum S, et al. Dopamine D2 receptor imaging and measurement with SPECT. Adv Neurol 1993;60:494–500.

[39] Brucke T, Asenbaum S, Pirker W, et al. Measurement of the dopaminergic degeneration in Parkinson's disease with [123I]beta-CIT and SPECT: correlation with clinical findings and comparison with multiple system atrophy and progressive supranuclear palsy. J Neural Transm Suppl 1997;50:9–24.

[40] van Royen E, Verhoeff NF, Speelman JD, et al. Multiple system atrophy and progressive supranuclear palsy: diminished striatal D2 dopamine receptor activity demonstrated by 123I-IBZM single photon emission computed tomography. Arch Neurol 1993;50(5):513–6.

[41] Buck A, Westera G, Sutter M, et al. Iodine-123-IBF SPECT evaluation of extrapyramidal diseases. J Nucl Med 1995;36(7):1196–200.

[42] Pirker W, Asenbaum S, Wenger S, et al. Iodine-123-epidepride-SPECT: studies in Parkinson's disease, multiple system atrophy and Huntington's disease. J Nucl Med 1997;38(11):1711–7.

[43] Verhoeff NPLG, Speelman JD, Kuiper MA, et al. Clinical significance of dopamine D2-receptor imaging with [123I]-iodobenzamide SPECT in patients with parkinsonian syndromes. In: De Deyn PP, Dierckx RA, Alavi A, et al, editors. A textbook of SPECT in neurology and psychiatry. London: Libbey; 1997. p. 149–65.

[44] Thobois S, Guillouet S, Broussolle E. Contributions of PET and SPECT to the understanding of the pathophysiology of Parkinson's disease. Neurophysiol Clin 2001;31(5):321–40.

[45] Chabriat H, Levasseur M, Vidailhet M, et al. In vivo SPECT imaging of D2 receptor with iodine-iodolisuride: results in supranuclear palsy. J Nucl Med 1992;33(8):1481–5.

[46] Churchyard A, Donnan GA, Hughes A, et al. Dopa resistance in multiple-system atrophy: loss of postsynaptic D2 receptors. Ann Neurol 1993;34(2):219–26.

[47] Schulz JB, Klockgether T, Petersen D, et al. Multiple system atrophy: natural history, MRI

morphology, and dopamine receptor imaging with 123IBZM-SPECT. J Neurol Neurosurg Psychiatry 1994;57(9):1047–56.

[48] Verhoeff NP. Radiotracer imaging of dopaminergic transmission in neuropsychiatric disorders. Psychopharmacology (Berl) 1999;147(3):217–49.

[49] Stoffers D, Booij J, Bosscher L, et al. Early stage [123I]beta-CIT SPECT and long-term clinical follow-up in patients with an initial diagnosis of Parkinson's disease. Eur J Nucl Med Mol Imaging 2005;32(6):689–95.

[50] Brooks DJ, Ibanez V, Sawle GV, et al. Differing patterns of striatal 18F-dopa uptake in Parkinson's disease, multiple system atrophy, and progressive supranuclear palsy. Ann Neurol 1990;28(4):547–55.

[51] Brooks DJ, Salmon EP, Mathias CJ, et al. The relationship between locomotor disability, autonomic dysfunction, and the integrity of the striatal dopaminergic system in patients with multiple system atrophy, pure autonomic failure, and Parkinson's disease, studied with PET. Brain 1990;113(Pt 5):1539–52.

[52] Broussolle E, Dentresangle C, Landais P, et al. The relation of putamen and caudate nucleus 18F-dopa uptake to motor and cognitive performances in Parkinson's disease. J Neurol Sci 1999;166(2):141–51.

[53] Leenders KL, Palmer AJ, Quinn N, et al. Brain dopamine metabolism in patients with Parkinson's disease measured with positron emission tomography. J Neurol Neurosurg Psychiatry 1986;49(8):853–60.

[54] Vingerhoets FJ, Schulzer M, Calne DB, et al. Which clinical sign of Parkinson's disease best reflects the nigrostriatal lesion? Ann Neurol 1997;41(1):58–64.

[55] Marek K, Jennings D, Seibyl J. Dopamine agonists and Parkinson's disease progression: what can we learn from neuroimaging studies. Ann Neurol 2003;53(Suppl 3):S160–6 [discussion: S166–9].

[56] Nurmi E, Ruottinen HM, Bergman J, et al. Rate of progression in Parkinson's disease: a 6-[18F]fluoro-L-dopa PET study. Mov Disord 2001;16(4):608–15.

[57] Morrish PK, Rakshi JS, Bailey DL, et al. Measuring the rate of progression and estimating the preclinical period of Parkinson's disease with [18F]dopa PET. J Neurol Neurosurg Psychiatry 1998;64(3):314–9.

[58] Eshuis SA, Maguire RP, Leenders KL, et al. Comparison of FP-CIT SPECT with F-DOPA PET in patients with de novo and advanced Parkinson's disease. Eur J Nucl Med Mol Imaging 2006;33(2):200–9.

[59] Piccini P. Neurodegenerative movement disorders: the contribution of functional imaging. Curr Opin Neurol 2004;17(4):459–66.

[60] Piccini P, Pavese N, Brooks DJ. Endogenous dopamine release after pharmacological

challenges in Parkinson's disease. Ann Neurol 2003;53(5):647–53.

[61] Whone AL, Moore RY, Piccini PP, et al. Plasticity of the nigropallidal pathway in Parkinson's disease. Ann Neurol 2003;53(2):206–13.

[62] Strafella AP, Ko JH, Grant J, et al. Corticostriatal functional interactions in Parkinson's disease: a rTMS/[11C]raclopride PET study. Eur J Neurosci 2005;22(11):2946–52.

[63] Brooks DJ. Positron emission tomography imaging of transplant function. NeuroRx 2004;1(4):482–91.

[64] Anderson KE. Huntington's disease and related disorders. Psychiatr Clin North Am 2005;28(1):275–90.

[65] Rosas HD, Feigin AS, Hersch SM. Using advances in neuroimaging to detect, understand, and monitor disease progression in Huntington's disease. NeuroRx 2004;1(2):263–72.

[66] Rego AC, de Almeida LP. Molecular targets and therapeutic strategies in Huntington's disease. Curr Drug Targets CNS Neurol Disord 2005;4(4):361–81.

[67] Lawrence AD, Weeks RA, Brooks DJ, et al. The relationship between striatal dopamine receptor binding and cognitive performance in Huntington's disease. Brain 1998;121(Pt 7):1343–55.

[68] Turjanski N, Weeks R, Dolan R, et al. Striatal D1 and D2 receptor binding in patients with Huntington's disease and other choreas: a PET study. Brain 1995;118(Pt 3):689–96.

[69] Backman L, Farde L. Dopamine and cognitive functioning: brain imaging findings in Huntington's disease and normal aging. Scand J Psychol 2001;42(3):287–96.

[70] van Oostrom JC, Maguire RP, Verschuuren-Bemelmans CC, et al. Striatal dopamine D2 receptors, metabolism, and volume in preclinical Huntington disease. Neurology 2005;65(6):941–3.

[71] Antonini A, Leenders KL, Spiegel R, et al. Striatal glucose metabolism and dopamine D2 receptor binding in asymptomatic gene carriers and patients with Huntington's disease. Brain 1996;119(Pt 6):2085–95.

[72] Ichise M, Toyama H, Fornazzari L, et al. Iodine-123-IBZM dopamine D2 receptor and technetium-99m-HMPAO brain perfusion SPECT in the evaluation of patients with and subjects at risk for Huntington's disease. J Nucl Med 1993;34(8):1274–81.

[73] Olanow CW, Goetz CG, Kordower JH, et al. A double-blind controlled trial of bilateral fetal nigral transplantation in Parkinson's disease. Ann Neurol 2003;54(3):403–14.

[74] Nakamura T, Dhawan V, Chaly T, et al. Blinded positron emission tomography study of dopamine cell implantation for Parkinson's disease. Ann Neurol 2001;50(2):181–7.

[75] Freed CR, Greene PE, Breeze RE, et al. Transplantation of embryonic dopamine neurons

for severe Parkinson's disease. N Engl J Med 2001;344(10):710–9.

[76] Lindvall O, Hagell P. Clinical observations after neural transplantation in Parkinson's disease. Prog Brain Res 2000;127:299–320.

[77] Furtado S, Sossi V, Hauser RA, et al. Positron emission tomography after fetal transplantation in Huntington's disease. Ann Neurol 2005; 58(2):331–7.

[78] Seeman P, Lee T. Antipsychotic drugs: direct correlation between clinical potency and presynaptic action on dopamine neurons. Science 1975; 188(4194):1217–9.

[79] Parsey RV, Mann JJ. Applications of positron emission tomography in psychiatry. Semin Nucl Med 2003;33(2):129–35.

[80] Abi-Dargham A, Laruelle M. Mechanisms of action of second generation antipsychotic drugs in schizophrenia: insights from brain imaging studies. Eur Psychiatry 2005;20(1): 15–27.

[81] Sedvall G, Pauli S, Karlsson P, et al. PET imaging of neuroreceptors in schizophrenia. Eur Neuropsychopharmacol 1995;5(Suppl):25–30.

[82] Abi-Dargham A, Mawlawi O, Lombardo I, et al. Prefrontal dopamine D1 receptors and working memory in schizophrenia. J Neurosci 2002; 22(9):3708–19.

[83] Seeman P, Bzowej NH, Guan HC, et al. Human brain D1 and D2 dopamine receptors in schizophrenia, Alzheimer's, Parkinson's, and Huntington's diseases. Neuropsychopharmacology 1987;1(1):5–15.

[84] Czudek C, Reynolds GP. Binding of [11C]SCH 23390 to post-mortem brain tissue in schizophrenia. Br J Pharmacol 1988;93(Suppl):166P.

[85] Knable MB, Hyde TM, Herman MM, et al. Quantitative autoradiography of dopamine-D1 receptors, D2 receptors, and dopamine uptake sites in postmortem striatal specimens from schizophrenic patients. Biol Psychiatry 1994; 36(12):827–35.

[86] Hirvonen J, van Erp TG, Huttunen J, et al. Increased caudate dopamine D2 receptor availability as a genetic marker for schizophrenia. Arch Gen Psychiatry 2005;62(4):371–8.

[87] Seeman P, Chau-Wong M, Tedesco J, et al. Brain receptors for antipsychotic drugs and dopamine: direct binding assays. Proc Natl Acad Sci USA 1975;72(11):4376–80.

[88] Creese I, Burt DR, Snyder SH. Dopamine receptor binding predicts clinical and pharmacological potencies of antischizophrenic drugs. Science 1976;192(4238):481–3.

[89] Farde L, Wiesel FA, Halldin C, et al. Central D2-dopamine receptor occupancy in schizophrenic patients treated with antipsychotic drugs. Arch Gen Psychiatry 1988;45(1):71–6.

[90] Laruelle M, Kegeles LS, Abi-Dargham A. Glutamate, dopamine, and schizophrenia: from pathophysiology to treatment. Ann N Y Acad Sci 2003;1003:138–58.

[91] Laruelle M, Frankle WG, Narendran R, et al. Mechanism of action of antipsychotic drugs: from dopamine D(2) receptor antagonism to glutamate NMDA facilitation. Clin Ther 2005; 27(Suppl A):S16–24.

[92] Farde L, Nordstrom AL, Nyberg S, et al. D1-, D2-, and 5-HT2-receptor occupancy in clozapine-treated patients. J Clin Psychiatry 1994; 55(Suppl B):67–9.

[93] Kessler RM, Ansari MS, Riccardi P, et al. Occupancy of striatal and extrastriatal dopamine D2/D3 receptors by olanzapine and haloperidol. Neuropsychopharmacology 2005;30(12): 2283–9.

[94] Laruelle M, Abi-Dargham A, van Dyck CH, et al. Single photon emission computerized tomography imaging of amphetamine-induced dopamine release in drug-free schizophrenic subjects. Proc Natl Acad Sci USA 1996;93(17):9235–40.

[95] Abi-Dargham A, Gil R, Krystal J, et al. Increased striatal dopamine transmission in schizophrenia: confirmation in a second cohort. Am J Psychiatry 1998;155(6):761–7.

[96] Breier A, Su TP, Saunders R, et al. Schizophrenia is associated with elevated amphetamine-induced synaptic dopamine concentrations: evidence from a novel positron emission tomography method. Proc Natl Acad Sci USA 1997;94(6): 2569–74.

[97] Bertolino A, Breier A, Callicott JH, et al. The relationship between dorsolateral prefrontal neuronal N-acetylaspartate and evoked release of striatal dopamine in schizophrenia. Neuropsychopharmacology 2000;22(2):125–32.

[98] Abi-Dargham A, Rodenhiser J, Printz D, et al. Increased baseline occupancy of D2 receptors by dopamine in schizophrenia. Proc Natl Acad Sci USA 2000;97(14):8104–9.

[99] Reith J, Benkelfat C, Sherwin A, et al. Elevated dopa decarboxylase activity in living brain of patients with psychosis. Proc Natl Acad Sci USA 1994;91(24):11651–4.

[100] Hietala J, Syvalahti E, Vuorio K, et al. Presynaptic dopamine function in striatum of neuroleptic-naive schizophrenic patients. Lancet 1995; 346(8983):1130–1.

[101] Hietala J, Syvalahti E, Vilkman H, et al. Depressive symptoms and presynaptic dopamine function in neuroleptic-naive schizophrenia. Schizophr Res 1999;35(1):41–50.

[102] Lindstrom LH, Gefvert O, Hagberg G, et al. Increased dopamine synthesis rate in medial prefrontal cortex and striatum in schizophrenia indicated by L-(beta-11C) DOPA and PET. Biol Psychiatry 1999;46(5):681–8.

[103] Meyer-Lindenberg A, Miletich RS, Kohn PD, et al. Reduced prefrontal activity predicts exaggerated striatal dopaminergic function in schizophrenia. Nat Neurosci 2002;5(3): 267–71.

[104] Dao-Castellana MH, Paillere-Martinot ML, Hantraye P, et al. Presynaptic dopaminergic

function in the striatum of schizophrenic patients. Schizophr Res 1997;23(2):167–74.

[105] Elkashef AM, Doudet D, Bryant T, et al. 6-(18)F-DOPA PET study in patients with schizophrenia: positron emission tomography. Psychiatry Res 2000;100(1):1–11.

[106] Brunswick DJ, Amsterdam JD, Mozley PD, et al. Greater availability of brain dopamine transporters in major depression shown by [99m Tc]TRODAT-1 SPECT imaging. Am J Psychiatry 2003;160(10):1836–41.

[107] Argyelan M, Szabo Z, Kanyo B, et al. Dopamine transporter availability in medication free and in bupropion treated depression: a 99mTc-TRODAT-1 SPECT study. J Affect Disord 2005; 89(1–3):115–23.

[108] Szabo Z, Argyelan M, Kanyo B, et al. [Change of dopamine transporter activity (DAT) during the action of bupropion (in depression)]. Neuropsychopharmacol Hung 2004;6(2):79–81.

[109] Meyer JH, Goulding VS, Wilson AA, et al. Bupropion occupancy of the dopamine transporter is low during clinical treatment. Psychopharmacology (Berl) 2002;163(1): 102–5.

[110] Kugaya A, Seneca NM, Snyder PJ, et al. Changes in human in vivo serotonin and dopamine transporter availabilities during chronic antidepressant administration. Neuropsychopharmacology 2003;28(2):413–20.

[111] Dougherty DD, Bonab AA, Spencer TJ, et al. Dopamine transporter density in patients with attention deficit hyperactivity disorder. Lancet 1999;354(9196):2132–3.

[112] Krause KH, Dresel SH, Krause J, et al. The dopamine transporter and neuroimaging in attention deficit hyperactivity disorder. Neurosci Biobehav Rev 2003;27(7):605–13.

[113] Cheon KA, Ryu YH, Kim YK, et al. Dopamine transporter density in the basal ganglia assessed with [123I]IPT SPET in children with attention deficit hyperactivity disorder. Eur J Nucl Med Mol Imaging 2003;30(2):306–11.

[114] van Dyck CH, Quinlan DM, Cretella LM, et al. Unaltered dopamine transporter availability in adult attention deficit hyperactivity disorder. Am J Psychiatry 2002;159(2):309–12.

[115] Jucaite A, Fernell E, Halldin C, et al. Reduced midbrain dopamine transporter binding in male adolescents with attention-deficit/hyperactivity disorder: association between striatal dopamine markers and motor hyperactivity. Biol Psychiatry 2005;57(3):229–38.

[116] Vles JS, Feron FJ, Hendriksen JG, et al. Methylphenidate down-regulates the dopamine receptor and transporter system in children with attention deficit hyperkinetic disorder (ADHD). Neuropediatrics 2003;34(2):77–80.

[117] Dresel S, Krause J, Krause KH, et al. Attention deficit hyperactivity disorder: binding of [99mTc]TRODAT-1 to the dopamine transporter before and after methylphenidate

treatment. Eur J Nucl Med 2000;27(10): 1518–24.

[118] Spencer TJ, Biederman J, Madras BK, et al. In vivo neuroreceptor imaging in attention-deficit/hyperactivity disorder: a focus on the dopamine transporter. Biol Psychiatry 2005;57(11): 1293–300.

[119] Madras BK, Miller GM, Fischman AJ. The dopamine transporter and attention-deficit/hyperactivity disorder. Biol Psychiatry 2005;57(11): 1397–409.

[120] Volkow ND, Wang GJ, Fowler JS, et al. Dopamine transporter occupancies in the human brain induced by therapeutic doses of oral methylphenidate. Am J Psychiatry 1998;155(10): 1325–31.

[121] Schneier FR, Liebowitz MR, Abi-Dargham A, et al. Low dopamine D(2) receptor binding potential in social phobia. Am J Psychiatry 2000; 157(3):457–9.

[122] Tiihonen J, Kuikka J, Bergstrom K, et al. Dopamine reuptake site densities in patients with social phobia. Am J Psychiatry 1997;154(2): 239–42.

[123] Coupland NJ. Social phobia: etiology, neurobiology, and treatment. J Clin Psychiatry 2001; 62(Suppl 1):25–35.

[124] Farde L, Gustavsson JP, Jonsson E. D2 dopamine receptors and personality traits. Nature 1997;385(6617):590.

[125] Breier A, Kestler L, Adler C, et al. Dopamine D2 receptor density and personal detachment in healthy subjects. Am J Psychiatry 1998; 155(10):1440–2.

[126] Laakso A, Vilkman H, Kajander J, et al. Prediction of detached personality in healthy subjects by low dopamine transporter binding. Am J Psychiatry 2000;157(2):290–2.

[127] Sekine Y, Minabe Y, Ouchi Y, et al. Association of dopamine transporter loss in the orbitofrontal and dorsolateral prefrontal cortices with methamphetamine-related psychiatric symptoms. Am J Psychiatry 2003;160(9):1699–701.

[128] Volkow ND, Chang L, Wang GJ, et al. Low level of brain dopamine D2 receptors in methamphetamine abusers: association with metabolism in the orbitofrontal cortex. Am J Psychiatry 2001;158(12):2015–21.

[129] Volkow ND, Chang L, Wang GJ, et al. Association of dopamine transporter reduction with psychomotor impairment in methamphetamine abusers. Am J Psychiatry 2001;158(3): 377–82.

[130] Volkow ND, Chang L, Wang GJ, et al. Loss of dopamine transporters in methamphetamine abusers recovers with protracted abstinence. J Neurosci 2001;21(23):9414–8.

[131] Malison RT, Best SE, Wallace EA, et al. Euphorigenic doses of cocaine reduce [123I]beta-CIT SPECT measures of dopamine transporter availability in human cocaine addicts. Psychopharmacology (Berl) 1995;122(4):358–62.

[132] Volkow ND, Wang GJ, Fowler JS, et al. Relationship between psychostimulant-induced "high" and dopamine transporter occupancy. Proc Natl Acad Sci USA 1996;93(19):10388–92.

[133] Volkow ND, Wang GJ, Fischman MW, et al. Relationship between subjective effects of cocaine and dopamine transporter occupancy. Nature 1997;386(6627):827–30.

[134] Volkow ND, Fowler JS, Ding YS, et al. Imaging the neurochemistry of nicotine actions: studies with positron emission tomography. Nicotine Tob Res 1999;1(Suppl 2):S127–32. [discussion: S139–140].

[135] Volkow ND, Wang GJ, Fischman MW, et al. Effects of route of administration on cocaine induced dopamine transporter blockade in the human brain. Life Sci 2000;67(12):1507–15.

[136] Howell LL, Wilcox KM. The dopamine transporter and cocaine medication development: drug self-administration in nonhuman primates. J Pharmacol Exp Ther 2001;298(1):1–6.

[137] Volkow ND, Wang GJ, Fowler JS, et al. Decreases in dopamine receptors but not in dopamine transporters in alcoholics. Alcohol Clin Exp Res 1996;20(9):1594–8.

[138] Laine TP, Ahonen A, Torniainen P, et al. Dopamine transporters increase in human brain after alcohol withdrawal. Mol Psychiatry 1999;4(2):189–91.

[139] Tiihonen J, Kuikka J, Bergstrom K, et al. Altered striatal dopamine re-uptake site densities in habitually violent and non-violent alcoholics. Nat Med 1995;1(7):654–7.

[140] Hietala J, West C, Syvalahti E, et al. Striatal D2 dopamine receptor binding characteristics in vivo in patients with alcohol dependence. Psychopharmacology (Berl) 1994;116(3):285–90.

[141] Repo E, Kuikka JT, Bergstrom KA, et al. Dopamine transporter and D2-receptor density in late-onset alcoholism. Psychopharmacology (Berl) 1999;147(3):314–8.

[142] Heinz A, Ragan P, Jones DW, et al. Reduced central serotonin transporters in alcoholism. Am J Psychiatry 1998;155(11):1544–9.

[143] Volkow ND, Wang GJ, Maynard L, et al. Effects of alcohol detoxification on dopamine D2 receptors in alcoholics: a preliminary study. Psychiatry Res 2002;116(3):163–72.

[144] Wang GJ, Volkow ND, Logan J, et al. Brain dopamine and obesity. Lancet 2001;357(9253):354–7.

[145] Yasuno F, Suhara T, Sudo Y, et al. Relation among dopamine D(2) receptor binding, obesity and personality in normal human subjects. Neurosci Lett 2001;300(1):59–61.

[146] Kuikka JT, Tammela L, Karhunen L, et al. Reduced serotonin transporter binding in binge eating women. Psychopharmacology (Berl) 2001;155(3):310–4.

[147] Matochik JA, London ED, Yildiz BO, et al. Effect of leptin replacement on brain structure in genetically leptin-deficient adults. J Clin Endocrinol Metab 2005;90(5):2851–4.

[148] Pannacciulli N, Del Parigi A, Chen K, et al. Brain abnormalities in human obesity: a voxel-based morphometric study. Neuroimage 2006;31(4):1419–25.

[149] Hesse S, Muller U, Lincke T, et al. Serotonin and dopamine transporter imaging in patients with obsessive-compulsive disorder. Psychiatry Res 2005;140(1):63–72.

[150] Malison RT, McDougle CJ, van Dyck CH, et al. [123I]beta-CIT SPECT imaging of striatal dopamine transporter binding in Tourette's disorder. Am J Psychiatry 1995;152(9):1359–61.

[151] Singer HS, Hahn IH, Moran TH. Abnormal dopamine uptake sites in postmortem striatum from patients with Tourette's syndrome. Ann Neurol 1991;30(4):558–62.

[152] Singer HS, Szymanski S, Giuliano J, et al. Elevated intrasynaptic dopamine release in Tourette's syndrome measured by PET. Am J Psychiatry 2002;159(8):1329–36.

[153] Wolf SS, Jones DW, Knable MB, et al. Tourette syndrome: prediction of phenotypic variation in monozygotic twins by caudate nucleus D2 receptor binding. Science 1996;273(5279):1225–7.

[154] Wong DF, Singer HS, Brandt J, et al. D2-like dopamine receptor density in Tourette syndrome measured by PET. J Nucl Med 1997;38(8):1243–7.

[155] Albin RL, Koeppe RA, Bohnen NI, et al. Increased ventral striatal monoaminergic innervation in Tourette syndrome. Neurology 2003;61(3):310–5.

[156] George MS, Robertson MM, Costa DC, et al. Dopamine receptor availability in Tourette's syndrome. Psychiatry Res 1994;55(4):193–203.

[157] Turjanski N, Sawle GV, Playford ED, et al. PET studies of the presynaptic and postsynaptic dopaminergic system in Tourette's syndrome. J Neurol Neurosurg Psychiatry 1994;57(6):688–92.

[158] Meyer P, Bohnen NI, Minoshima S, et al. Striatal presynaptic monoaminergic vesicles are not increased in Tourette's syndrome. Neurology 1999;53(2):371–4.

[159] Acton PD, Meyer PT, Mozley PD, et al. Simplified quantification of dopamine transporters in humans using [99mTc]TRODAT-1 and single-photon emission tomography. Eur J Nucl Med 2000;27(11):1714–8.

[160] Bao SY, Wu JC, Luo WF, et al. Imaging of dopamine transporters with technetium-99m TRODAT-1 and single photon emission computed tomography. J Neuroimaging 2000;10(4):200–3.

[161] Weng YH, Kao PF, Tsai CH, et al. Dopamine deficiency in rubral tremor caused by midbrain hemangioma: case report. Chang Gung Med J 2000;23(8):485–91.

[162] Huang WS, Lin SZ, Lin JC, et al. Evaluation of early-stage Parkinson's disease with

99mTc-TRODAT-1 imaging. J Nucl Med 2001; 42(9):1303–8.

[163] Shyu WC, Lin SZ, Chiang MF, et al. Early onset Parkinson's disease in a Chinese population: 99mTc-TRODAT-1 SPECT, Parkin gene analysis and clinical study. Parkinsonism Relat Disord 2005;11(3):173–80.

[164] Krause KH, Dresel SH, Krause J, et al. Increased striatal dopamine transporter in adult patients with attention deficit hyperactivity disorder: effects of methylphenidate as measured by single photon emission computed tomography. Neurosci Lett 2000;285(2):107–10.

[165] Soyka M, Dresel S, Horak M, et al. PET and SPECT findings in alcohol hallucinosis: case report and super-brief review of the pathophysiology of this syndrome. World J Biol Psychiatry 2000;1(4):215–8.

[166] Tzen KY, Lu CS, Yen TC, et al. Differential diagnosis of Parkinson's disease and vascular parkinsonism by (99m)Tc-TRODAT-1. J Nucl Med 2001;42(3):408–13.

[167] Yen TC, Lu CS, Tzen KY, et al. Decreased dopamine transporter binding in Machado-Joseph disease. J Nucl Med 2000;41(6):994–8.

[168] Yen TC, Tzen KY, Chen MC, et al. Dopamine transporter concentration is reduced in asymptomatic Machado-Joseph disease gene carriers. J Nucl Med 2002;43(2):153–9.

[169] Krause KH, Dresel S, Krause J, et al. Elevated striatal dopamine transporter in a drug naive patient with Tourette syndrome and attention deficit/hyperactivity disorder: positive effect of methylphenidate. J Neurol 2002;249(8):1116–8.

[170] Lu CS, Chang HC, Kuo PC, et al. The parkinsonian phenotype of spinocerebellar ataxia type 3 in a Taiwanese family. Parkinsonism Relat Disord 2004;10(6):369–73.

[171] Lu CS, Wu Chou YH, Kuo PC, et al. The parkinsonian phenotype of spinocerebellar ataxia type 2. Arch Neurol 2004;61(1):35–8.

[172] Huang CC, Yen TC, Weng YH, et al. Normal dopamine transporter binding in dopa responsive dystonia. J Neurol 2002;249(8):1016–20.

[173] Huang CC, Weng YH, Lu CS, et al. Dopamine transporter binding in chronic manganese intoxication. J Neurol 2003;250(11):1335–9.

[174] Ku MC, Huang CC, Kuo HC, et al. Diffuse white matter lesions in carbon disulfide intoxication: microangiopathy or demyelination. Eur Neurol 2003;50(4):220–4.

[175] Huang CC. Carbon disulfide neurotoxicity: Taiwan experience. Acta Neurol Taiwan 2004; 13(1):3–9.

[176] Hsiao MC, Lin KJ, Liu CY, et al. Dopamine transporter change in drug-naive schizophrenia: an imaging study with 99mTc-TRODAT-1. Schizophr Res 2003;65(1):39–46.

[177] Yang YK, Yu L, Yeh TL, et al. Associated alterations of striatal dopamine D2/D3 receptor and transporter binding in drug-naive patients with schizophrenia: a dual-isotope SPECT study. Am J Psychiatry 2004;161(8):1496–8.

[178] Huang CC, Chu NS, Yen TC, et al. Dopamine transporter binding in Wilson's disease. Can J Neurol Sci 2003;30(2):163–7.

[179] Lai SC, Weng YH, Yen TC, et al. Imaging early-stage corticobasal degeneration with [99mTc]TRODAT-1 SPET. Nucl Med Commun 2004;25(4):339–45.

[180] Lu CS, Weng YH, Chen MC, et al. 99mTc-TRODAT-1 imaging of multiple system atrophy. J Nucl Med 2004;45(1):49–55.

[181] Swanson RL, Newberg AB, Acton PD, et al. Differences in [99mTc]TRODAT-1 SPECT binding to dopamine transporters in patients with multiple system atrophy and Parkinson's disease. Eur J Nucl Med Mol Imaging 2005;32(3): 302–7.

[182] Mozley PD, Acton PD, Barraclough ED, et al. Effects of age on dopamine transporters in healthy humans. J Nucl Med 1999;40(11): 1812–7.

[183] Mozley LH, Gur RC, Mozley PD, et al. Striatal dopamine transporters and cognitive functioning in healthy men and women. Am J Psychiatry 2001;158(9):1492–9.

[184] Krause KH, Dresel SH, Krause J, et al. Stimulant like action of nicotine on striatal dopamine transporter in the brain of adults with attention deficit hyperactivity disorder. Int J Neuropsychopharmacol 2002;5(2):111–3.

[185] Gardiner SA, Morrison MF, Mozley PD, et al. Pilot study on the effect of estrogen replacement therapy on brain dopamine transporter availability in healthy postmenopausal women. Am J Geriatr Psychiatry 2004;12(6): 621–30.

NEUROIMAGING
CLINICS
OF NORTH AMERICA

Neuroimag Clin N Am 16 (2006) 575–589

ELSEVIER
SAUNDERS

Single Photon Emission Computed Tomography and Positron Emission Tomography Imaging of Multi-drug Resistant P-glycoprotein—Monitoring a Transport Activity Important in Cancer, Blood–Brain Barrier Function and Alzheimer's Disease

David Piwnica-Worms, MD, PhD*, Aparna H. Kesarwala, AB, Andrea Pichler, PhD, Julie L. Prior, BA, Vijay Sharma, PhD

- Radiopharmaceuticals for imaging P-glycoprotein transport activity: survey of single-photon emission computed tomography and positron emission tomography agents
  Single-photon emission computed tomography agents for molecular imaging of P-glycoprotein transport activity
- Positron emission tomography agents for molecular imaging of P-glycoprotein transport activity

- Clinical studies: multi-drug resistance in cancer
- Future clinical studies: analysis of P-glycoprotein at the blood-brain barrier
- Future clinical studies: analysis of P-glycoprotein in Alzheimer's disease
- Summary
- Acknowledgments
- References

Resistance of malignant tumors to chemotherapeutic agents is a major cause of treatment failure in patients who have cancer [1,2]. The phenotype, known as multi-drug resistance, is characterized by a lack of response to various drugs. Classically, such refractory behavior to multiple chemotherapeutic agents was thought to occur in recurring tumors following initial treatment with a single agent; it appears, however, that tumors at the time of presentation also may exhibit multi-drug

This educational project was funded by the NIH Molecular Imaging Center grant P50 CA94056 and DOE contract DE FG02 94ER61885.
Washington University Medical School, 510 South Kingshighway Boulevard, Box 8225, St. Louis, MO 63110, USA
* Corresponding author.
E-mail address: piwnica-wormsd@mir.wustl.edu (D. Piwnica-Worms).

doi:10.1016/j.nic.2006.06.007

resistance a priori as a reflection of an aggressive phenotype [3]. One of the first biochemically characterized mechanisms of multi-drug resistance was transporter-mediated resistance conferred by the ATP-binding cassette (ABC) superfamily of transporters [2,4]. Biochemical and clinical data implicate P-glycoprotein (Pgp; ABCB1), a 170 kD plasma membrane protein product of the MDR1 gene [2,5], the multi-drug resistant-associated protein (MRP1, ABCC1), a related 190 kD transporter protein [6,7], along with other selected members of the MRP subfamily (MRP1-13, ABCC1-13) in mediating multi-drug resistance. Pgp confers resistance by outward transport of various structurally and functionally unrelated, generally cationic xenobiotics, thereby reducing their intracellular content. Similarly, MRPs are thought to outwardly transport generally anionic compounds, conjugated or unconjugated, and selected neutral hydrophobic chemotherapeutic agents. In addition, other ABC half transporters, such as the breast cancer resistance protein (BCRP/MXR; ABCG2), also are known to confer resistance to selected chemotherapeutic agents [8–10].

In addition to the standard paradigm of Pgp as an ATP-dependent efflux transporter of xenobiotics and chemotherapeutic drugs, several studies provide evidence for additional mechanisms for diminished drug accumulation in multi-drug resistant (MDR) cells. For example, a flippase model has been proposed to explain the broad specificity of Pgp [11]. This model suggests that Pgp either flips hydrophobic cytotoxic compounds from the inner to outer leaflet of the lipid bilayer, allowing the agents to diffuse away, or acts as a phospholipid flippase that alters membrane permeability, thereby accounting for the observed decrease in intracellular concentration of drug. Some studies have shown a more alkaline internal pH and decreased membrane potential in selected cells transfected with MDR1 compared with normal cells [12,13], suggesting that Pgp may alter indirectly partitioning of substrates within cells through effects on intracellular pH or membrane potential. This, however, has not been observed uniformly in all MDR cells [14]. In addition, cells expressing Pgp may have intracellular compartments that are more acidic than non-Pgp expressing cells, thereby altering intracellular distribution of drug [15,16]. They also may show altered membrane permeability resulting in decreased drug influx [14,17], or interfere with pathways of apoptosis (programmed cell death) [18,19]. Thus, the observed combined effect of Pgp expression is a decreased intracellular concentration of cytotoxic drugs, thereby rendering chemotherapeutic treatment ineffective in cancer.

Pgp expression correlates with a poor response to treatment [3] and has been a target for cancer therapy on several fronts. First, reversal of multi-drug resistance in tumor cells has been an important target for pharmaceutical development of nontoxic agents that block the transport activity of Pgp [2]. When coadministered with a cytotoxic agent, these inhibitors, known as MDR modulators, enhance net accumulation of cytotoxic compounds within tumor cells. Second, transgenic expression of MDR1 has been explored for hematopoietic cell protection in the context of cancer chemotherapy [20], wherein Pgp could protect hematopoietic progenitor cells from chemotherapy-induced myelotoxicity. In addition, both Pgp and MRP transporters are normally present in various tissues including intestinal epithelium, choroid plexus epithelium, testes, kidney, liver, adrenal, placenta, and capillary endothelial cells of the blood–brain barrier (BBB) [7,21,22]. Since ABC transporters affect the pharmacokinetics of many common pharmaceuticals, Pgp modulation has been evaluated as a means to improve oral absorption and BBB penetration of drugs such as chemotherapeutics and HIV protease inhibitors [23,24].

Because Pgp is expressed highly on the luminal surface of brain capillary endothelial cells, Pgp functionally comprises a major component of the BBB by limiting central nervous system (CNS) penetration of various chemotherapeutic agents, small peptides, antibiotics, HIV protease inhibitors, antidepressants, antiarrhythmics, and new molecular therapeutics such as Gleevec [2,25]. Recently, the authors also demonstrated using Pgp gene deleted mice that amyloid-beta (Aβ) removal from the brain is at least partially mediated by Pgp on the BBB [26]. Consequently, the lack of Pgp expression exacerbates Aβ deposition and accelerates plaque formation in a mouse model of Alzheimer's disease (AD). Therefore, Pgp-mediated drug transport activity could be a novel diagnostic imaging target in AD. It also could be important in predicting oral absorptivity, pharmacokinetics, and penetrance of many common drugs into tumors and the brain.

Radiopharmaceuticals for imaging P-glycoprotein transport activity: survey of single-photon emission computed tomography and positron emission tomography agents

Single-photon emission computed tomography agents for molecular imaging of P-glycoprotein transport activity

Significant effort has been directed toward the non invasive detection of transporter-mediated resistance using planar scintigraphy or single-photon emission computed tomography (SPECT) employing radiolabeled metal complexes characterized as transport substrates for Pgp. These include ^{99m}Tc-Sestamibi, ^{99m}Tc-Tetrofosmin, ^{99m}Tc-Furifosmin, [99m]TcQ-58, [99m]TcQ-63 and ^{99m}Tc-CO-MIBI [27–29] (Fig. 1).

Hexakis(2-methoxyisobutylisonitrile)technetium-99m (commonly known as ^{99m}Tc-Sestamibi), although originally developed as a radiopharmaceutical for myocardial perfusion imaging [30,31], subsequently was the first metal complex shown to be a Pgp transport substrate [32]. Characterized by octahedral geometry around the central technetium(I) core [30,33], the radiopharmaceutical possesses a cationic charge and modest hydrophobicity similar to many chemotherapeutic agents in the MDR substrate phenotype. In the absence of Pgp expression, this ^{99m}Tc-isonitrile complex accumulates within the interior of cells [34,35]. In Pgp-expressing MDR tumor cells, however, net cellular accumulation levels of ^{99m}Tc-Sestamibi are low [32,36–39]. Furthermore, complete reversal of the Pgp-mediated exclusion of ^{99m}Tc-Sestamibi

has been induced by treatment with conventional Pgp inhibitors such as verapamil, cyclosporin A, and quinidine, and newer, more potent reversal agents such as GF120918, LY335979, PSC 833, or VX710 [32,36,37,40–47], and more recently, XR-9576 [2,47,48].

The mechanisms of uptake and retention of hydrophobic cationic ^{99m}Tc-based complexes have been studied extensively in various cellular and subcellular preparations in vitro, and a model of cationic metal complex transport-mediated by Pgp is shown in Fig. 2. Net cell content of these ^{99m}Tc-based cationic agents generally is determined by the balance of passive potential-dependent influx and Pgp transporter-mediated efflux [32]. For example, biophysical analysis has shown that ^{99m}Tc-Sestamibi is a high fidelity probe of transmembrane potential [49], with passive inward movement of this lipophilic cation being driven (in the absence of cell surface transporters) by the inside-negative transmembrane potentials generated in living cells

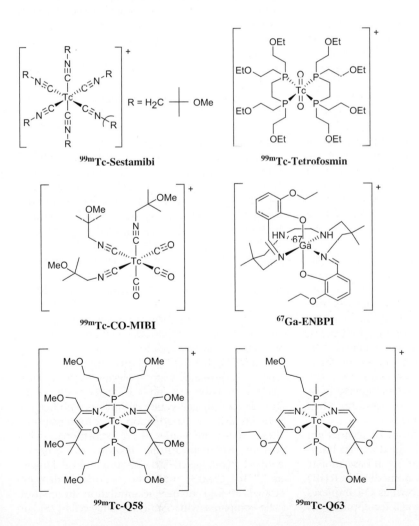

Fig. 1. Structures of SPECT radiopharmaceuticals characterized as transport substrates for Pgp.

[99m]Tc-Sestamibi

[99m]Tc-Tetrofosmin

R = H_2C—OMe

^{99m}Tc-CO-MIBI

^{67}Ga-ENBPI

[99m]Tc-Q58

[99m]Tc-Q63

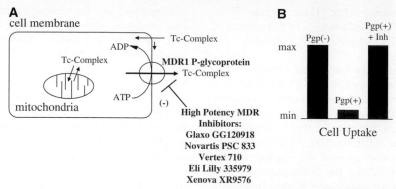

Fig. 2. Model of cationic metal-complex transport mediated by Pgp. *(A)* Net cell content of these [99mTc]-based cationic SPECT agents is determined by the balance of passive inward movement of these lipophilic cation agents driven by the inside-negative plasma membrane and mitochondrial inner membrane potentials generated in living cells versus active outward transport mediated by Pgp. *(B)* Cells with high mitochondrial content and lacking Pgp (Pgp(-)) will show high tracer accumulation levels, while cells with high levels of Pgp (Pgp(+)) will pump the tracer to low levels. Blockade of Pgp-mediated extrusion by treatment with Pgp inhibitors (+ Inh) produces an increase in cell tracer content as the agent can concentrate once again into mitochondria.

[34,35]. The complex is sequestered reversibly within mitochondria by the serial thermodynamic driving forces of the negative plasma membrane and mitochondrial inner membrane potentials [35,50]. This explains why the tracer has excellent properties as a perfusion tracer. [99mTc]-Sestamibi has rapid first-pass extraction and retention in the heart, a tissue with high mitochondrial content and negative membrane potential, but lacking Pgp. Opposing passive influx is the action of active transporters such as Pgp [32]. For example, baculo-viral expression of recombinant human MDR1 in insect cells confers decreased accumulation of [99mTc]-Sestamibi [51], and MDR cells expressing Pgp accumulate decreased [99mTc]-Sestamibi [36]. Overall, when Pgp is present in a tissue, net cellular accumulation of the tracer is decreased in proportion to the level of Pgp expression.

[99mTc]-Sestamibi also is recognized to a lesser degree as a transport substrate for the multi-drug resistance-associated protein (MRP1) [52–54], a close homolog of Pgp [55]. On the one hand, cross-reactivity with MRP1 may reduce the specificity of the tracer for functional imaging of Pgp in tumors, but alternatively, this property may enable [99mTc]-Sestamibi to be a more general probe of transporter-mediated multi-drug resistance in some cancers. These low MRP1-mediated signals, however, appear to be lost in the background when imaging patients in vivo (see below).

Several entirely different classes of technetium complexes also have been identified as Pgp transport substrates. Using a planar Schiff-base moiety and hydrophobic phosphines, nonreducible Tc(III) monocationic compounds known as Q-complexes were developed over a decade ago for applications in myocardial perfusion imaging [56,57]. The lead complex for clinical development was [99mTc]-Furifosmin [58], while various novel [99mTc]-Q-complexes with subtle structural differences have been evaluated for features conferring enhanced Pgp-mediated transport properties [40,59]. Of these, [99mTc]-Q58 and [99mTc]-Q63 were nearly identical to [99mTc]-Sestamibi in their Pgp recognition properties in cellulo [40,59].

In addition, a Tc(V) complex known as [99mTc]-Tetrofosmin [60] has been identified as another [99mTc]-complex with highly favorable Pgp-mediated transport properties [59,61]. Although these metal complexes do not share any obvious structural homology, they do share the common features of a delocalized cationic charge and modest hydrophobicity, and all are handled by cancer cells similar to [99mTc]-Sestamibi (see **Fig. 1**). Overall, these [99mTc]-complexes may be clinically useful in evaluating the Pgp status of tumors by SPECT imaging, and they remain under intense investigation.

Another class of technetium-based radiopharmaceuticals has emerged on the basis of pioneering work done on the development of an air- and water-stable organometallic aqua complex $[^{99m}Tc(OH_2)_3(CO)_3]^+$ [62]. Because it was shown that the coordinated water molecules were labile, it became possible to replace water with other ligands, thereby generating complexes with heterogeneous ligands. Based upon these observations, these water molecules were substituted with methoxy-isobutylisonitrile ligands to generate a novel Pgp-targeted radiopharmaceutical known as [99mTc]-CO-MIBI [63]. The radiotracer demonstrated 60-fold higher accumulation in control cells compared with Pgp-expressing cells [28]. In

Pgp-expressing cells, tracer enhancement (multidrug resistance reversal) was observed with the potent modulator LY335979.

Organic scaffolds capable of coordinating other metals also have been explored. Multi-dentate ligands containing an N_4O_2 donor core have the ability to form stable monomeric, monocationic, hydrophobic complexes with various metals [64–68]. Specifically, gallium (Ga) complexes previously were reported as radiopharmaceuticals with potential utility as myocardial perfusion imaging agents [69,70]. These complexes, exemplified by ^{67}Ga-ENBPI, later were shown to demonstrate pharmacological profiles consistent with their potential utility as SPECT probes of Pgp activity [71–75]. Accumulation of ^{67}Ga-ENBPI complexes in cancer cells was inversely proportional to Pgp expression. Furthermore, low uptake levels in MDR cells were reversed to that of control cells in the presence of potent multi-drug resistance inhibitors, further demonstrating Pgp-mediated transport of the complex [29,73–75].

Positron emission tomography agents for molecular imaging of P-glycoprotein transport activity

Positron emission tomography (PET) radiopharmaceuticals may offer enhanced spatial resolution and quantification capabilities compared with SPECT agents. To probe Pgp transport activity, PET-based radiopharmaceuticals have been investigated on three fronts:

- **Use of SPECT scaffolds capable of accommodating PET radionuclides**
- **Employing bioinorganic radiochemistry to develop PET-specific metal-complexes**
- **Conventional PET strategies of organic radiochemistry (Fig. 3)**

Regarding use of scaffolds that coordinate both SPECT and PET radionuclides, two validated examples make use of the PET radionuclides [94m]Tc and [68]Ga. To this end, the radiosynthesis and biochemical validation of [94m]Tc-Sestamibi and ^{68}Ga-ENBPI complexes have been reported [73,75,76]. As expected chemically, the highly favorable Pgp-targeting properties of these complexes were retained upon transformation from SPECT-based to PET-based imaging agents. Thus, these nonmetabolized PET radiopharmaceuticals offer alternative probes with enhanced quantitative capacity for molecular imaging of Pgp activity in tissues in vivo. Indeed, the high steady-state nontarget/target cellular accumulation ratios of the ^{68}Ga-ENBPI complexes [75] exceeded [94m]Tc-Sestamibi [76–78] and thus demonstrate the potential superior sensitivity of ^{68}Ga-ENBPI in detecting the outward transport

activity of Pgp by PET. Furthermore, in considering alternative radiolabels apart from conventional cyclotron-produced PET isotopes, generator-produced ^{68}Ga complexes may offer practical radiopharmacy and on-site distribution advantages, a property being exploited at many European sites.

On another front, organic scaffolds capable of accommodating PET radionuclides that generate novel metallo-radiopharmaceuticals through short synthetic routes have been reported. Thus, based upon rigorous prior contributions [79,80], a stable, monocationic complex of copper(II) was reported as a potential ^{64}Cu PET radiopharmaceutical targeting Pgp [81]. Cellular accumulation studies demonstrated significantly more accumulation of the radiolabeled compound in drug-sensitive MES-SA compared with Pgp-expressing MES-SA/DX5 human uterine sarcoma cells in vitro. Addition of the MDR reversal agent cyclosporin A completely reversed the accumulation profile in MES-SA/DX5 cells, rendering uptake comparable to control cells.

Bidentate tertiary phosphine ligands have the ability to generate stable copper(I) complexes through a one-step synthesis in quantitative yields [82,83] and represent another class of potential ^{64}Cu PET radiopharmaceuticals targeting Pgp. These complexes previously demonstrated potent antitumor properties compared with their free ligands alone [84,85]. These potential PET radiopharmaceuticals show evidence of Pgp targeting properties [86,87]. Although several leads exist for a ^{64}Cu-based radiopharmaceutical for interrogation of Pgp by PET, these radiopharmaceuticals show only modest Pgp-targeting properties compared with [94m]Tc-Sestamibi or ^{68}Ga-ENBPI.

A third focus has been directed toward incorporation of conventional PET radionuclides ^{11}C or ^{18}F into existing substrates or inhibitors known to interact with Pgp [88–90]. Employing this strategy, various PET-labeled agents such as ^{11}C-colchicine, ^{11}C-verapamil, ^{11}C-daunomycin, and ^{11}C/^{18}F-paclitaxel have been reported [90–99]. Recently, the dopamine D_3 receptor antagonist ^{11}C-GR218231 also was identified as a PET tracer for P-glycoprotein [100]. Although promising data have been generated, some of these PET agents suffer from modest radiochemical yields and others from complex pharmacokinetics in vivo mediated, at least in part, by rapid metabolism of the radiolabeled compounds.

Clinical studies: multi-drug resistance in cancer

Originally developed for myocardial perfusion imaging, the clinically approved single photon agents ^{99m}Tc-Sestamibi and ^{99m}Tc-Tetrofosmin have been

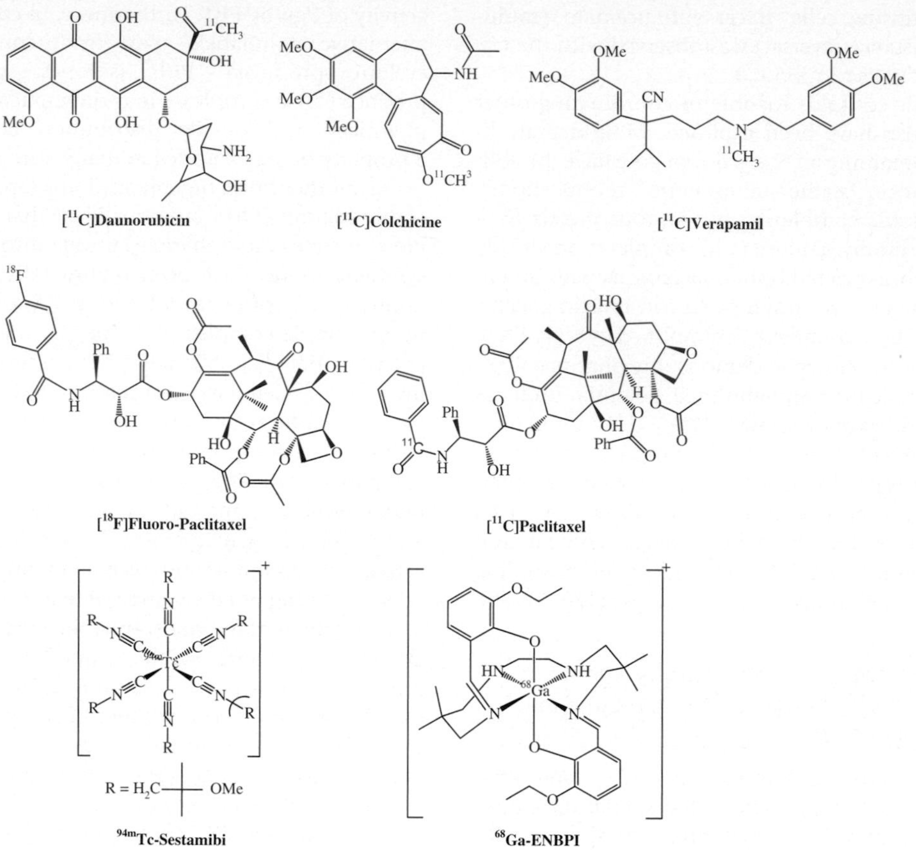

Fig. 3. Structures of selected PET radiopharmaceuticals characterized as transport substrates for Pgp.

tested off-label in patients and shown in many clinical studies to be robust substrates of Pgp. Probing Pgp transport function in vivo may guide chemotherapeutic choices, drug regimens, and gene therapy strategies before treatment. These clinical studies have documented the feasibility of interrogating Pgp transport activity in vivo with imaging cameras commonly available in nuclear medicine facilities [42–44,101–106]. In general, ^{99m}Tc-Sestamibi pharmacokinetic data are extracted from tumor images over time and correlated with immunohistochemical assessment of Pgp expression in the tumor specimen. For example, in a pioneering clinical study, Del Vecchio and colleagues determined rates of efflux of ^{99m}Tc-Sestamibi in 30 patients with untreated breast cancer [101]. Dynamic imaging of the primary tumor was performed for 4 hours following injection of ^{99m}Tc-Sestamibi, and tumor specimens were obtained for quantitative autoradiography of Pgp. Rates of efflux of ^{99m}Tc-Sestamibi were 2.7-fold greater in tumors overexpressing Pgp compared with tumors that expressed Pgp at a level comparable to benign breast lesions. Estimates of sensitivity and specificity for in vivo detection of Pgp using ^{99m}Tc-Sestamibi were 80% and 95%,

respectively. From these data, the authors concluded that efflux rate constants of ^{99m}Tc-Sestamibi may be used for noninvasive identification of Pgp in breast cancer [101].

Clinical studies have examined the relationship between tumor retention of ^{99m}Tc-complexes and multi-drug resistance in various tumor types [48,105–115]. The agents have been shown to detect transport activity of Pgp in normal human tissues, human tumors, and in patients treated with multi-drug resistance modulators, and indeed, may predict chemotherapeutic failure in breast cancer, lung cancer, lymphoma, multiple myeloma, and osteosarcoma.

For example, the prospective value of high-tumor clearance rates of ^{99m}Tc-Sestamibi to predict poor therapeutic outcomes has been evaluated in locally advanced breast cancer. In a study by Ciarmiello and colleagues [106], 39 patients with stage III disease were enrolled in a prospective clinical trial to receive pretreatment mammoscintigraphy with ^{99m}Tc-Sestamibi before neoadjuvant chemotherapy. Breast tumor clearance of ^{99m}Tc-Sestamibi was determined out to 4 hours after injection, and washout half-times were calculated from the image sets using monoexponential curve fitting. Patients subsequently were treated with standard chemotherapy (epirubicin) for 6 weeks and then underwent surgery within 3 weeks of completion of chemotherapy. Tumor burden was assessed by pathologic examination of the mastectomy specimens. Of the 39 patients, 17 showed a tumor clearance half time of less than 204 min, a value previously shown by this group to correspond to the mean tracer clearance rate minus 1 standard deviation in tumors with high Pgp content. Of these rapidly effluxing tumors, 15 of 17 showed a highly cellular residual tumor, indicating a lack of response to neoadjuvant chemotherapy. Conversely, 22 patients showed prolonged tumor clearance (half time of greater than 204 minutes) and of these, only eight showed highly cellular residual tumor at the time of surgery. As pointed out by the investigators, the fact that slow clearance rates were not necessarily predictive of a good response is consistent with the observation that mechanisms of drug resistance other than Pgp are relevant in breast cancer patients. No patient with a half time of less than 164 minutes, which was approximately two standard deviations faster the mean half time of high Pgp-expressing breast tumors [101], showed evidence of pathologic response to neoadjuvant chemotherapy. Thus, pretreatment scintigraphy of advanced breast tumor was highly predictive of subsequent response to neoadjuvant chemotherapy. Especially noteworthy was the ability of dynamic mammoscintigraphy to identify patients with very rapid clearance rates who failed chemotherapy.

Similar data also were reported by Kostakoglu and colleagues in a prospective study of 48 patients with either breast (30 patients) or lung (18 patients) cancer at the time of presentation (37 patients) or after therapy (11 patients) [104]. Scintigraphy was done with whole-body planar images and SPECT beginning 30 minutes after injection of 20 mCi of ^{99m}Tc-Sestamibi. Tumor-to-background ratios of radioactivity from regions of interest were correlated with immunohistochemistry of specimens obtained 3 to 5 days after imaging. Overall, tumor-to-background ratios of ^{99m}Tc-Sestamibi were correlated inversely with expression of Pgp. The authors also noted that strong, but focal expression of Pgp in a specimen did not alter ratios for uptake of ^{99m}Tc-Sestamibi.

Early uptake levels, delayed uptake levels, and washout rates of ^{99m}Tc-Sestamibi also have been obtained for correlation with Pgp, MRP1, and LRP protein levels determined by immunohistochemistry and mRNA levels determined by real-time reverse-transcription polymerase chain reaction [113]. These investigators found that increased levels of Pgp expression correlated with a low

accumulation of ^{99m}Tc-Sestamibi on delayed scans and a high washout rate of ^{99m}Tc-Sestamibi. Interestingly, neither MRP1 nor LRP expression on the level of either protein or mRNA correlated significantly with tumor accumulation or efflux of ^{99m}Tc-Sestamibi in lung cancer. Thus, although ^{99m}Tc-Sestamibi has been shown to modestly cross-react with MRP1 using cells in culture under ideal laboratory conditions [53,77], this lower level of MRP1 transport activity cannot be detected in patients in vivo, unlike Pgp. It would appear that the modest MRP1-dependent cross-reactivity observed with studies in cells is lost in the background in living patients. As a practical consequence, when used in patients, ^{99m}Tc-Sestamibi may be specific for detection of Pgp transport activity in vivo.

In general, analysis of washout rates by comparing early (less than 30 min) and delayed (180 to 240 min) SPECT and planar images have shown a strong correlation between tumor washout rates and levels of Pgp expression. The relation between therapeutic response and tumor retention of tracer also was analyzed in some studies and showed that most tumors with high tracer retention exhibited a favorable response to chemotherapy, whereas most tumors with low tracer retention did not respond to chemotherapy. Investigators have concluded that the clinical agents ^{99m}Tc-Sestamibi and ^{99m}Tc-Tetrofosmin are useful tools in vivo for predicting multidrug resistance in various cancers.

Furthermore, clinical blockade of Pgp-mediated extrusion of ^{99m}Tc-Sestamibi from tissues and tumors in patients has been imaged following treatment with highly selective and potent Pgp modulators such as PSC 833 (valspodar), VX-710 (biricodar), and XR-9576 (tariquidar) [2,42,43,46,48]. A two-step protocol for imaging multi-drug resistance reversal in patients is being evaluated. This protocol may provide a noninvasive method to determine the effectiveness of multi-drug resistance modulation. After baseline imaging, a potent modulating agent is administered, and the tracer is reinjected. Those tissues or tumors showing higher accumulation of the tracer or reduced washout rates would indicate specific blockade of MDR1 Pgp. Thus, these radiopharmaceuticals enable noninvasive mapping of specific transport processes in vivo and provide a basis for further exploration of targeted molecular imaging of Pgp in cancer and gene therapy.

Future clinical studies: analysis of P-glycoprotein at the blood–brain barrier

Pgp is expressed in capillary endothelial cells of the brain and forms a major component of the BBB to limit entry of amphipathic compounds into the

CNS [116–120], including various chemotherapeutic agents, small peptides, antibiotics, HIV protease inhibitors, and antidepressant drugs [2,121].

To initially characterize the potential use of ^{99m}Tc-Sestamibi as a marker of BBB transport function and modulation of Pgp in vivo, the biodistribution of ^{99m}Tc-Sestamibi in blood and brain tissue of wild-type FVB mice following intravenous injection of the tracer and the Pgp modulator GF120918 was reported [122]. Penetration of ^{99m}Tc-Sestamibi into brain tissue of vehicle-treated wild-type FVB mice was limited, demonstrating exclusion of the tracer relative to blood. By comparison, in mice treated with the modulator GF120918, the area-under-the-curve showed two-fold enhancement of brain uptake compared with vehicle-treated mice. These data provided evidence that ^{99m}Tc-Sestamibi can detect Pgp-mediated transport at the BBB.

Although mice have two isoforms of Pgp which confer multidrug resistance, only mdr1a is expressed in endothelial cells of capillaries at the BBB [118]. Thus, mdr1a (−/−) mice are thought to have no drug-transporting Pgp at the BBB, while doubly disrupted mdr1a/1b (−/−) mice offer a more general model to evaluate the utility of imaging agents as probes of Pgp transporter-mediated activity in vivo. To directly demonstrate that drug-transporting Pgp at the BBB excludes ^{99m}Tc-Sestamibi from brain, initial uptake and retention of the tracer were analyzed in untreated mdr1a (−/−) mice compared with wild-type FVB and mdr1a/1b (−/−) double knockout mice [78]. Relative to wild-type mice, mdr1a (−/−) mice showed approximately 3.5-fold more ^{99m}Tc-Sestamibi in brain parenchyma 5 min after injection of the tracer and an enhanced area-under-the-curve [78]. In mdr1a/1b (−/−) double knockout mice, the area-under-the-curve of ^{99m}Tc-Sestamibi in brain was 4.5-fold that

of wild-type mice (Fig. 4), but not significantly different from mdr1a (−/−) single knockout mice. By contrast, blood retention values of ^{99m}Tc-Sestamibi in mdr1a (−/−) and mdr1a/1b (−/−) mice were comparable to FVB control mice. Because blood flow to the brain does not differ between wild-type and mdr1a (−/−) mice [123], the observed enhancement in penetration and retention of ^{99m}Tc-Sestamibi in brains of mdr1a (−/−) and mdr1a/1b (−/−) mice compared with wild type could not be attributed to differences in cerebral perfusion. These data further support the hypothesis that ^{99m}Tc-Sestamibi is a substrate for drug-transporting Pgp isoforms in vivo and can be used as a marker of function and inhibition of these proteins at the BBB in vivo [78]. In addition, biodistribution analysis following tail vein injection of ^{99m}Tc-Tetrofosmin and ^{99m}Tc-CO-MIBI also show enhanced brain uptake and retention in mdr1a/1b(−/−) gene deleted mice versus wild-type mice, directly demonstrating that both ^{99m}Tc-Tetrofosmin and ^{99m}Tc-CO-MIBI are functional probes of Pgp transport activity at the BBB in vivo [28,77].

As expected, PET imaging agents exemplified by ^{11}C-verapamil [94,124] and ^{18}F-paclitaxel [98,99] also have shown potential for noninvasive imaging of Pgp-mediated drug transport at the BBB [125,126]. Although ^{11}C-verapamil demonstrated 10-fold enhanced activity in the brain of knockout mice compared with wild-type, the agent did not show any significant differences of activity in other Pgp-rich tissues, including the liver [124]. Another PET agent [18]F- paclitaxel, also displayed pharmacokinetic profiles consistent with Pgp-mediated transport at the BBB. Enhanced accumulation in the brains of knockout mice compared with wild-type mice was reported [98].

The Ga-complex ^{67}Ga-ENBPI also has shown potential to image Pgp activity at the BBB. ^{67}Ga-ENBPI

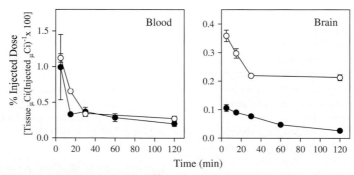

Fig. 4. Blood *(A)* and brain *(B)* pharmacokinetics of ^{99m}Tc-Sestamibi in wild-type (black circles) and mdr1a/1b (−/−) double knockout mice (open circles). Data are expressed as percent of injected dose of radioactivity per organ at each respective time point; bars represent ± SEM when larger than the symbol. (*Modified from* Slapak C, Dahlheimer J, Piwnica-Worms D. Reversal of multidrug resistance with LY335979: functional analysis of P–glycoprotein-mediated transport/activity and its modulation in vivo. J Clin Pharmacol 2001;41:29S–38S.)

displayed a large increase in brain uptake in knock-out mice compared with wild-type mice [75], three- to fivefold greater than ^{99m}Tc-Sestamibi [78] and ^{99m}Tc-Tetrofosmin [77], further documenting the high potential of ^{67}Ga-ENBPI for imaging Pgp activity in vivo.

To further demonstrate the potential utility of the gallium complex as a PET radiotracer in vivo, ^{68}Ga-ENBPI was injected through the tail vein into wild-type and mdr1a/1b(−/−) double knockout mice. Representative micro-PET images of brain tracer uptake at 5 min after injection are shown in Fig. 5. Increased penetration and retention of the PET radiotracer were apparent in the brain of knockout mice compared with wild-type consistent with expectations for imaging Pgp activity at the BBB.

Future clinical studies: analysis of P-glycoprotein in Alzheimer's disease

Recent estimates indicate that approximately 4 million Americans suffer from AD, a progressive neurodegenerative disorder [127]. The AD brain is associated with loss of neurons in regions of the brain responsible for learning and memory. AD

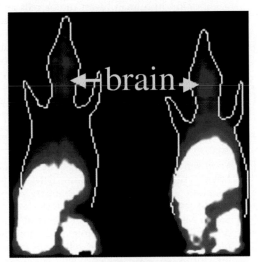

Fig. 5. MicroPET image of ^{68}Ga-ENBPI in brains of wild-type and mdr1a/1b (−/−) double knockout mice. Following injection of mice with an intravenous bolus of the radiopharmaceutical, images of the abdomen, thorax, and head were obtained with a microPET scanner. Representative coronal images of wild-type *(left)* and mdr1a/1b (−/−) *(right)* mice obtained 5 min after injection are shown. A body outline is included for orientation. (*Modified from* Sharma V, Prior J, Belinsky M, et al. Characterization of a gallium-67/gallium-68 radiopharmaceutical for SPECT and PET imaging of MDR1 P-glycoprotein transport activity in vivo: validation in multi-drug resistant tumors and at the blood–brain barrier. J Nucl Med 2005;46:354–64; with permission.)

involves the appearance of two distinct abnormal proteinaceous deposits: extracellular amyloid plaques, which are characteristic of AD, and intracellular neurofibrillary tangles that also are found in other neurodegenerative disorders [128–130]. AD amyloid plaques are comprised primarily of a family of proteins known collectively as Aβ proteins [131], derived from the ubiquitously expressed cell surface amyloid precursor protein (APP). Indeed, several lines of investigation suggest Aβ accumulation is an initiating event in the pathogenic cascade of AD [132–134]. Conversion of Aβ within the extracellular spaces of the brain into toxic forms is accelerated at higher concentrations, implying that pathways influencing Aβ production or elimination could modulate disease progression. Aβ is secreted from neurons into brain interstitial fluid, where it is eliminated by proteolytic degradation [135,136], passive bulk flow [137], and active transport across the BBB [138,139]. The latter, representing efflux across the BBB into the peripheral circulation, appears to be a substantial pathway for elimination of CNS-derived Aβ [139]. Recent studies demonstrated that low-density lipoprotein receptor-related protein (LRP1) is a major Aβ efflux transporter at the BBB [140], but other Aβ transporters have been suspected [141,142]. Region-specific levels of Aβ deposition in postmortem AD brains are correlated inversely to the local level of Pgp in brain capillaries as assessed by immunohistochemistry [143]. Using mdr1a/1b(−/−) double knockout mice, Aβ removal from the brain was reported to be mediated at least partially by Pgp activity at the BBB [26]. The study shows that acute inhibition of Pgp activity using a selective Pgp modulator increases Aβ levels in brain interstitial fluid within hours of treatment. Importantly, mdr1a/1b(−/−) double knockout mice show enhanced Aβ plaque formation in a mouse model of AD [26]. These data strongly suggest that Pgp normally transports Aβ out of the brain and that perturbation of Aβ efflux directly affects Aβ accumulation within the brain. Thus, there appears to be a direct link between Pgp and Aβ metabolism in vivo such that Pgp activity at the BBB could impact risk for developing AD and serve as a novel diagnostic imaging target.

Although deletion of Pgp has not been reported in people, several mechanisms for modulation of Pgp activity at the BBB could influence AD. For example, single nucleotide polymorphisms, such as the exon 26 3435T allele, have been described that decrease Pgp expression and result in functional differences in oral absorption and disposition of drugs [144]. Similar polymorphisms in Pgp could decrease Aβ transport out of the brain, thereby increasing the probability of plaque formation. In addition, many commonly used drugs and natural product medicinals alter Pgp function. For example, dexamethasone, morphine, rifampin, and St. John's Wort are reported to enhance Pgp activity, while verapamil, cyclosporine A, erythromycin, progesterone, HIV protease inhibitors, and several statins inhibit Pgp activity [2,121]. Typically, these medicinals only show modest impact on Pgp activity in short-term assays at clinically relevant concentrations, but with chronic use or in combination, these drugs may have a greater effect on Pgp function, and, consequently, on brain Aβ levels. Thus, it may be possible in the future to assess Pgp transport activity at the BBB using ^{99m}Tc-Sestamibi and related radiopharmaceuticals. Enhanced brain uptake would indicate a genetic or pharmacologically induced defect in Pgp transport activity, which may place these patients at higher risk for developing AD.

Summary

Several radiopharmaceuticals enable SPECT and PET monitoring of Pgp-mediated transport activity in tissues in vivo. There is significant promise for noninvasive assessment of Pgp to guide choices of chemotherapy regimens, monitor MDR gene therapy, and assess a potential risk factor for development of AD at the level of the BBB.

Acknowledgments

The authors thank colleagues past and present of the Molecular Imaging Center for insightful discussions.

References

[1] Endicott JA, Ling V. The biochemistry of P-glycoprotein-mediated multidrug resistance. Annu Rev Biochem 1989;58:137–71.

[2] Gottesman M, Fojo T, Bates S. Multi-drug resistance in cancer: role of ATP-dependent transporters. Nat Rev Cancer 2002;2:48–58.

[3] Clarke R, Leonessa F, Trock B. Multidrug resistance/P-glycoprotein and breast cancer: review and meta-analysis. Semin Oncol 2005;32(Suppl 7):S9–15.

[4] Juliano RL, Ling V. A surface glycoprotein modulating drug permeability in Chinese hamster ovary cell mutants. Biochim Biophys Acta 1976;455:152–62.

[5] Ambudkar S, Dey S, Hrycyna C, et al. Biochemical, cellular, and pharmacological aspects of the multidrug transporter. Annu Rev Pharmacol Toxicol 1999;39:361–98.

[6] Borst P, Evers R, Kool M, et al. A family of drug transporters: the multi-drug resistance-associated proteins. J Natl Cancer Inst 2000;92(16):1295–302.

[7] Kruh G, Belinsky M. The MRP family of drug efflux pumps. Oncogene 2003;22:7537–52.

[8] Miyake K, Mickley L, Litman T, et al. Molecular cloning of cDNAs which are highly overexpressed in mitoxantrone-resistant cells: demonstration of homology to ABC transport genes. Cancer Res 1999;59:8–13.

[9] Sarkadi B, Ozvegy-Laczka C, Nemet K, et al. ABCG2—a transporter for all seasons. FEBS Lett 2004;567:116–20.

[10] Doyle LA, Ross DD. Multidrug resistance mediated by the breast cancer resistance protein BCRP (ABCG2). Oncogene 2003;22(47):7340–58.

[11] Higgins CF, Gottesman MM. Is the multi-drug transporter a flippase? Trends Biochem Sci 1992;17:18–21.

[12] Hoffman M, Wei L, Roepe P. Are altered pHi and membrane potential in hu MDR 1 transfectants sufficient to cause MDR protein-mediated multidrug resistance? J Gen Physiol 1996;108:295–313.

[13] Hoffman M, Roepe P. Analysis of ion transport perturbations caused by huMDR1 protein overexpression. Biochemistry 1997;36:11153–68.

[14] Luker GD, Flagg TP, Sha Q, et al. MDR1 P-glycoprotein reduces influx of substrates without affecting membrane potential. J Biol Chem 2001;276(52):49053–60.

[15] Altan N, Chen Y, Schindler M, et al. Defective acidification in human breast tumor cells and implications for chemotherapy. J Exp Med 1998;187:1583–98.

[16] Hurwitz S, Terashima M, Mizunuma N, et al. Vesicular anthracycline accumulation in doxorubicin-selected U-937 cells: participation of lysosomes. Blood 1997;89:3745–54.

[17] Stein WD, Cardarelli C, Pastan I, et al. Kinetic evidence suggesting that the multi-drug transporter differentially handles influx and efflux of its substrates. Mol Pharmacol 1994;45:763–72.

[18] Robinson L, Roberts W, Ling T, et al. Human MDR1 protein overexpression delays the apoptotic cascade in Chinese hamster ovary fibroblasts. Biochemistry 1997;36:11169–78.

[19] Smyth MJ, Krasovskis E, Sutton VR, et al. The drug efflux protein P-glycoprotein additionally protects drug-resistant tumor cells from multiple forms of caspase-dependent apoptosis. Proc Natl Acad Sci U S A 1998;95:7024–9.

[20] Abonour R, Croop J, Cornetta K. Multi-drug resistance gene therapy in hematopoietic cell transplantation. 2nd edition. San Diego (CA): Academic Press; 2002.

[21] Cordon-Cardo C, O'Brien JP, Boccia J, et al. Expression of the multi-drug resistance gene product (P-glycoprotein) in human normal and tumor tissues. J Histochem Cytochem 1990;38(9):1277–87.

[22] Rao V, Dahlheimer J, Bardgett M, et al. Choroid plexus epithelial expression of MDR1 P-glycoprotein and multi-drug resistance-associated protein contribute to the blood–cerebrospinal

fluid drug–permeability barrier. Proc Natl Acad Sci U S A 1999;96:3900–5.

[23] van Asperen J, van Tellingen O, van der Valk M, et al. Enhanced oral absorption and decreased elimination of paclitaxel in mice cotreated with cyclosporin A. Clin Cancer Res 1998;4: 2293–7.

[24] Kim RB, Fromm MF, Wandel C, et al. The drug transporter P-glycoprotein limits oral adsorption and brain entry of HIV-1 protease inhibitors. J Clin Invest 1998;101:289–94.

[25] van der Sandt I, Vos C, Nabulsi L, et al. Assessment of active transport of HIV protease inhibitors in various cell lines and the in vitro blood-brain barrier. AIDS 2001;15:483–91.

[26] Cirrito JR, Deane R, Fagan AM, et al. P-glycoprotein deficiency at the blood-brain barrier increases amyloid-beta deposition in an Alzheimer's disease mouse model. J Clin Invest 2005;115:3285–90.

[27] Sharma V, Piwnica-Worms D. Metal complexes for therapy and diagnosis of drug resistance. Chem Rev 1999;99:2545–60.

[28] Dyszlewski M, Blake H, Dahlheimer J, et al. Characterization of a novel Tc-99m-carbonyl complex as a functional probe of MDR1 P-glycoprotein transport activity. Mol Imaging 2002;1:24–35.

[29] Sharma V. Radiopharmaceuticals for assessment of multidrug resistance P-glycoprotein-mediated drug transport activity. Bioconjugate Chem 2004;15:1464–74.

[30] Abrams MA, Davison A, Jones AG, et al. Synthesis and characterization hexakis(alkyl isocyanide) and hexakis(arylisocyanide) complexes of technetium(I). Inorg Chem 1983;22: 2798–800.

[31] Wackers FJ, Berman D, Maddahi J, et al. Tc-99m-hexakis 2-methoxy isobutylisonitrile: human biodistribution, dosimetry, safety and preliminary comparison to thallium-201 for myocardial perfusion imaging. J Nucl Med 1989;30:301–9.

[32] Piwnica-Worms D, Chiu M, Budding M, et al. Functional imaging of multidrug-resistant P-glycoprotein with an organotechnetium complex. Cancer Res 1993;53:977–84.

[33] Kronauge JF, Davison A, Roseberry AM, et al. Synthesis and identification of monocation Tc(CPI)$_6$ $^+$ in Tc(CNC(CH$_3$)$_2$COOCH$_3$)$_6$Cl and its hydrolysis products. Inorg Chem 1991;30: 4265–71.

[34] Piwnica-Worms D, Kronauge J, Chiu M. Uptake and retention of hexakis (2-methoxy isobutyl isonitrile) technetium(I) in cultured chick myocardial cells: mitochondrial and plasma membrane potential dependence. Circulation 1990; 82:1826–38.

[35] Backus M, Piwnica-Worms D, Hockett D, et al. Microprobe analysis of Tc-MIBI in heart cells: calculation of mitochondrial potential. Am J Physiol Cell Physiol 1993;265:C178–87.

[36] Piwnica-Worms D, Rao V, Kronauge J, et al. Characterization of multidrug-resistance P-glycoprotein transport function with an organotechnetium cation. Biochemistry 1995;34: 12210–20.

[37] Ballinger J, Hua H, Berry B, et al. ^{99m}Tc-Sestamibi as an agent for imaging P-glycoprotein-mediated multi-drug resistance: in vitro and in vivo studies in a rat breast tumour cell line and its doxorubicin-resistant variant. Nucl Med Commun 1995;16:253–7.

[38] Ballinger JR, Sheldon KM, Boxen I, et al. Differences between accumulation of Tc-99m-MIBI and Tl-201-thallous chloride in tumor cells: Role of P-glycoprotein. Q J Nucl Med 1995; 39:122–8.

[39] Cordobes M, Starzec A, Delmon-Moingeon L, et al. Technetium-99m-Sestamibi uptake by human benign and malignant breast tumor cells: correlation with *mdr* gene expression. J Nucl Med 1996;37:286–9.

[40] Luker G, Rao V, Crankshaw C, et al. Characterization of phosphine complexes of technetium (III) as transport substrates of the multidrug resistance (MDR1) P-glycoprotein and functional markers of P-glycoprotein at the blood-brain barrier. Biochemistry 1997; 36:14218–27.

[41] Bosch I, Crankshaw C, Piwnica-Worms D, et al. Characterization of functional assays of P-glycoprotein transport activity. Leukemia 1997;11: 1131–7.

[42] Luker GD, Fracasso PM, Dobkin J, et al. Modulation of the multidrug resistance P-glycoprotein: detection with Tc-99m-Sestamibi in vivo. J Nucl Med 1997;38:369–72.

[43] Chen C, Meadows B, Regis J, et al. Detection of in vivo P-glycoprotein inhibition by PSC 833 using Tc-99m-Sestamibi. Clin Cancer Res 1997; 3:545–52.

[44] Barbarics E, Kronauge J, Cohen D, et al. Characterization of P-glycoprotein transport and inhibition in vivo. Cancer Res 1998;58:276–82.

[45] Luker G, Nilsson K, Covey D, et al. MDR1 P-glycoprotein enhances esterification of plasma membrane cholesterol. J Biol Chem 1999;274: 6979–91.

[46] Peck R, Hewett J, Harding M, et al. Phase I and pharmacokinetic study of the novel MDR1 and MRP1 inhibitor biricodar administered alone and in combination with doxorubicin. J Clin Oncol 2001;19:3130–41.

[47] Pichler A, Prior J, Piwnica-Worms D. Imaging reversal of multidrug resistance in living mice with bioluminescence: MDR1 P-glycoprotein transports coelenterazine. Proc Natl Acad Sci U S A 2004;101:1702–7.

[48] Agrawal M, Abraham J, Balis F, et al. Increased Tc-99m-Sestamibi accumulation in normal liver and drug-resistant tumors after the administration of the glycoprotein inhibitor, XR9576. Clin Cancer Res 2003;9:650–6.

[49] Chernoff DM, Strichartz GR, Piwnica-Worms D. Membrane potential determination in large unilamellar vesicles with hexakis(2-methoxyisobutyl isonitrile) technetium(I). Biochim Biophys Acta 1993;1147:262–6.

[50] Piwnica-Worms D, Kronuage JF, LeFurgey A, et al. Mitochondrial localization and characterization of 99-Tc-SESTAMIBI in heart cells by electron probe X-ray microanalysis and 99-Tc-NMR spectroscopy. Magn Reson Imaging 1994;12:641–52.

[51] Rao VV, Chiu ML, Kronauge JF, et al. Expression of recombinant human multidrug resistance P-glycoprotein in insect cells confers decreased accumulation of technetium-99m-SESTAMIBI. J Nucl Med 1994;35:510–5.

[52] Crankshaw C, Piwnica-Worms D. Tc-99-Sestamibi may be a transport substrate of the human multidrug resistance-associated protein (MRP). J Nucl Med 1996;37:247P.

[53] Hendrikse N, Franssen E, van der Graaf W, et al. ^{99m}Tc-sestamibi is a substrate for P-glycoprotein and the multidrug resistance-associated protein. Br J Cancer 1998;77:353–8.

[54] Moretti J-L, Cordobes M, Starzec A, et al. Involvement of glutathione in loss of technetium-99m-MIBI accumulation related to membrane MDR protein expression in tumor cells. J Nucl Med 1998;39:1214–8.

[55] Cole SPC, Bhardwaj G, Gerlach JH, et al. Overexpression of a transporter gene in a multidrug-resistant human lung cancer cell line. Science 1992;258:1650–4.

[56] Jurisson S, Berning D, Jia W, Ma DS. Coordination compounds in nuclear medicine. Chem Rev 1993;93:1137–56.

[57] Deutsch E, Vanderheyden JL, Gerundini P, et al. Development of nonreducible technetium-99m(III) cations as myocardial perfusion imaging agents: initial experience in humans. J Nucl Med 1987;28:1870–80.

[58] Rossetti C, Vanoli G, Paganelli G, et al. Human biodistribution, dosimetry and clinical use of technetium(III)-99m-Q12. J Nucl Med 1994;35:1571–80.

[59] Crankshaw C, Marmion M, Luker G, et al. Novel Tc(III)-Q-complexes for functional imaging of the multidrug resistance (MDR1) P-glycoprotein. J Nucl Med 1998;39:77–86.

[60] Kelly J, Forster A, Higley B, et al. Technetium-99m-tetrofosmin as a new radiopharmaceutical for myocardial perfusion imaging. J Nucl Med 1993;34:222–7.

[61] Ballinger JR, Bannerman J, Boxen I, et al. Technetium-99m-Tetrofosmin as a substrate for P-glycoprotein: in vitro studies in multidrug-resistant breast tumor cells. J Nucl Med 1996; 37:1578–82.

[62] Alberto R, Schibli R, Egli A, et al. A novel organometallic aqua complex of technetium for the labeling of biomolecules: synthesis of $[^{99m}Tc(OH_2)_3(CO)_3]^+$ from $[^{99m}TcO_4]-$ in aqueous solution and its reaction with a bifunctional ligand. J Am Chem Soc 1998;120: 7987–8.

[63] Marmion M, MacDonald J. Preparation and biodistribution of ^{99m}Tc(I)-tricarbonyl complexes containing isonitrile and phosphine ligands. J Nucl Med 2000;41:40P.

[64] Wong E, Liu S, Lugger T, et al. Hexadentate N_4O_2 amine phenol complexes of gallium and indium. Inorg Chem 1995;34:93–101.

[65] Yang LW, Liu S, Wong E, Rettig SJ, Orvig C. Complexes of trivalent metal ions with potentially heptadentate N_4O_3 Schiff base and amine phenol ligands of variable rigidity. Inorg Chem 1995;34:2164–78.

[66] Sarma BD, Bailar JC. The stereochemistry of metal complexes with polydentate ligands. Part I. J Am Chem Soc 1955;77:5476–80.

[67] Sarma BD, Ray KR, Sievers RE, et al. The stereochemistry of metal chelates with multi-dentate ligands. Part II. J Am Chem Soc 1964;86:14–6.

[68] Tweedle MF, Wilson LJ. Variable spin iron(III) chelates with hexadentate ligands derived from triethylenetetramine and various salicylaldehydes. J Am Chem Soc 1976;98:4824–34.

[69] Tsang B, Mathias C, Green M. A gallium-68 radiopharmaceutical that is retained in myocardium: ^{68}Ga-$[(4,6-MeO)_2sal)_2BAPEN]^+$. J Nucl Med 1993;34:1127–31.

[70] Tsang B, Mathias C, Fanwick P, et al. Structure–distribution relationship for metal-labeled myocardial imaging agents: comparison of a series of cationic gallium(III) complexes with hexadentate bis(salicylaldimine) ligands. J Med Chem 1994;37:4400–6.

[71] Sharma V, Crankshaw C, Piwnica-Worms D. Effects of multi-drug resistance (*MDR1*) P-glycoprotein expression levels and coordination metal on the cytotoxic potency of multi-dentate (N_4O_2) ethylenediamine-bis[propyl(R-benzylimino)]metal(III) cations. J Med Chem 1996; 39:3483–90.

[72] Sharma V, Wey SP, Bass L, et al. Monocationic N_4O_2 Schiff-Base phenolate complexes of gallium(III): novel PET imaging agents of the human multidrug resistance (MDR1) P-glycoprotein. J Nucl Med 1996;37:51P.

[73] Sharma V, Beatty A, Wey SP, et al. Novel gallium(III) complexes transported by MDR1 P-glycoprotein: potential PET imaging agents for probing P-glycoprotein-mediated transport activity in vivo. Chem Biol 2000;7:335–43.

[74] Sharma V, Piwnica-Worms D. Monitoring multidrug resistance P-glycoprotein drug transport activity with single-photon emission computed tomography and positron emission tomography radiopharmaceuticals. Top Curr Chem 2005;252:155–78.

[75] Sharma V, Prior J, Belinsky M, et al. Characterization of a gallium-67/gallium-68 radiopharmaceutical for SPECT and PET imaging of MDR1 P-glycoprotein transport activity in vivo:

validation in multi-drug resistant tumors and at the blood-brain barrier. J Nucl Med 2005; 46:354–64.

[76] Bigott HM, Prior JL, Piwnica-Worms DR, et al. Imaging multidrug resistance P-glycoprotein transport function using micro-PET with technetium-94m-Sestamibi. Mol Imaging 2005;4: 30–9.

[77] Chen W, Luker K, Dahlheimer J, et al. Effects of MDR1 and MDR3 P-glycoproteins, MRP1 and BCRP/MXR/ABCP on transport of Tc-99m-Tetrofosmin. Biochem Pharmacol 2000;60: 413–26.

[78] Slapak C, Dahlheimer J, Piwnica-Worms D. Reversal of multi-drug resistance with LY335979: functional analysis of P-glycoprotein-mediated transport activity and its modulation in vivo. J Clin Pharmacol 2001;41:29S–38S.

[79] Anderson O, Packard A. Structure variations in macrocyclic copper(II) complexes: crystal and molecular structure of cyano(difluoro-3, 3-(trimethylenedinitrilo)bis(2-butanone oximato)-borato)copper II-methanol[Cu(cyclops)CN]. CH₃OH. Inorg Chem 1980;19:2941–5.

[80] Anderson O, Packard A. Structural variations in macrocyclic copper(II) complexes: Crystal and molecular structures of [Cu(cyclops)H₂O] (ClO₄) and [Cu(PreH)H₂O](ClO₄).H₂O. Inorg Chem 1979;18:1940–7.

[81] Packard A, Kronauge J, Barbarics E, et al. Synthesis and biodistibution of a lipophilic ^{64}Cu-labeled monocationic copper(II) complex. Nucl Med Biol 2002;29:289–94.

[82] Lewis J, Zweit J, Dearling J, et al. Copper(I) bis diphosphine complexes as basis for radiopharmaceuticals for positron emission tomography and targeted radiotherapy. Chem Commun 1996; 1093–4.

[83] Blower P. Small coordination compounds as radiopharmaceuticals for cancer targeting. Transition Metal Chemistry 1998;23:109–12.

[84] Camus A, Marsich N, Nardin G. Transition Metal Chemistry 1976;1:205.

[85] Berners-Price S, Johnson R, Mirabelli C, et al. Copper(I) complexes with bidentate tertiary phosphine ligands: solution chemistry and antitumor activity. Inorg Chem 1987;26:3383–7.

[86] Zweit J, Lewis J, Dearling J, et al. Copper-64-diphosphine complexes: potential PET tracers for the assessment of multidrug resistance in tumors [abstract]. J Nucl Med 1997;38:133P.

[87] Lewis J, Dearling J, Sosabowski J, et al. Copper bis(diphosphine)complexes: radiopharmaceuticals for detection of multidrug resistance in tumors by PET. Eur J Nucl Med 2000;27: 638–46.

[88] Mehta BM, Rosa E, Fissekis JD, et al. In-vivo identification of tumor multidrug resistance with tritum-3-colchicine. J Nucl Med 1992;33: 1373–7.

[89] Mehta B, Rosa E, Biedler J, Larson S. In vivo uptake of carbon-14-colchicine for identification of tumor multidrug resistance. J Nucl Med 1994;35:1179–84.

[90] Elsinga PH, Franssen JF, Hendrikse NH, et al. Carbon-11-labeled daunorubicin and verapamil for probing P-glycoprotein in tumors with PET. J Nucl Med 1996;37:1571–5.

[91] Hendrikse N, Franssen E, van der Graaf W, et al. Visualization of multidrug resistance in vivo. Eur J Nucl Med 1999;26:283–93.

[92] Hendrikse N, de Vries EG, Eriks-Fluks L, et al. A new in vivo method to study P-glycoprotein transport in tumors and the blood-brain barrier. Cancer Res 1999;59:2411–6.

[93] Levchenko A, Mehta B, Lee J-B, et al. Evaluation of ^{11}C-colchicine for PET imaging of multiple drug resistance. J Nucl Med 2000;41:493–501.

[94] Luurtsema G, Molthoff C, Windhorst A, et al. (R)- and (S)-[11C] Verapamil as PET-tracers for measuring P-glycoprotein function: in vitro and in vivo evaluation. Nucl Med Biol 2003;30: 747–51.

[95] Hendrikse N, Vaalburg W. Imaging of P-glycoprotein function in vivo with PET. Novartis Found Symp 2002;243:137–45.

[96] Ravert H, Klecker R, Collins J, et al. Radiosynthesis of [C-11]paclitaxel. J Labelled Comp Radiopharm 2002;45(6):471–7.

[97] Kiesewetter D, Eckelman W. Radiochemical synthesis of [18F]fluoropaclitaxel [abstract]. J Labelled Comp Radiopharm 2001;44:S903–5.

[98] Kiesewetter D, Jagoda E, Kao C, et al. Fluoro-, bromo-, and iodopaclitaxel derivatives: synthesis and biological evaluation. Nucl Med Biol 2003;30:11–24.

[99] Kurdziel K, Kiesewetter D, Carson R, et al. Biodistribution, radiation dose estimates, and in vivo Pgp modulation studies of ^{18}F-paclitaxel in nonhuman primates. J Nucl Med 2003;44: 1330–9.

[100] de Vries EFJ, Kortekaas R, van Waarde A, et al. Synthesis and evaluation of dopamine D₃ receptor antagonist ^{11}C GR218231 as PET tracer for P-glycoprotein. J Nucl Med 2005;46:1384–92.

[101] Del Vecchio S, Ciarmiello A, Potena MI, et al. In vivo detection of multidrug resistance (MDR1) phenotype by technetium-99m-sestamibi scan in untreated breast cancer patients. Eur J Nucl Med 1997;24:150–9.

[102] Del Vecchio S, Ciarmiello A, Pace L, et al. Fractional retention of technetium-99m-sestamibi as an index of P-glycoprotein expression in untreated breast cancer patients. J Nucl Med 1997; 38:1348–51.

[103] Bom H, Kim Y, Lim S, et al. Dipyridamole modulated Tc-99m-sestamibi (mibi) scintigraphy: a predictor of response to chemotherapy in patients with small cell lung cancer [abstract]. J Nucl Med 1997;38:240P.

[104] Kostakoglu L, Elahi N, Kirarli P, et al. Clinical validation of the influence of P-glycoprotein on technetium-99m-Sestamibi uptake in malignant tumors. J Nucl Med 1997;38:1003–8.

[105] Kostakoglu L, Kirath P, Ruacan S, et al. Association of tumor washout rates and accumulation of technetium-99m-MIBI with expression of P-glycoprotein in lung cancer. J Nucl Med 1998; 39:228–34.

[106] Ciarmiello A, Del Vecchio S, Silvestro P, et al. Tumor clearance of technetium-99m-Sestamibi as a predictor of response to neoadjuvant chemotherapy for locally advanced breast cancer. J Clin Oncol 1998;16:1677–83.

[107] Fukumoto M, Yoshida D, Hayase N, et al. Scintigraphic prediction of resistance to radiation and chemotherapy in patients with lung carcinoma: technetium 99m-tetrofosmin and thallium-201 dual single photon emission computed tomography study. Cancer 1999;86:1470–9.

[108] Nagamachi S, Jinnouchi S, Ohnishi T, et al. The usefulness of Tc-99m-MIBI for evaluating brain tumors: comparative study with Tl-201 and relation with P-glycoprotein. Clin Nucl Med 1999;24:765–72.

[109] Kao C, Hsieh J, Tsai S, et al. Paclitaxel-based chemotherapy for non-small cell lung cancer: predicting the response with 99mtc-tetrofosmin chest imaging. J Nucl Med 2001;42:17–20.

[110] Shiau Y, Tsai S, Wang J, et al. Technetium-99m tetrofosmin chest imaging related to p-glycoprotein expression for predicting the response with paclitaxel-based chemotherapy for non-small cell lung cancer. Lung Cancer 2001;179: 197–207.

[111] Sciuto R, Pasqualoni R, Bergomi S, et al. Prognostic value of 99mTc-Sestamibi washout in predicting response of locally advanced breast cancer to neoadjuvant chemotherapy. J Nucl Med 2002;43:745–51.

[112] Shih C, Shiau Y, Wang J, et al. Using technetium-99m tetrofosmin chest imaging to predict taxol-based chemotherpy response in non-small cell lung cancer but not related to lung resistance protein expression. Lung 2003;181: 103–11.

[113] Zhou J, Higashi K, Ueda Y, et al. Expression of multidrug resistance protein and messenger RNA correlate with ^{99m}Tc-MIBI imaging in patients with lung cancer. J Nucl Med 2001;42: 1476–83.

[114] Ding H, Huang W, Tsai C, et al. Usefulness of technetium-99m tetrofosmin liver imaging to detect hepatocellular carcinoma and related to expression of P-glycoprotein or multidrug resistance associated protein - a preliminary report. Nucl Med Biol 2003;30:471–5.

[115] Pace L, Catalano L, Del Vecchio S, et al. Washout of [99mTc]Sestamibi in predicting response to chemotherapy in patients with multiple myeloma. Q J Nucl Med Mol Imaging 2005;49: 281–5.

[116] Cordon-Cardo C, OBrien J, Casals D, et al. Multidrug-resistance gene (P-glycoprotein) is expressed by endothelial cells at blood-brain barrier sites. Proc Natl Acad Sci U S A 1989; 86(2):695–8.

[117] Thiebaut F, Tsuruo T, Hamada H, et al. Immunohistochemical localization in normal tissues of different epitopes in the multidrug transport protein P170: evidence for localization in brain capillaries and cross-reactivity of one antibody with a muscle protein. J Histochem Cytochem 1989;37(2):159–64.

[118] Schinkel A, Smit J, van Tellingen O, et al. Disruption of the mouse *mdr1a* P-glycoprotein gene leads to a deficiency in the blood-brain barrier and to increased sensitivity to drugs. Cell 1994;77:491–502.

[119] Schinkel AH. P-glycoprotein, a gatekeeper in the blood-brain barrier. Adv Drug Deliv Rev 1999;36(2–3):179–94.

[120] Demeule M, Regina A, Jodoin J, et al. Drug transport to the brain: key roles for the efflux pump P-glycoprotein in the blood-brain barrier. Vascul Pharmacol 2002;38(6):339–48.

[121] Marzolini C, Paus E, Buclin T, et al. Polymorphisms in human MDR1 (P-glycoprotein): recent advances and clinical relevance. Clin Pharmacol Ther 2004;75:13–33.

[122] Dahlheimer J, Crankshaw C, Marmion M, et al. Modulation of the pharmacokinetics of P-glycoprotein-targeted Tc-99m-complexes by GW0918 (GG918) in wild-type and mdr1a P-glycoprotein knock-out mice. Proc Am Assoc Cancer Res 1997;38:590.

[123] Franssen E, Hendrikse N, Elsinga P, et al. P-glycoprotein monitoring of carbon-11 daunorubicin and verapamil in P-glycoprotein gene knock-out and wild type mice with PET. J Nucl Med 1996;37:355P.

[124] Hendrikse N, Vaalburg W. Dynamics of multidrug resistance P-glycoprotein analyses with positron emission tomography. Methods 2002;27:228–33.

[125] Elsinga P, Hendrikse N, Bart J, et al. PET studies on P-glycoprotein in the blood-brain barrier; how it effects uptake and binding of drugs in the CNS. Curr Pharm Des 2004;10: 1493–503.

[126] Vaalburg W, Hendrikse N, Elsinga P, et al. P-glycoprotein activity and biological response. Toxicol Appl Pharmacol 2005;207(Suppl 2): 257–60.

[127] Schumock G. Economic considerations in the treatment and management of Alzheimer's disease. Am J Health Syst Pharm 1998; 55(Suppl.2):S17–22.

[128] McKhann G, Drachman D, Folstein M, et al. Clinical diagnosis of Alzheimer's disease: a report of the NINCDS-ADRDA work group under the auspices of Department of Health and Human Services Task Force on Alzheimer's Disease. Neurology 1984;34(7):939–44.

[129] Weiner M. Alzheimer's disease: diagnosis and treatment. Harv Rev Psychiatry 1997;4:306–16.

[130] Yanker B. Mechanisms of neuronal degeneration in Alzheimer's disease. Neuron 1996;16: 921–32.

[131] Lansbury PJ. A reductionist view of Alzheimer's disease. Acc Chem Res 1996;29:317–21.

[132] Teller J. Presence of soluble amyloid β-peptide precedes amyloid plaque formation in Down's syndrome. Nat Med 1996;2:93–5.

[133] Games D, Adams D, Alessandrini R, et al. Alzheimer-type neuropathology in transgenic mice overexpressing V717F β-amyloid precursor protein. Nature 1995;373:523–7.

[134] Hsiao K, Chapman P, Nilsen S, et al. Correlative memory deficits, Aß elevation, and amyloid plaques in transgenic mice. Science 1996;274: 99–102.

[135] Farris W, Mansourian S, Chang Y, et al. Insulin-degrading enzyme regulates the levels of insulin, amyloid β, and β-amyloid precursor protein intyracellular domain in vivo. Proc Natl Acad Sci U S A 2003;100:4162–7.

[136] Iwata N, Mizukami H, Shirotani K, et al. Presynaptic localization of neprilysin contributes to efficient clearance of amyloid-beta peptide in mouse brain. J Neurosci 2004;24:991–8.

[137] Weller R, Massey A, Newman T, et al. Cerebral amyloid angiopathy: amyloid beta accumulates in putative interstitial fluid drainage pathways in Alzheimer's disease. Am J Pathol 1998;153: 725–33.

[138] DeMattos R, Bales K, Cummins D, et al. Brain to plasma amyloid-β efflux: a measure of brain amyloid burden in a mouse model of Alzheimer's disease. Science 2002;295:2264–7.

[139] Shibata M, Yamada S, Kumar S, et al. Clearance of Alzheimer's amyloid-ss(1–40) peptide from brain by LDL receptor-related protein-1 at the blood-brain barrier. J Clin Invest 2000;106: 1489–99.

[140] Zlokovic B. Neurovascular mechanisms of Alzheimer's neurodegeneration. Trends Neurosci 2005;28:202–8.

[141] Deane R, Wu Z, Sagare A, et al. LRP/amyloid β peptide interaction mediates differential brain efflux of Aβ isoforms. Neuron 2004;43:333–44.

[142] Zlokovic B, Yamada S, Holtzman D, et al. Clearance of amyloid β peptide from brain: transport or metabolism? Nat Med 2000;6: 718–9.

[143] Vogelgesang S, Cascorbi I, Schroeder R, et al. Deposition of Alzheimer's β amyloid is inversely correlated with P-glycoprotein expression in the brains of elderly non-demented humans. Pharmacogenetics 2002;12:535–41.

[144] Hoffmeyer S, Burk O, von Richter O, et al. Functional polymorphisms of the human multidrug-resistance gene: multiple sequence variations and correlation of one allele with P-glycoprotein expression and activity in vivo. Proc Natl Acad Sci U S A 2000;97:3473–8.

NEUROIMAGING CLINICS OF NORTH AMERICA

Neuroimag Clin N Am 16 (2006) 591–603

Positron Emission Tomography of the Brain

Homer A. Macapinlac, MD

- 2[^{18}F]fluoro-2-deoxy-D-glucose positron emission tomography
- Positron emission tomography image acquisition
- Other positron emission tomography tracers

- DNA precursors
- Tumor hypoxia
- Blood flow
- Amyloid imaging
- Summary
- References

Positron emission tomography (PET) is a technique that allows imaging of the temporal and spatial distribution of positron-emitting radionuclides. The purpose of this article is to outline the current clinical use for PET imaging in the brain and other radiopharmaceuticals used for assessing various physiologic parameters pertaining to tumor metabolism.

Positron emission tomography (PET) is a technique that allows imaging of the temporal and spatial distribution of positron-emitting radionuclides. After the advent of CT imaging in the early 1970s, PET and MR imaging were developed, producing an excellent opportunity to examine neurobiological function. PET has been in existence for nearly 30 years, and much of the initial work with this method focused on analysis of the function of the brain, with some emphasis on the heart. In the past 20 years, it has been recognized that PET has clinical value for managing patients who have cancer. More recently the combination PET/CT hybrid imaging has demonstrated synergistic improvements in the accuracy of staging cancer patients and assessing response to treatment. Like all nuclear medicine imaging procedures, PET not only demonstrates physiology, but is able to do so more quantitatively than other nuclear medicine tests.

The power of the technique rests on the use of cyclotron-produced positron-emitting radionuclides like ^{18}F, ^{11}C, ^{13}N, and ^{15}O. Another source would be generator-produced radionuclides including ^{68}Ga and ^{82}Rb. These radionuclides are tagged to specific pharmaceuticals, allowing in vivo assessment of various physiologic processes such as perfusion, glucose metabolism, amino acid transport, DNA synthesis, various receptors. They also may be used as surrogate markers for gene expression. The purpose of this article is to outline the current clinical use for PET imaging in the brain and other radiopharmaceuticals used for assessing various physiologic parameters pertaining to tumor metabolism.

2[^{18}F]fluoro-2-deoxy-D-glucose positron emission tomography

The most commonly used tracer is 2[^{18}F]fluoro-2-deoxy-D-glucose (FDG). Deoxyglucose (DG) initially was developed as a chemotherapy agent to block the accelerated glycolysis of tumor cells, but its central nervous system (CNS) toxicity was

Department of Nuclear Medicine, Division of Diagnostic Imaging, University of Texas, M.D. Anderson Cancer Center, 1515 Holcombe Boulevard, Box 83, Houston, TX 77030, USA
E-mail address: hmacapinlac@di.mdacc.tmc.edu

doi:10.1016/j.nic.2006.08.001

limiting [1]. The current use of FDG was derived from the [^{14}C]deoxyglucose method for measuring glucose use in the rat brain described by Sokoloff [1,2]. FDG initially follows the same metabolic pathway as glucose. Like glucose, 2- deoxyglucose is taken into the brain by glucose transporters, where it is phosphorylated like glucose by hexokinase to yield DG -6-phosphate. Whereas glucose-6-phosphate subsequently is used for energy, ending up as CO_2 and water, DG- 6- phosphate is trapped and accumulates. This trapping of DG is enhanced further by low levels of the reverse enzyme glucose 6 phosphatase in the brain, making the phosphorylation an essentially irreversible step (Fig. 1). There are multiple assumptions in the Sokoloff model, including the lumped constant accounting for the differences in transport and phosphorylation between glucose and DG. The Sokoloff model assumes that DG-6-PO4 is trapped, because the activity of phosphatase is low in brain tissue. Phelps and colleagues take into account the possible dephosphorylation, to incorporate a fourth rate constant k4, representing the slow process of dephosphorylation, or, more generally, the loss of labeled metabolic product [3]. Part of this controversy is that in altered states such as the presence of pathology, this correction is variable; hence multiple proposals for normalization methods have been done. PET imaging can be used to derive local cerebral metabolic rates of glucose (CMRGlc) from a series of measured tissue activities over time by a multiple time graphical analysis, which was derived by Patlak and Blasberg [4]. This would require a dynamic acquisition over time with arterial blood sampling. Subsequent methods have sought to use fewer blood samples, a population-based arterial blood curve with venous sampling. Nonquantitative methods are more popular clinically, as they are easier to perform, requiring no blood sampling, a single static scan, and use of a calculated attenuation correction, negating the need of a transmission scan.

Most of the energy consumed by the brain for function is by the catabolism of glucose to CO_2 and water, which is by glycolysis and oxidative phosphorylation. Hence, glucose use reflects neuronal synaptic activity. This makes FDG PET imaging a useful tool in imaging regional cerebral metabolism and reflecting the state of cerebral activation [5]. This has allowed its application in neurology, neuro-oncology, and psychiatry. A stereotactic PET atlas by Minoshima provides a very good reference and aid for visual interpretation of brain images, as one needs to recognize the limitation of FDG PET for identifying the anatomy of the brain accurately [6].

Most recently, the Center for Medicare and Medicaid Services (CMS) approved the use of FDG PET imaging in the diagnosis for a select group of Medicare beneficiaries with suspected Alzheimer's disease (AD). This has fostered increasing use of FDG PET in a clinically relevant and increasing problem. A recent review by Silverman outlines improvements in the ability of FDG PET to identify very early changes associated with AD and other neurodegenerative dementias [7]. The clinical need for early diagnosis aided by imaging has been reinforced by the recent US Food and Drug Administration (FDA) approval of drugs like rivastigmine tartrate for mild-to-moderate AD. This drug also has been recommended for approval for treating Parkinson's disease (PD), as up to 40% of these patients also develop dementia. These drugs reduce the rate of cognitive decline in patients diagnosed with AD. The typical FDG PET images of AD show decreased cerebral metabolism involving the posterior cingulate and neocortical association cortices, while largely sparing the basal ganglia, thalamus, cerebellum, and cortex-mediating primary sensory and motor functions. This would

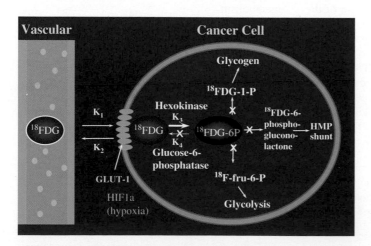

Fig. 1. Mechanism of uptake of FDG into tumor cells.

differentiate AD from vascular dementia, which usually would have focal lesions affecting cortical subcortical and cerebellar areas. Fronto-temporal dementias like Pick's disease will affect the frontal and anterior/mesial temporal areas earlier. PD is similar to AD but may show less sparing of the visual cortex and mesiotemporal areas. Huntington's disease will demonstrate hypometabolism of the lenticular and caudate nuclei early. Dementia with Lewy bodies will be similar to AD and may show more involvement of the cerebellum and occipital cortex. Earlier studies using FDG PET have been applied to patients with AIDS dementia complex for diagnosis and monitoring of response to zidovudine therapy [8]. Pretreatment scans demonstrated large focal cortical abnormalities, with increase in FDG metabolism accompanying immunologic and neurologic improvement following treatment.

FDG PET imaging also is covered by CMS for patients with intractable seizures being considered for possible surgery. Interictal imaging identifies an area of hypometabolism in the epileptogenic zone. If the scan is acquired during the ictal state, these reveal complex patterns of increased and decreased FDG metabolism. FDG PET is able to lateralize and regionalize potentially epileptogenic regions in patients who have normal MR imaging [9]. Table 1 illustrates the indications covered by CMS.

FDG PET imaging has been applied to tumor imaging. This is based on the abnormal metabolism of tumors that have increased rates of anaerobic and aerobic glycolysis over most normal tissues. This observation first was made by Warburg over 60 years ago [10]. This means that many tumors have greater rates of glucose use than normal tissues. These alterations are fairly common across a range of tumor types. The accelerated glycolysis is usually greater in more aggressive tumors. Box 1 illustrates common tumors that are FDG avid and nonavid. Some demonstrated that FDG accumulated into

Box 1: 2[¹⁸F]fluoro-2-deoxy-D-glucose avidity of tumors

FDG avid tumors
- Nonsmall cell lung ca
- Colorectal cancer
- Intraductal breast Ca
- Anaplastic meningioma
- Glioblastoma multiforme
- Neuroendocrine tumors–poorly differentiated
- Malignant melanoma
- Osteosarcoma

Non-FDG avid tumors
- Bronchoalveolar cancer
- Mucinous tumors
- Lobular Breast Ca
- Meningioma
- Low-grade gliomas
- Carcinoid
- Hepatocellular Ca
- Low-grade chondrosarcoma

rodent tumors in 1980, and 2 years later, the first imaging of human tumors was reported, both in brain tumors and colorectal cancer metastatic to the liver [11,12].

In the past decade, the uptake of FDG into various human cancers has been shown to occur, with high tumor/background uptake ratios at just 1 to 2 hours after intravenous injection [13,14]. The mechanisms for this increased FDG 6 phosphate accumulation in many cancer cells have been shown to be caused by:

- **Increased expression of glucose transporter molecules at the tumor cell surface**
- **Increased levels or activity of hexokinase in tumor cells**
- **Reduced levels of glucose 6 phosphatase versus most normal tissues in tumor cells**

Autoradiographic studies have shown that there is greater FDG uptake into areas of viable tumor than areas of frank necrosis, but in some rodent tumor models and in people, it has been shown that the uptake of FDG can be high in inflammatory cells, although the bulk of activity generally is into tumors [15].

A recent review by Macheda [16] further elucidates the transport of glucose into malignant cells. Increased glucose transport in malignant cells has been associated with increased and deregulated expression of GLUT1 or GLUT3. Macheda also showed that in human studies, high levels of GLUT1 expression in tumors have been associated with a worse prognosis. Uptake of FDG in breast and prostate cancer at presentation appears less than other cancers. More recently, GLUT12 has

Table 1: 2[¹⁸F] fluoro-2-deoxy-D-glucose positron emission tomography clinical indications approved by the Center for Medicare and Medicaid Services

Alzheimer's disease	Yes
Seizure localization	Yes
Brain tumor grading	No
Radiation necrosis versus recurrent brain tumor	No
Brain biopsy localization	No
Preoperative functional assessment	No
Stroke evaluation	No
Parkinson's disease and other neurodegenerative	No

been found in breast and prostate cancers. Trafficking of GLUT12 to the plasma membrane therefore could contribute to glucose uptake in these tumors. Several factors have been implicated in the regulation of glucose transporter expression such as hypoxia and epidermal growth factor (EGFR). Bos and colleagues have shown that breast cancers vary in FDG uptake, and the low uptake in lobular breast cancer is a function of various parameters, such as microvasculature for delivering nutrients, Glut-1 receptors, hexokinase, the number of tumor cells/volume, proliferation rate, number of lymphocytes (not macrophages), and hypoxia-inducible factor-1alpha (HIF-1a) for upregulating Glut-1 [17].

Brain tumors are the most extensively studied of any tumor type using PET, mainly because many of the first dedicated type PET scanners were designed in size and shape to be well-suited to brain imaging. Indeed, in several countries, the use of FDG and PET has been validated sufficiently that these are routine clinical procedures reimbursed by insurance carriers.

DiChiro and colleagues recognized the potential of FDG for imaging brain tumors and reported on this approach in 1982 [18]. Several studies have demonstrated the ability of FDG PET to distinguish histologically aggressive from less aggressive brain tumors [19,20], and to separate viable tumor from scar or necrosis [21]. It is also possible to use FDG PET imaging to identify transformation of a low-grade glioma to a more aggressive type [22]. The reason FDG uptake appears to correlate with survival and tumor grade is not clear, but it may be related to the increased cellular density seen in high-grade tumors (ie, the larger quantity of viable tumor cells would correlate with a poorer prognosis) [23].

There is controversy concerning the ability of FDG PET to identify brain tumors of various grades, and uptake of FDG in low-grade tumors is inadequate for reliable detection [24]. This is particularly true if the lesions are in white matter, wherein less of the low background FDG uptake can mimic the activity in these low-grade tumors. In other cases, high uptake of FDG can be seen in tumors that have evidence of contrast enhancement on CT, but which are associated with a reasonably good prognosis. This has been seen in juvenile pilocytic astrocytomas [25]. Other tumors such as choroid plexus papillomas and pleomorphic xanthoastrocytoma also have shown high FDG uptake with low malignancy potential [26,27]. Quantitative criteria for separating high- and low-grade gliomas from one another by FDGPET have been reported. A tumor/white matter uptake ratio of greater than 1.5 was reported to provide a sensitivity/specificity in separating tumor types (untreated) of 94% and

77%, respectively [28,29]. This quantitative assessment approach can be viewed as supplemental to traditional qualitative assessments, in which high-grade tumors typically have more FDG uptake than normal gray matter, and low-grade tumors have uptake greater than normal white matter, but less than normal gray matter. Some series, however, indicate that visual evaluation may prove superior to semiquantitative methods [30]. A more recent study in a pediatric brain tumor population demonstrated that FDG PET imaging of the brain with MRI coregistration can be used to obtain a more specific diagnosis with respect to malignancy grading, but difficulties arise with respect to low-grade malignancies [31].

Following the completion of radiation therapy, FDG uptake into a contrast-enhancing lesion on MR imaging or CT suggests the presence of viable tumor, while lack of FDG uptake suggests that radiation necrosis is present, presuming high FDG uptake before therapy [32]. In clinical practice, qualitative visual analysis, in which FDG uptake is compared with normal white or gray matter, generally is used for analysis, in preference to quantitative analysis. This approach generally means that any focus of FDG activity that is more intense in tracer uptake than normal brain white matter is considered to represent viable tumor. It generally is recognized that FDG PET has substantial difficulty in detecting low-grade gliomas and some intermediate-grade gliomas, as their FDG uptake can be quite low. Despite some concerns about the sensitivity of FDG PET in low-grade brain tumors, DiChiro showed that radiation necrosis can identify correctly 10 cases in a group of 95 patients with suspected tumor recurrence after brain tumor therapy [33]. Similarly, Doyle reported 84% accuracy of PET in determining if necrosis was present following interstitial brachytherapy for brain tumors [34]. Thus, PET with FDG is fairly reliable in separating residual viable tumor from scar. It should be noted, however, that the actual number of cases and well-controlled studies is small. Recent reviews acknowledge the methodological flaws and wide criticism, but overall, if FDG uptake is noted in MR-enhancing lesions, recurrence is likely. Better interpretation is aided by MR fusion or coregistration. Furthermore, the prognostic value of FDG PET is established clinically [35].

In the situation of low-grade gliomas, ^{11}C-L-methionine (MET), a good marker or amino acid transport, would be a better agent, as it has low background brain uptake (Fig. 2). The use of MET in cancer imaging is based on the observation of increased amino acid transport and the increased activity of the transmethylation pathways in some cancers. There is normally high uptake of this tracer

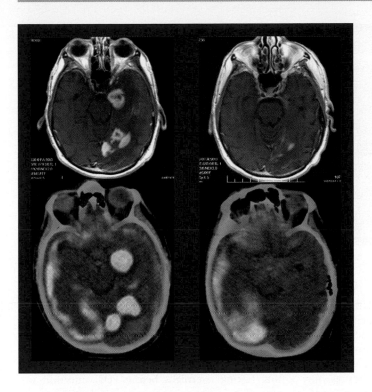

Fig. 2. Lymphoma FDG. A 62-year-old man with primary CNS large B-cell lymphoma by biopsies of the brain. Upper left MR T1 with GdDTPA showing multiple enhancing lesions in the left parietooccipital and inferomedial temporal lobes. Lower left fused PET/CT image showing FDG avid lesions corresponding to the MR findings. Upper right MR image showing residual enhancement in left parietooccipital and inferomedial temporal lobes after five courses of high-dose methotrexate and procarbazine. Lower right PET/CT showing in post-treatment hypometabolism in the left hemisphere consistent with metabolic response to therapy.

in the pancreas, salivary glands, liver, and kidneys [36,37]. The smaller amount of excretion in the urine is an advantage of imaging cancers such as prostate cancer [38]. As a natural amino acid, there is some metabolism of L-methionine in the bloodstream. This tracer is taken up by tumor in a matter of minutes, allowing early imaging, and it has stereospecific activity [39]. MET has been used in imaging brain tumors, including pituitary adenomas [40,41]. Although there is some level of methionine accumulation in the normal pituitary, this should not be confused with an adenoma. The response of pituitary adenomas to therapy also has been evaluated by PET. Although diagnosis of pituitary disease has been made much easier in the past decade through the availability of CT and MR imaging, PET may have a role in selected instances. It is of interest that nonfunctional adenomas are reported to generally have higher FDG uptake than functional adenomas [40].

MET has been shown not to accumulate into focal radiation necrosis in the relatively small number of patients studied; however, it does accumulate into many low-grade gliomas. Bergström and colleagues reported that 7 of 11 low-grade gliomas had an increased uptake of ^{11}C-methionine versus normal brain [42]. More recent studies in 27 pediatric patients have demonstrated that the accumulation of MET and FDG is substantially higher in high-grade tumors versus low grade-gliomas [43].

Low-grade tumor tumors can, on sequential studies, develop sites of increased FDG uptake, indicating malignant transformation [44]. Hence a clinical application would be to monitor low-grade gliomas with FDG PET, particularly when they develop new symptoms, and perform intervention when there is interval appearance of FDG hypermetabolism evidence suggesting malignant change. This aspect of patient management needs more study, as surgical resection of low-grade gliomas can be potentially curative.

Metastatic brain tumors are the most common tumors, Griffeth reported that FDG uptake into untreated metastases from various cancers can, in a significant fraction of cases (up to one-third of patients in his study), be insufficient to produce satisfactory images of the metastases [45]. A more recent series in 40 patients screened for cerebral metastases demonstrated that FDG PET had a sensitivity of only 75% and specificity of 83%. Only 61% of metastatic lesions in the brain were identified by PET in contrast to MR imaging. Overall, contrast enhanced MR imaging appears to be the better imaging modality in detecting brain metastases [46].This is particularly the case when small lesions are located in close proximity to gray matter folds in the brain that have high FDG uptake (**Fig. 3**).

It should be noted that CNS lymphomas, both intra-axial and extra-axial, have been reported to

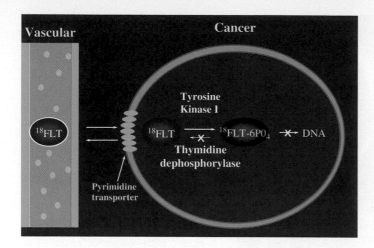

Fig. 3. Mechanism of uptake of FLT into tumor cells.

be visualized well by PET using FDG. The intensity of FDG uptake into lymphomas has been reported to be comparable to that seen in high-grade gliomas and is significantly more than that reported in low-grade gliomas [47]. Kawai demonstrated that in patients who had primary CNS lymphomas, the metabolic rate of glucose uptake and phosphorylation rate in lymphoma was significantly higher than that observed in the normal cortex in 14 control patients [48]. The K1 rate of lymphoma, however, was the same as normal cortex. They also studied these patients after methotrexate-based therapy, demonstrating response as marked reduction of K1 and K3 (see Fig. 3). FDG PET also was shown to be capable of accurately detecting the presence of CNS lymphoma in patients with AIDS, and in differentiating this pattern from that seen in CNS infectious processes, as infections such as toxoplasmosis tend to be hypometabolic or have less FDG uptake than CNS lymphomas [49–51].

Among extra-axial tumors, meningiomas can be imaged with FDG PET. DiChiro showed that FDG uptake was highest in the most aggressive tumors on histology, while lower FDG uptake wais noted in patients with a less aggressive histology in a series of 17 patients [52]. In this series, FDG uptake correlated with the growth rate of the meningiomas, and the tumors with the lowest FDG uptake were found to have the better likelihood for survival. Lippitz, in a larger series of 62 meningiomas, demonstrated that the glucose metabolism was significantly different between the groups with high versus low cellularity ($P < .01$), increased versus normal proliferation rates ($P < .025$) and low (World Health Organization [WHO] grade I) versus higher (WHO grades II, III) graded tumors [53]. The data supported the fact that FDG PET is suitable as a noninvasive predictor of tumor growth characteristics in

meningiomas. It is uncertain if low FDG uptake in a meningioma would suggest that surgery could be delayed, but such prognostic information may be a useful adjunct in such challenging cases. Cremerius, in a series of 75 patients, demonstrated that fasting overnight before FDG injection improved the diagnostic accuracy of FDG PET for noninvasive metabolic grading of meningioma. PET correctly identified eight of nine atypical or malignant meningiomas and 58 of 66 grade 1 meningiomas in this retrospective series [54].

FDG PET may be used in directing biopsy in patients who have complex lesions on CT or MR imaging. In view of the coexistence of low- and high-grade components of some brain tumors, FDG PET can assist in selection of biopsy site and allow more appropriate therapy to be implemented. Numerous studies have confirmed the improvement in accuracy of biopsy when using FDG PET in conjunction with CT or MR imaging [55,56]. The increasing availability of hybrid PET/CT scanners, however, may allow better use of FDG PET for this purpose, allowing a stereotactic frame attached to the bed of the scanner, making it a more practical clinical procedure [57]. This is particularly relevant in lesions where mixed low- and high-grade tumors can coexist. The use of $H_2^{15}O$ water activation studies to define motor or language cortex areas also can assist in the direction of biopsies and surgery for brain tumors that permits adequate resection of tumor while sparing the closely adjacent functional cortical areas [58].

Positron emission tomography image acquisition

Although multiple tracers have been developed for brain PET imaging, the most widely used tracer remains FDG. See Table 2 for tracers used in clinical studies. The acquisition of FDG PET images of the brain in patients is similar in preparation to most oncology PET studies, with patients studied after a 6-hour fast. The usual dose of FDG should be 5.18 to 7.77 MBq (0.14 to 0.21 mCi)/kg of body-weight, with a typical range of 370 to 740 MBq (10 to 20 mCi). Brain imaging, however, could be done with less FDG than oncologic imaging, usually with a dose of at least 5 mCi for adults, and weight adjusted for children. After injection, patients must be allowed to rest in a quiet, darkened environment to minimize stimulation and subsequent changes in normal brain on the FDG PET scan. Data acquisition normally is performed after a minimum 30-min uptake period. The images may be acquired in a dynamic or static mode. Dynamic images are done for pediatric patients to allow flexibility for patient motion (ie, discard datasets with motion and sum-up images with minimal motion). The type of imaging is scanner-dependent, and usually three-dimensional imaging with calculated attenuation is performed. If preferred, the CT acquired with hybrid machines also could be used for attenuation correction and reference for localization during interpretation. In pediatric patients, a general anesthetic may be required. In patients with known seizures, electroencephalogram (EEG) recording during the uptake period, and during the PET image acquisition, also may be required. The attenuation correction, either with CT or a transmission source like ^{68}Ge, is mathematically necessary for image quantification. The deeper structures are attenuated by the overlying tissues, giving an inaccurate distribution of tracer if the observed lower counts from central body parts are not corrected for losses by attenuation. Likewise, more superficial structures with little attenuation from overlying tissues may show too much activity; therefore, attenuation correction is necessary for accurate image representation. Most imaging is performed in three-dimensional mode for the brain, which means that the septa between detectors is retracted, allowing greater sensitivity to acquire images. In the three-dimensional setting, all collumation is done electronically by means of the simultaneity detection circuitry. Two-dimensional imaging is performed with lead septae between the detectors acting as a collimator for scatter and random events. Widely used three-dimensional reconstruction techniques have overcome the scatter and random events with the advantage of greater counts acquired over the same or shorter period. Most clinical brain studies therefore are acquired in three-dimensional mode, allowing better image quality and shorter acquisition times.

The interpretation of PET scans in patients is dependent on the anatomy of the brain shown on CT/MR imaging, the patterns of FDG uptake in normal brain tissue, the clinical history of the patient, and concomitant medications. Normal gray matter shows high FDG uptake, as the brain uses glucose almost exclusively for energy requirements. Uptake of FDG in brain tumors normally is evaluated qualitatively by comparison with normal gray matter. Medications such as corticosteroids, anticonvulsant medications, and sedatives/anesthetics may reduce normal gray matter glucose metabolism, which may degrade image quality [59–61]. Surgery and prior radiotherapy also may produce structural changes in brain anatomy, which need to be evaluated carefully in interpreting FDG PET scans of the brain. Additionally, post-therapy metabolic changes (principally hypometabolism) may appear more extensive than anatomic changes on MR/CT imaging. Also, the intrinsic resolution limitations of PET scanners make small (ie, less than 5 to 7 mm) lesions difficult to identify, particularly when they may be adjacent to an area of normal gray matter with high FDG uptake. A strong recommendation would be to coregister image sets of PET and MR imaging or CT if possible to allow better image interpretation taking into reference the anatomic changes. Various vendor-provided programs are available and widely used.

One finding commonly seen in patients with supratentorial brain tumors is reduced FDG uptake in the contralateral cerebellum, referred to as crossed cerebellar diaschisis. This occurs as a result of a disruption of the normal corticopontocerebellar pathway from the cerebral hemispheres afferent input into the contralateral cerebellar cortex [62]. This PET scan finding also is seen following stroke and trauma, but in patients who have brain tumors, it may persist indefinitely. This also has been studied and verified using O-15 perfusion imaging with PET [63]. Fulham described the preservation of FDG metabolism in the contralateral dentate

Table 2: Positron emission tomography tracers for brain imaging

11C-thymidine	DNA synthesis
18F-3'-deoxy-3'-fluorothymidine	DNA synthesis
124I-iododeoxyuridine	DNA synthesis
11C-methionine	Amino acid transport
18F-alpha methyl tyrosine	Amino acid transport
60C-ATSM	Hypoxia
18F-fluoromisonidazole	Hypoxia
15O water	Perfusion
18F-DOPA	Dopamine transport
18F-FDG	Glycolysis

nucleus, indicating preservation of afferent input to the largest of the deep cerebellar nuclei from the Purkinje cells in the cortex, despite interruption of the major excitatory input to the Purkinje cells [62]. The diminution in uptake over the contralateral cerebellar cortex reflects the pathology not evaluable by MR or CT scanning and sometimes accounts for the neurologic deficits encountered in these patients.

The evaluation of FDG uptake in brain tumors may be qualitative or quantitative through the use of regions of interest comparing tumor with white matter metabolism, or calculation of SUVs. Simple quantification can be performed by measuring tumor/nontumor uptake ratios or by determining the standardized uptake value. Standard vendor-provided software now allows easy calculation of SUV. This latter value often is used to reflect the uptake of the tracer in tumor or normal tissues. Generally, the higher the value, the more likely it is that tumor is present.

$$SUV = \frac{\text{decay-corrected dose/cm}^3 \text{ tumor}}{\text{injected dose/patient weight in g}}$$

It should be noted that there is variation in SUV with the time following tracer injection, with the SUV increasing over time in most untreated tumors. Thus, standardization of imaging time for SUV determination is important in serial studies, particularly for response evaluation. Most investigators use a small region of interest (relative to the tumor size) and attempt to quantify activity in the most metabolically active portion of the tumor, but there is some variability in practice, and SUV from one institution with one type of scanning device cannot necessarily be compared directly with the SUV from another institution with another type of scanning device as acquisition parameters (two- or three-dimensional), correction (calculated, rod source, CT), and time of scanning are all variables. Care in the consistency of scanning technique is vital for multi-center trial comparisons, particularly in response evaluations. A recent guideline was published for treatment response evaluation using FDG PET with similar recommendations as described previously [64]. It is also important to note that body weight-based SUV may not be the best measure, particularly for pediatric patients, as they may benefit from using body surface area SUV calculation, and in adults, lean body mass may be better than body weight-based SUV [65].

In some centers, arterial sampling, or arterialized venous sampling, also is used to provide more accurate measurement of tumor metabolism. The use of blood sampling techniques is important in clinical scenarios where precise changes in tumor metabolism are evaluated (eg, to monitor therapy changes) or where new PET ligands are being evaluated. In view of the increasing use of FDG PET in monitoring brain tumors from initial diagnosis through various treatment regimes, a standardized imaging protocol and method of semiquantitative analysis of tumor metabolism should be adopted for all PET sties in this patient population [64].

Other positron emission tomography tracers

DNA precursors

Increased rates of DNA synthesis are typical of many fast-growing tumors and rapidly proliferating normal tissues. Early response evaluation to provide an alternative for FDG is a promising application of PET, particularly with the advent of novel therapies. Thymidine is an attractive tracer in that it targets only tissues with ongoing DNA synthesis. The use of thymidine is made difficult by the rapid metabolism in the blood, meaning that only a small fraction of the labeled material in the blood is ^{11}C-thymidine [66,67]. This technique also is made very difficult because of the short half life of ^{11}C, and quantification is complex because of various metabolites like C-11 CO2 [68]. Labeling an alternative tracer with _I-124 (4.2-day half-life) also was done, using I-124 IUdR. The same complex and rapid catabolism in the blood made this tracer difficult to quantify and makes it impractical for wider clinical application [69]. [18]F-3′-deoxy-3′-fluorothymidine (FLT) is a new tracer that images cellular proliferation by entering the salvage pathway of DNA synthesis, but is not a direct marker of DNA proliferation [70]. A review by Shields highlights the fact that the greatest unmet need for PET imaging is in further developing and validating its use in the measurement of treatment response. FLT is one of the more promising tracers, and further clinical trials are warranted. An advantage of the tracer is the low uptake in the normal brain and the half-life of an F-18 labeled tracer [71]. A recent pilot study by Chen compared FDG with FLT in 18 patients [72], showing that FLT was more sensitive than FDG to image recurrent high-grade tumors. Additionally, it correlated better with Ki-67 values and was a more powerful predictor of tumor progression and survival. Thus, FLT appears to be a promising tracer as a surrogate marker of proliferation in high-grade gliomas (Fig. 4).

Tumor hypoxia

Tumor hypoxia plays an important role in the biology of cancer cells through effects on signal transduction pathways and the regulation and transcription of various genes involved in malignant growth and metastases. Well-oxygenated cells are more sensitive to the cytotoxic effects of

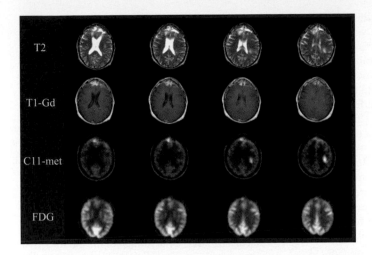

Fig. 4. This is a patient with low-grade glioma by biopsy in the left deep frontal lobe. (*Top*) T2 weighted MR image showing abnormal signal in the tumor. (*Second row*) T1 with GdDTPA MR showing no enhancement in tumor. (*Third row*) C-11 methionine PET showing uptake in the tumor. (*Fourth row*) FDG PET showing no FDG uptake.

ionizing radiation compared with hypoxic cells, and there is preclinical evidence indicating that hypoxic cells are also resistant to the effects of chemotherapy (eg, by amplification of genes conferring drug resistance) [73,74].

The PET tracer most widely used in a clinical setting of hypoxia is ^{18}F-fluoromisonidazole (^{18}F-FMISO). ^{18}F-FMISO PET scanning has been used for noninvasive assessment of hypoxia in tumors, including gliomas. Scott and colleagues used ^{18}F-FMISO PET studies in 13 patients who had suspected gliomas before surgery and demonstrated that hypoxia measured noninvasively is related to tumor grade and ^{18}F-FDG uptake (although the areas of maximal uptake were often discordant). Additionally, this also may predict the site of relapse [75]. A comparison of FMISO PET with O-15 water PET studies in 11 patients demonstrated that delayed FMISO PET images provide a spatial description of hypoxia in brain tumors that is independent of BBB disruption and tumor perfusion [76]. Several other radiolabeled markers of hypoxia have been developed that can be measured by PET scanning, including ^{60}Cu-ATSM and ^{62}Cu-ATSM [77]. Cu-ATSM has been studied and shown to have rapid uptake and selective retention in hypoxic cells. Clinical studies have been done for head and neck, cervical, and lung cancers [78–80]. The intent was to identify the hypoxic and presumed radio resistant volume of tumor, which potentially may benefit from more intense or higher doses of radiation to this tumor fraction with the hope of improving patient response or outcome. Further studies are required to define the role of hypoxia imaging in brain tumors.

Blood flow

Various fundamental physical properties of tumor physiology can be defined by PET imaging. Tumor blood flow can be measured using ^{15}O H$_2$O or ^{15}O CO$_2$ inhalation with image quantification. Tumor blood volume can be estimated by using ^{15}CO inhalation. Tumor volume of distribution (ie, that portion of the tumor that freely communicates with the blood) can be imaged using ^{15}O H$_2$O. These parameters can be determined quantitatively using mathematical modeling techniques. In some instances, the increased blood flow in a tumor may be sufficient to allow it to be defined as cancer versus normal tissues, although this is quite variable, as some cancers do not have increased flow versus normal tissues. It should be pointed out that these could be performed in a research setting with fairly restrictive technical demands. CT and MR techniques rival this traditional method, particularly in ease of acquisition and need of a proximal cyclotron/radiochemistry chemistry facility.

Amyloid imaging

AD is characterized by the presence of beta-amyloid plaques in the brain. Substantial evidence indicates that the presence of increased beta-amyloid peptide is neurotoxic and may initiate the pathogenesis observed in AD, including neurofibrillary tangles, synaptic loss and dysfunction, and neurodegeneration. The use of brain PET imaging in patients with or at risk for AD has increased understanding of the pathophysiology of the disease and may potentially aid in diagnosis. The development of new therapeutics that reduce beta-amyloid peptide in the brain also has indicated a potential use for amyloid imaging in monitoring response to treatment [81]. University of California Los Angeles investigators developed 2-(1-(6-[(2-[^{18}F]fluoroethyl)(methyl)amino]-2-naphthyl)ethylidene) malononitrile (F-18 FDDNP), a probe that crosses the blood–brain barrier and determines the localization and load of SPs and NFTs in vivo in patients who have

AD [82]. In a study of nine patients who had AD compared with control subjects, there was greater accumulation, and slower clearance was noted in brain regions affected by AD [83]. Limitations of this FDDNP include high nonspecific binding (can bind to tau protein), low brain uptake, no validated quantitation method, and interference by nonsteroidal anti-inflammatory drugs [81]. Klunk and colleagues described the first human study of Pittsburgh compound-B (PIB), in 16 patients who had diagnosed mild AD and nine controls [84]. Patients who had AD typically showed marked retention of PIB in areas of association cortex known to contain large amounts of amyloid deposits in AD. In cortical areas, PIB retention correlated inversely with cerebral glucose metabolism determined with FDG [82]. These pilot studies suggest that PET radiotracers for amyloid may allow for the early diagnosis of AD, and provide a means of assessing response to novel therapies.

Summary

There are multiple tracers developed for the brain to assess various functions, including metabolic activity, neurotransmitter function, hormone receptors, and gene expression. The great discord is the lack of transfer from the radiochemistry and in vivo/animal studies to clinical applications. PET imaging has been around for decades, and most clinical experience is with FDG. Expanding PET with other tracers beyond FDG, however, may reap rewards that hopefully would end up saving money instead of wasting it. Multiple applications in neurology, cardiology, and oncology await the wider use of novel tracers.

The unmet needs of PET tumor imaging are for a more selective tracer for tumor with low background activity. Most tracers that have been used clinically are indirect surrogates of transport or nonselective general metabolic surrogates. Tracers are needed that have fairly long half-life label such as ^{18}F to allow ease of distribution, with very good labeling efficiency, allowing high-quality, high- volume synthesis for wider clinical availability. Finally, clinical trials demonstrating significant improvement in outcome need to be proven with the use of such tracers. This could facilitate CMS approval and insurance coverage to pay for these studies.

References

[1] Sokoloff L, Reivich M, Kennedy C, et al. The [14C]deoxyglucose method for the measurement of local glucose utilization: theory, procedure and normal values in the conscious and anesthetized albino rat. J Neurochem 1977;28:897–916.

[2] Reivich M, Kuhl D, Wolf A, et al. Measurement of local cerebral glucose metabolism in man with 18F–2-fluoro-2-deoxy-d-glucose. Acta Neurol Scand Suppl 1977;64:190–1.

[3] Phelps ME, Huang SC, Hoffman EJ, et al. Tomographic measurement of local cerebral glucose metabolic rate in humans with (F-18)2-fluoro-2-deoxy-D-glucose: validation of method. Ann Neurol 1979;6:371–88.

[4] Wienhard K. Measurement of glucose consumption using [^{18}F]fluorodeoxglucose. Methods 2002;27:218–22.

[5] Raichle ME, Mintun MA. Brain work and brain imaging. Annu Rev Neurosci 2006;29:449–76.

[6] Minoshima S, Koeppe RA, Frey KA, et al. Stereotactic PET atlas of the human brain: aid for visual interpretation of functional brain images. J Nucl Med 1994;35(6):949–54.

[7] Silverman DH. Brain 18F-FDG PET in the diagnosis of neurodegenerative dementias: comparison with perfusion SPECT and with clinical evaluations lacking nuclear imaging. Nucl Med 2004;45(4):594–607.

[8] Brunetti A, Berg G, Di Chiro G, et al. Reversal of brain metabolic abnormalities following treatment of AIDS dementia complex with 3′-azido-2′, 3′-dideoxythymidine (AZT, zidovudine): a PET-FDG study. J Nucl Med 1989;30(5):581–90.

[9] Juhasz C, Chugani HT. Imaging the epileptic brain with positron emission tomography. Neuroimaging Clin N Am 2003;13(4):705–16.

[10] Warburg O. The metabolism of tumors. New York: Richard R. Smith; 1931. p. 29–169.

[11] Some P, Atkins HK, Bandoypadhyay D, et al. A fluorinated glucose analog, 2-fluoro-2-deoxy-D-glucose (F-18): nontoxic tracer for rapid tumor detection. J Nucl Med 1980;21:670–5.

[12] Wahl RL, et al. ^{18}F-2-deoxy-2-fluoro-D-glucose uptake into human tumor xenografts. Feasibility studies for cancer imaging with positron emission tomography. Cancer 1991;67:1544–50.

[13] Brown RS, Wahl RL. Overexpression of Glut-1 glucose transporter in human breast cancer. An immunohistochemical study. Cancer 1993;72: 2979–85.

[14] Brown RS, et al. Intratumoral distribution of titrated- FDG in breast carcinoma: correlation between Glut-1 expression and FDG uptake. J Nucl Med 1996;37:1042–7.

[15] Kubota R, et al. Intratumoral distribution of fluorine-18-fluorodeoxyglucose in vivo: high accumulation in macrophages and granulation tissues studied by microautoradiography. J Nucl Med 1992;33:1972–80.

[16] Macheda ML, Rogers S, Best JD. Molecular and cellular regulation of glucose transporter (glut) proteins in cancer. J Cell Physiol 2005;202:654–62.

[17] Bos R, van Der Hoeven JJ, van Der Wall E, et al. Biologic correlates of (18)fluorodeoxyglucose uptake in human breast cancer measured by

positron emission tomography. J Clin Oncol 2002;20(2):379–87.

[18] Di Chiro G, et al. Glucose utilization of cerebral gliomas measured by [18F] fluorodeoxyglucose and positron emission tomography. Neurology 1982;32:1323–9.

[19] Alavi JB, Alavi A, Chawluk J, et al. Positron emission tomography in patients with glioma. A predictor of prognosis. Cancer 1988;62(6):1074–8.

[20] Schifter T, et al. Serial FDG-PET studies in the prediction of survival in patients with primary brain tumors. J Comput Assist Tomogr 1993;17:509–61.

[21] Patronas NJ, Di Chiro G, Brooks RA, et al. Work in progress: [18F] fluorodeoxyglucose and positron emission tomography in the evaluation of radiation necrosis of the brain. Radiology 1982;144:885–9.

[22] Francavilla TL, Miletich RS, Di Chiro G, et al. Positron emission tomography in the detection of malignant degeneration of low-grade gliomas. Neurosurgery 1989;24:1–5.

[23] Herholz K, Pietrzyk U, Voges J, et al. In vivo imaging of glucose consumption and lactate concentration in human gliomas. Ann Neurol 1992;31:319–27.

[24] Janus TJ, et al. Use of [18F]fluorodeoxyglucose positron emission tomography in patients with primary malignant brain tumors. Ann Neurol 1993;33:540–8.

[25] Fulham MJ, Melisi JW, Nishimiya J, et al. Neuroimaging of juvenile pilocytic astrocytomas: an enigma. Radiology 1993;189:221–5.

[26] Sunada I, Tsuyuguchi N, Hara M, et al. 18F-FDG and 11C-methionine PET in choroid plexus papilloma: report of three cases. Radiat Med 2002;20:97–100.

[27] Tsuyuguchi N, Matsuoka Y, Sunada I, et al. Evaluation of pleomorphic xanthoastrocytoma by use of positron emission tomography with. AJNR Am J Neuroradiol 2001;22:311–3.

[28] Di Chiro G. Positron emission tomography using [18F]fluorodeoxyglucose in brain tumors. A powerful diagnostic and prognostic tool. Invest Radiol 1987;22:360–71.

[29] Delbeke D, Meyerowitz C, Lapidus RL, et al. Optimal cutoff levels of F-18 fluorodeoxyglucose uptake in the differentiation of low-grade from high-grade brain tumors with PET. Radiology 1995;195:47–52.

[30] Hustinx R, Smith RJ, Benard F, et al. Can the standardized uptake value characterize primary brain tumors on FDG-PET? Eur J Nucl Med 1999;26:1501–9.

[31] Borgwardt L, Hojgaard L, Carstensen H, et al. Increased fluorine-18 2-fluoro-2-deoxy-D-glucose (FDG) uptake in childhood CNS tumors is correlated with malignancy grade: a study with FDG positron emission tomography/magnetic resonance imaging coregistration and image fusion. J Clin Oncol 2005;23(13):3030–7.

[32] Ishikawa M, et al. Glucose consumption in recurrent gliomas. Neurosurgery 1993;33:28–33.

[33] Di Chiro G, Oldfield E, Wright DC, et al. Cerebral necrosis after radiotherapy and/or intra-arterial chemotherapy for brain tumors: PET and neuropathologic studies. AJR Am J Roentgenol 1988;150(1):189–97.

[34] Doyle WK, Budinger TF, Valk PE, et al. Differentiation of cerebral radiation necrosis from tumor recurrence by [18F]FDG and 82Rb positron emission tomography. J Comput Assist Tomogr 1987;11:563–70.

[35] Hustinx R, Pourdehnad M, Kaschten B, et al. PET imaging for differentiating recurrent brain tumor from radiation necrosis. Radiol Clin North Am 2005;43(1):35–47.

[36] Kubota K, Yamada K, Fukada H, et al. Tumor detection with carbon-11-labelled amino acids. Eur J Nucl Med 1984;9:136–40.

[37] Kubota K, et al. Lung tumor imaging by positron emission tomography using C-11 L-methionine. J Nucl Med 1985;26:37–42.

[38] Bergström M, et al. Comparison of the accumulation kinetics of L-(methyl-11C)-methionine and D-(methyl-11C)-methionine in brain tumors studied with positron emission tomography. Acta Radiol 1987;28:225–9.

[39] Macapinlac HA, Humm JJ, Akhurst T, et al. Differential metabolism and pharmacokinetics of L-[1-(11)C]-methionine and 2-[(18)F] fluoro-2-deoxy-D-glucose (FDG) in androgen-independent prostate cancer. Clin Positron Imaging 1999;2(3):173–81.

[40] Francavilla TL, Miletich RS, DeMichele D, et al. Positron emission tomography of pituitary macroadenomas: hormone prediction and effects of therapy. Neurosurgery 1991;28:826–33.

[41] Bergström M, et al. Rapid decrease in amino acid metabolism in prolactin-secreting pituitary adenomas after bromocriptine treatment: a PET study. J Comput Assist Tomogr 1987;11:815–81.

[42] Bergström M, et al. Discrepancies in brain tumor extent as shown by computed tomography and positron emission tomography using [68Ga]ED-TA, [11C]glucose, and [11C]methionine. J Comput Assist Tomogr 1983;7:1062–6.

[43] Utriainen M, Metsahonkala L, Salmi TT, et al. Metabolic characterization of childhood brain tumors: comparison of 18F-fluorodeoxyglucose and 11C-methionine positron emission tomography. Cancer 2002;95(6):1376–86.

[44] Francavilla TL, Miletich RS, Di Chiro G, et al. Positron emission tomography in the detection of malignant degeneration of low-grade gliomas. Neurosurgery 1989;24:1–5.

[45] Griffeth LK, et al. Brain metastases from non-central nervous system tumors: evaluation with PET. [see comments]. Radiology 1993;186:37–44.

[46] Rohren EM, Provenzale JM, Barboriak DP, et al. Screening for cerebral metastases with FDG PET in patients undergoing whole-body staging of

noncentral nervous system malignancy. Radiology 2003;226(1):181–7.

[47] Rosenfeld SS, et al. Studies of primary central nervous system lymphoma with fluorine-18-fluorodeoxyglucose positron emission tomography. J Nucl Med 1992;33:532–6.

[48] Kawai N, Nishiyama Y, Miyake K, et al. Evaluation of tumor FDG transport and metabolism in primary central nervous system lymphoma using [18F]fluorodeoxyglucose (FDG) positron emission tomography (PET) kinetic analysis. Ann Nucl Med 2005;19(8):685–90.

[49] Hoffman JM, et al. FDG-PET in differentiating lymphoma from nonmalignant central nervous system lesions in patients with AIDS. J Nucl Med 1993;34:567–75.

[50] Pierce MA, et al. Evaluating contrast-enhancing brain lesions in patients with AIDS by using positron emission tomography. Ann Intern Med 1995;123:594–8.

[51] Roelcke U, Leenders KL. Positron emission tomography in patients with primary CNS lymphomas. J Neurooncol 1999;43(3):231–6.

[52] Di Chiro G, et al. Glucose utilization by intracranial meningiomas as an index of tumor aggressivity and probability of recurrence: a PET study. Radiology 1987;164:521–6.

[53] Lippitz B, Cremerius U, Mayfrank L, et al. PET study of intracranial meningiomas: correlation with histopathology, cellularity and proliferation rate. Acta Neurochir Suppl (Wien) 1996;65: 108–11.

[54] Cremerius U, Bares R, Weis J, et al. Fasting improves discrimination of grade 1 and atypical or malignant meningioma in FDG-PET. J Nucl Med 1997;38(1):26–30.

[55] Massager N, David P, Goldman S, et al. Combined magnetic resonance imaging- and positron emission tomography-guided stereotactic biopsy in brainstem mass lesions: diagnostic yield in a series of 30 patients. J Neurosurg 2000;93(6):951–7.

[56] Hanson MW, Glantz MJ, Hoffman JM, et al. FDG-PET in the selection of brain lesions for biopsy. J Comput Assist Tomogr 1991;15(5):796–801.

[57] Picozzi P, Rizzo G, Landoni C, et al. A simplified method to integrate metabolic images in stereotactic procedures using a PET/CT scanner. Stereotact Funct Neurosurg 2005;83:208–12.

[58] Meyer PT, Sturz L, Schreckenberger M, et al. Preoperative mapping of cortical language areas in adult brain tumour patients using PET and individual nonnormalised SPM analyses. Eur J Nucl Med Mol Imaging 2003;30(7):951–60.

[59] Fulham MJ, Brunetti A, Aloj L, et al. Decreased cerebral glucose metabolism in patients with brain tumors: an effect of corticosteroids. J Neurosurg 1995;83(4):657–64.

[60] Blacklock JB, Oldfield EH, Di Chiro G, et al. Effect of barbiturate coma on glucose utilization in normal brain versus gliomas. Positron emission tomography studies. J Neurosurg 1987;67(1): 71–5.

[61] Gaillard WD, Zeffiro T, Fazilat S, et al. Effect of valproate on cerebral metabolism and blood flow: an 18F-2-deoxyglucose and 15O water positron emission tomography study. Epilepsia 1996;37(6):515–21.

[62] Fulham MJ, Brooks RA, Hallett M, et al. Cerebellar diaschisis revisited: pontine hypometabolism and dentate sparing. Neurology 1992;42(12): 2267–73.

[63] Sobesky J, Thiel A, Ghaemi M, et al. Crossed cerebellar diaschisis in acute human stroke: a PET study of serial changes and response to supratentorial reperfusion. J Cereb Blood Flow Metab 2005;25(12):1685–91.

[64] Shankar LK, Hoffman JM, Bacharach S, et al. Consensus Recommendations for the Use of 18F-FDG PET as an indicator of therapeutic response in patients in National Cancer Institute trials. J Nucl Med 2006;47(6):1059–66.

[65] Yeung HW, Sanches A, Squire OD, et al. Standardized uptake value in pediatric patients: an investigation to determine the optimum measurement parameter. Eur J Nucl Med Mol Imaging 2002;29(1):61–6.

[66] Shields AF, Larson SM, Grunbaum, et al. Short-term thymidine uptake in normal and neoplastic tissues: studies for PET. J Nucl Med 1984;25:759–64.

[67] Shields AF, et al. Cellular sources of thymidine nucleotides: studies for PET. J Nucl Med 1987; 28:1435–40.

[68] Eary JF, Mankoff DA, Spence AM, et al. 2-[C-11]thymidine imaging of malignant brain tumors. Cancer Res 1999;59(3):615–21.

[69] Blasberg RG, Roelcke U, Weinreich R, et al. Imaging brain tumor proliferative activity with [124I]iododeoxyuridine. Cancer Res 2000; 60(3):624–35.

[70] Shields AF, Grierson JR, Dohmen BM, et al. Imaging proliferation in vivo with [F-18]FLT and positron emission tomography. Nat Med 1998; 4(11):1334–6.

[71] Shields AF. Positron emission tomography measurement of tumor metabolism and growth: its expanding role in oncology. Mol Imaging Biol 2006;8(3):141–50.

[72] Chen W, Cloughesy T, Kamdar N, et al. Imaging proliferation in brain tumors with 18F-FLT PET: comparison with 18F-FDG. J Nucl Med 2005; 46(6):945–52.

[73] Teicher BA, Lazo JS, Sartorelli AC. Classification of antineoplastic agents by their selective toxicities toward oxygenated and hypoxic tumor cells. Cancer Res 1981;41(1):73–81.

[74] Rice GC, Hoy C, Schimke RT. Transient hypoxia enhances the frequency of dihydrofolate reductase gene amplification in Chinese hamster ovary cells. Proc Natl Acad Sci U S A 1986;83(16): 5978–82.

[75] Scott AM, Ramdave S, Hannah A, et al. Correlation of hypoxic cell fraction with glucose metabolic rate in gliomas with [18F]-fluoromisonidazole (FMISO) and [18F]-fluorodexyglucose (FDG)

positron emission tomography. J Nucl Med 2001; 42(5):678.

[76] Bruehlmeier M, Roelcke U, Schubiger PA, et al. Assessment of hypoxia and perfusion in human brain tumors using PET with 18F-fluoromisonidazole and 15O–H2O. J Nucl Med 2004; 45(11):1851–9.

[77] Lewis JS, Welch MJ. PET imaging of hypoxia. Q J Nucl Med 2001;45(2):183–8.

[78] Chao KS, Bosch WR, Mutic S, et al. A novel approach to overcome hypoxic tumor resistance: Cu-ATSM-guided intensity-modulated radiation therapy. Int J Radiat Oncol Biol Phys 2001; 49(4):1171–82.

[79] Dehdashti F, Grigsby PW, Mintun MA, et al. Assessing tumor hypoxia in cervical cancer by positron emission tomography with 60Cu-ATSM: relationship to therapeutic response-a preliminary report. Int J Radiat Oncol Biol Phys 2003;55(5):1233–8.

[80] Dehdashti F, Mintun MA, Lewis JS, et al. In vivo assessment of tumor hypoxia in lung cancer with 60Cu-ATSM. Eur J Nucl Med Mol Imaging 2003; 30(6):844–50.

[81] Nichols L, Pike VW, Cai L, et al. Imaging and in vivo quantitation of beta-amyloid: an exemplary biomarker for Alzheimer's disease? Biol Psychiatry 2006;59(10):940–7.

[82] Agdeppa ED, Kepe V, Liu J, et al. Binding characteristics of radiofluorinated 6-dialkylamino-2-naphthylethylidene derivatives as positron emission tomography imaging probes for beta-amyloid plaques in Alzheimer's disease. J Neurosci 2001;21(24):RC189.

[83] Shoghi-Jadid K, Small GW, Agdeppa ED, et al. Localization of neurofibrillary tangles and beta-amyloid plaques in the brains of living patients with Alzheimer's disease. Am J Geriatr Psychiatry 2002;10(1):24–35.

[84] Klunk WE, Engler H, Nordberg A, et al. Imaging brain amyloid in Alzheimer's disease with Pittsburgh compound B. Ann Neurol 2004;55(3): 306–19.

NEUROIMAGING
CLINICS
OF NORTH AMERICA

Neuroimag Clin N Am 16 (2006) 605–618

ELSEVIER
SAUNDERS

MR Spectroscopy: Truly Molecular Imaging; Past, Present and Future

Mark E. Mullins, MD, PhD

- Past
  Nuclear MR
  MR spectroscopy history
  Molecular imaging
- Present
  MR spectroscopy techniques
  MR spectroscopy applications
  Disease processes

- *Interpretation*
  MR spectroscopy performance literature
  Potential pitfalls
- Future
  MR spectroscopy future applications
  Outlook for the future
- Summary
- References

MR imaging has its origins in nuclear MR (NMR) examinations. NMR examinations give typically one- and two-dimensional maps of peaks, which represent a manifestation of the underlying molecular structure. In this way, it is like a map or jigsaw puzzle that suggests the structure of the molecule(s) within the sample chamber. After years of study and innumerable technical innovations, NMR begat MR imaging, and images of organs such as the brain could be obtained. The legendary story goes that patients did not like the word nuclear in the description of the examination, and thus the name changed to MR imaging. For awhile, one- and two-dimensional spectra were no longer obtained or provided with clinical MR imaging examinations. In recent years, it became evident that further characterization of tissues evaluated on MR imaging with such techniques as classical NMR may be useful. That is, MR imaging provided anatomical data and the NMR data may be useful to determine what may be the dominant molecular structure in a region examined clinically. Thus, NMR technology became attractive to clinicians yet again, and its resurgence is manifested as MR spectroscopy.

This is MR spectroscopy's past. Its present use involves a plethora of technical variations and predominant use in neuroimaging to complement anatomical data provided by the conventional and functional clinical MR imaging examinations. Its future is uncertain, but many are optimistic that technological advances will continue to make the examination work more universally and provide more clinical impact to a greater number of patients.

Past

Nuclear MR

History

NMR involves the analysis of one-, two-, or three-dimensional spectra produced when a sample is placed into an external magnetic field. Electromagnetic pulses are applied to the sample, and a probe is used to obtain the resultant signal emitted by the sample using complicated mathematical, physical, and engineering principles. In theory, the signal produced by the sample is indicative of the substance being examined. In practice, pure chemical

Department of Radiology/B-115, Emory University Hospital, 1364 Clifton Road Northeast, Atlanta, GA 30322, USA
E-mail address: mark.mullins@emoryhealthcare.org

samples under strict conditions may be shown to have characteristic spectra; however, living systems are, by their very nature, chemically complex. Thus, most living tissues and systems produce spectra that are a combination of their chemical constituents, overlapping one another and with relative intensities that reflect their inherent signal strength (this may vary from substance to substance) and their relative concentrations (ratios). Techniques have been derived to improve solid-state tissue analysis, such as magic angle spinning (HR-MAS) [1]. Despite these improvements, engineering requirements obviated scanning people in traditional NMR scanners, and thus MR imaging was developed specifically so that patients may be imaged safely and with resultant anatomical images that reflect their internal structures. Commercially available 1.5 Tesla field strength magnets intended for clinical use have been available since 1985 [2].

Several journal articles have been written on the history and application of MR spectroscopy [3–8]. For example, Burt and colleagues have made an excellent table regarding the chronology of events of interest in MR spectroscopy [3], and Gillies and Morse have a table of MR spectroscopy-relevant isotopes and some of their characteristics [6].

Basic technology

Some atomic nuclei are susceptible to perturbations when placed in a magnetic field. When the field is varied in a predictable pattern, some structural or chemical information may be available from how the nuclei react to the changes. This was the basis of NMR.

Historically, NMR has been performed routinely with a standard electromagnet maintained by a liquid coolant system, either nitrogen or helium. This necessitates safety considerations for both magnetic effects and also for the potential of quenching a magnet, which refers to potential dangers of liquid gas release or the effects of the magnet and system heating up too quickly or too much. The sample is placed into a container and placed into the sample cavity at the center of the magnet. A probe and other electronic equipment connect the magnet and sample to a computer that performs electromagnetic pulsations to interrogate the sample. Commercially available NMR set-ups have been around almost as long as the technology itself.

On a one-dimensional NMR spectrum, the peaks represents signal from a particular type of nucleus. In most instances, the Y axis is denoted as intensity; this could be given absolute measurements of spins (NMR-active nuclei) or concentration if an external or internal standard is available to calibrate. The X axis denotes magnetic field. Area under a peak

thus relates to the number of nuclei that have similar physical characteristics (both inherent and caused by adjacent structures).

Basic applications

Most frequently, NMR was performed to assess the signal associated with protons within a sample as a means of assessing some aspect of structure, usually chemical identity. The choice of protons for primary NMR was simple. Hydrogen and carbon were the most common atoms in most human tissues. The active isotope in hydrogen NMR (proton) was also the most common, approximating 100%, and the inherent signal strength of the proton was excellent. The latter two reasons contributing to strong signal—at least compared with other atoms and isotopes that could be considered. Thus, protons became the workhorse of human NMR, as they are for most living systems.

Historically, NMR was used to interrogate chemicals to ascertain chemical structure and purity. Initially, only one-dimensional NMR technology was available and detailed evaluations of complicated systems were challenging. Two and three-dimensional techniques spread out the peaks and accentuated their interactions, thus improving the resolution of the NMR examination.

Thus began the trend toward analyzing complicated chemical systems. By its very nature, human tissues fell into this category. Research was performed to assess whether NMR could determine reliably important chemical or structural aspects of biological systems in an ex vivo fashion. Several studies have shown promise but have not been amenable to universal validation, at least not yet.

The relationship of nuclear MR to clinical MR imaging

The fundamental physical principles of NMR and MR imaging were the same. Atoms of interest (typically protons, even more so in MR imaging) were placed into an external magnetic field. Electromagnetic variations were applied, and signal emitted from the patient (source) gave data that related to its structure and chemical composition. In MR imaging, position data were obtained through magnetic gradients; this localization was unavailable in NMR. Thus, NMR and MR imaging are truly molecular imaging examinations. Historically, MR imaging added anatomic data, because the position information in the examination allowed formation of images instead of peaks. This made it more generally interpretable than an NMR spectrum. Pathology data could be obtained by using different MR imaging sequences, thus adding at least simple functional data to the interpretation.

MR spectroscopy history

In this manner MR imaging had developed to make the NMR data simpler to interpret for the general viewer; it was on an anatomical framework in a picture that could be viewed akin to dissecting a patient in the plane of interest. Some clinicians and researchers wondered if it was simplified it too much. Otherwise, were there some data in the NMR spectrum that could be overlooked by using the routine MR imaging alone? Many researchers worked on performance and interpretation of single-voxel (one-dimensional spectra performed within a single volume/cube of interest) and multiple voxel (similar but using many adjacent voxels, also called chemical shift imaging [CSI] [9] to allude to the fact that the individual peaks have an effect on each other, thus resulting in a hopefully characteristic spectrum) spectroscopy during MR examinations. This was essentially the start of clinical MR spectroscopy.

Molecular imaging

MR spectroscopy is truly molecular imaging; molecular structure is interrogated by an electromagnetic field and some very complicated technology to elucidate the relative presence, absence, and ratio of certain metabolites. Once the location of the area to be interrogated is set by the MR scanner controller (usually the MR technologist in concert with the radiologist), a screen save of the area of the voxel overlaid on a conventional MR image will allow all subsequent viewers to see what portions of the body are being evaluated. After the examination is performed, and the data are presented in a one-dimensional spectrum, it may be presented by itself or overlaid on conventional MR images; the latter is, again, called CSI. One step further is to have a computer assess ratios of one or more metabolites and place this on a color-coded overlay superimposed upon a conventional MR imaging. This is a metabolite map, and it makes it easier to illustrate distribution of metabolite abnormalities. A primary goal of molecular imaging is to image particular images to determine their distribution and thus pathology that may be associated with their presence, absence, or relative ratio compared with other metabolites. MR spectroscopy addresses this primary goal specifically. The classical example is in brain tumor imaging.

Present

MR spectroscopy techniques
Sequences
Single-voxel acquisition is usually cubic in its overall shape and encompasses 2 to 3 cc volume [10].

Multiple-voxel MR spectroscopy may be performed by a series of one-dimensional examinations or slab, simultaneous two-dimensional examinations; it usually encompasses 0.5 to 1 cc per voxel [10].

Long echo time sequences tend to provide a better (less noise) baseline than short echo time sequences on MR spectroscopy, but there are several molecules that are detected better with short echo time imaging, most notably myoinositol [10]. As a result, some MR centers acquire long echo time images as a default and add or replace long echo time with short echo time sequences if there is a known or suspected issue that may be elucidated better on short echo time MR spectroscopy.

Full discussion of techniques such as point-resolved spectroscopy (PRESS), stimulated echo acquisition mode (STEAM), magnetic resonance spectroscopy imaging (MRSI), image-selected in vivo spectroscopy (ISIS), OSIRIS (modified ISIS) and spectral editing are available elsewhere [4,6].

Equipment
Theoretically, practically any strength MR scanner may be used to perform MR spectroscopy. As signal strength varies directly with the square root of the magnetic field, however, there is an improvement in signal-to-noise ratio (SNR) as MR scanner magnetic field strength is increased [2]. Typically, 1.5 and 3 Tesla MR scanners are used. One added benefit of increased magnet strength is the ability to spread out the peaks; this in turn makes it easier to discern what metabolites are present within the sample [2]. At this point, there are insufficient data to assess whether additional increases in magnetic field strength will make any difference for clinical MR spectroscopy.

Most MR spectroscopy packages are simply additional software to add to modern MR scanners. Older scanners may have to be refitted with additional hardware, and one should check with MR technologists and vendors as to the details of one's particular system(s). The cost of these upgrades is widely variable. When deciding how to outfit new equipment purchases, consideration of single and multiple voxel capability should be entertained.

Patient preparation
No specific additional patient preparation beyond that for the MR examination itself is usually necessary. Confirmation from local MR staff is recommended.

Time
The length of time necessary to perform the additional MR spectroscopy sequences varies, but most modern MR systems can perform routinely adequate scanning in 5 to 15 min. The author

recommends spending time carefully shimming before MR spectroscopy as he has found that some instances of failed or technically indeterminate MR spectroscopy results may be salvaged by improved shimming. This typically is done routinely just before MR spectroscopy. Postprocessing typically is automated on many modern systems and is commercially available.

MR physicist

In the author's experience, having a physicist who is assigned the primary duty of optimizing and troubleshooting the MRS process is invaluable. In some cases, this can be the difference between success and failure for one's MR spectroscopy program(s). Depending on the size of one's practice, however, this may not be feasible. Consideration of continued and dedicated vendor support may be another option.

Controversies of technique

Pre- versus postcontrast imaging It is generally preferable that MR spectroscopy be performed before contrast material administration. The reasoning behind this is largely theoretical and suggests that the MR spectroscopy results may be biased by the presence of the contrast material and thus potentially misleading. For practical purposes, this potential bias has not been proven; thus this remains a controversial issue. In many instances, however, it is of clinical interest that a particular area be targeted for MR spectroscopy, and this is performed best after contrast material has been given when postcontrast T1-weighted imaging helps to identify areas of interest for interrogation (MR spectroscopy voxel placement). When multiple voxel technology is used, this becomes less of an issue, because more of the brain is evaluated during the MR spectroscopy examination, thus decreasing the chance that an area would not be evaluated adequately. In terms of practicality, many commercial vendors use the same head coil for the remainder of the MR imaging examination as they do for MR spectroscopy, thus reducing the need for interrupting the scan to change a coil for MR spectroscopy before finishing with post-contrast imaging.

Single versus multiple voxel MR spectrscopy Some radiologists prefer single-voxel MR spectroscopy, whereas others prefer multiple-voxel MR spectroscopy. Some decide on which technique to use depending upon what the clinical question is at hand. For example, the author performs single-voxel MR spectroscopy placed at the lentiform nucleus (deep gray matter), centrum semiovale (white matter), and bilateral parafalcine cortex (gray matter) to evaluate for potential metabolic disorders

such as mitochondrial disorder. In a postoperative and post-radiation brain tumor patient, however, the author may perform focused single-voxel MR spectroscopy if there is a particular area of interest such as a new nodule at the resection cavity margin. Alternatively, the author may perform multiple-voxel MRS to survey for a recurrent or progressive tumor that may appear in an area that otherwise would not suggest significant pathology (normal-appearing white matter or unenhancing T2 and fluid-attenuated inversion recovery [FLAIR] hyper-intensity). Depending on the vendor, single- and multiple-voxel MR spectroscopy may take different times to perform and process. This varies, and one should check with MR technologists about the potential times for each. This may have an effect on whether the examination is effective, as patients may tend to move more during longer examinations. MR spectroscopy typically is performed at the end of a lengthy MR imaging examination in any case; any time saved may benefit the patient and should at least be a consideration. Technical adequacy has been cited by some as being better with one or the other approaches; however, the author's experience has been that with adequate shimming for both single and multiple voxel MRS that there appears to be no particular trend favoring one or the other. Thus, this is an issue probably best assessed on an individual basis until further study and technological advances are available.

MR spectroscopy applications

Peaks on proton MR scanning [11] (Fig. 1)
Myoinositol (MI): 3.56 ppm This is believed to be an osmolyte that is found primarily in astrocytes [12]. Castillo and colleagues have observed that myoinositol is relatively higher in low-grade gliomas and lower in higher grade tumors such as anaplastic astrocytoma and glioblastoma multiforme [12].

Choline (CHO): 3.2 ppm This generally is related to the synthesis of cellular membranes and thus a metabolic sign of membrane molecular breakdown when abnormal on MR spectroscopy. Croteau and colleagues have said that "choline-containing compounds seem to correlate with alteration in phospholipids membrane turnover, cellular density, and possibly proliferative activity [13]." This being said, Gillies and Morse contradict that choline is a marker for proliferation, and thus, this is controversial [6]. This peak is actually a combination of several resonant peaks for molecules containing choline including phospholipids [11].

Creatine (CRE): 3.0 ppm This generally is related to cellular energy states and intracellular

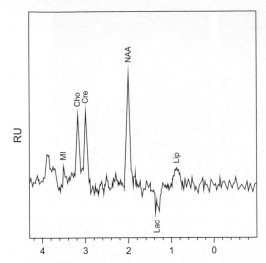

Fig. 1. Idealized one-dimensional spectrum showing the most commonly encountered peaks in clinical practice and their relative positions. Note: for illustrative purposes only, it would be very unusual to encounter such a spectrum in real life. See **Figs. 2–6** for examples of actual patient data.

metabolism [11]. Thus, it is a sign of intracellular energy stores and what the author calls "chemical health." Like CHO, this peak is actually a combination of several resonant peaks for molecules containing creatine including phosphocreatine [9].

N-acetylaspartate (NAA): 2.0 ppm This is believed to be located primarily within neurons [11,14] although some believe that oligodendrocytes may contain some NAA. In general, normal NAA is a sign of neuronal mass and integrity [14] or neuronal viability [9]. The converse is believed to be true also; that is, absence of normal NAA signal is a sign of neuronal degradation. It also may play some part in lipid synthesis [9].

Lactate (LAC): 1.3 ppm This is a product of anaerobic metabolism (glycolysis [11]) and thus a sign of nonoxidative metabolism. Although this can be seen in small amounts normally in some physiological states of the central nervous system (CNS) (such as newborn brains, if everything else appears normal on the conventional imaging and remainder of the MR spectroscopy examination), it can be a sign of abnormal blood flow (including hypoxia, anoxia, or infarct), abnormal metabolism (lactic acidosis or lactate-producing genetic metabolic disorders), and necrosis (tumor, treatment, and combined tumor and treatment).

Lipids (LIP): 0.9 ppm Lipids are found normally within cell walls and usually not evident on normal spectra. When evident, they are generally thought to be related to cellular membrane breakdown [11].

Disease processes

In general, MR spectroscopy is used much more specifically for imaging of the brain than for any other part of the body; this strongly affects the physiologies and pathophysiologies that have been studied and that are evaluated routinely. There are several reasons for this, including but not limited to:

- The brain remains relatively stationary (as compared with the heart, for example).
- Pulsation artifact from blood flow is minimal.
- There is a paucity of fat and gas juxtaposed against the brain parenchyma (these tend to artifactually degrade the MR spectroscopy signal and may make it uninterruptible).

One of the benefits of MR spectroscopy may be that its added diagnostic influence may help to avoid some staged surgeries (eg, brain biopsy followed by brain surgery or aspiration of an intracranial collection [Fig. 2] followed by a more invasive debridement).

Brain lesion characterization before treatment

MR spectroscopy may assist in the preoperative characterization of intracranial lesions [11]. For example, a lesion may be nonspecific on conventional MR imaging with a differential diagnosis of tumor versus encephalitis versus direct seizure effect or low-grade gliomas versus demyelinating plaque (Fig. 3) [5,10,11,15–17]. In many instances, the MRS may be of assistance to identify molecular signatures that suggest one particular diagnosis from the differential diagnosis or consideration of a diagnosis not heretofore considered.

In particular, MR spectroscopy is useful to characterize high- and low-grade primary brain tumors or gliomas [11,13,17,18]. The classical MR spectroscopy signature for a low-grade primary brain tumor is slightly elevated choline:creatine peak ratio at about 3:1, decreased NAA, and no lactate. The classical MR spectroscopy signature for a high-grade primary brain tumor is markedly elevated choline:creatine peak ratio at 3 to 10:1, decreased NAA, and possible lactate (Figs. 4 and 5). Krieger and colleagues have reported that MI detected within an intraventricular tumor in a pediatric patient suggests choroid plexus papilloma and that this observation is not only useful for preoperative evaluation, but also for follow-up surveillance [19]. Metastases are more variable on MR spectroscopy but tend to have decreased NAA and no lactate. It is important to remember that choline elevation in and of itself is quite nonspecific and may be seen in various disorders including malignancy and inflammation.

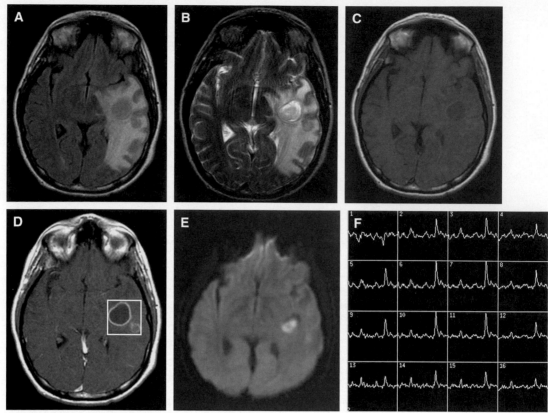

Fig. 2. 56-year-old man with headache, otherwise normal history, physical examination, and laboratory work-up. MR examination of the brain without and with contrast material reveals extensive axial FLAIR (*A*) and axial T2-weighted imaging (*B*) hyperintensity most consistent with vasogenic edema, abnormality on axial T1-weighted imaging (*C*) that is clarified as ring-enhancement with a satellite lesion on axial postcontrast T1-weighted imaging (*D*). There is central hyperintensity on axial diffusion-weighted imaging map (*E*) and hypointensity on apparent diffusion coefficient map (not shown). Multiple voxel MR spectroscopy (*F*) is remarkable for markedly decreased creatine and NAA, decreased choline, elevated lipids, and some lactate (voxel 1). See the text for expected clinical implications of these peaks. This constellation of findings is most consistent with a pyogenic abscess, and pus containing *Staphylococcus aureus* was aspirated at surgery.

Preliminary work with MR spectroscopy also has been used to identify potential abnormalities within the mesial temporal lobe in patients who have epilepsy [20].

Brain tumor imaging after treatment, especially radiation

After surgery, chemotherapy, and radiation therapy, it may be difficult to determine what areas on the follow-up imaging of the brain represent predominantly tumor (Fig. 6), predominantly radiation necrosis, or a combination [13,21]. This has implications for the patient's clinical management, and surgery may be contemplated to obtain pathological proof if the imaging and clinical scenarios are unclear. On MR spectroscopy, necrosis most classically is manifested as a decrease in all peaks, perhaps with some added lactate. Thus, the addition of MR spectroscopy, placed at appropriate

locations as governed by the conventional imaging, may help the radiologist and thus the treatment team to assign a more accurate diagnosis to new or persistent lesions and to help guide surgical biopsy, if that option remains viable and indicated after the imaging work-up [13,18,21]. Anecdotally, the author found that MR perfusion data are complementary to this type of differentiation also.

Metabolic diseases

Metabolic derangements sometimes result in particular characteristic MR spectroscopy signatures. Occasionally, there is an overabundance of a metabolite such as lactate, which suggests a mitochondrial disorder when located at the basal ganglia, or NAA, which suggests Canavan's disease [8]. Decrease in normal metabolites such as NAA also may signify a metabolic disorder, but they are typically more nonspecific until other peaks are

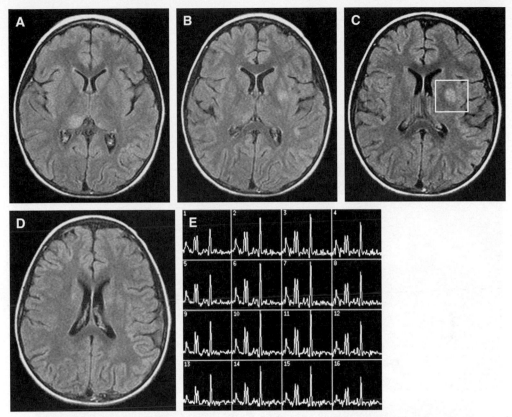

Fig. 3. 27-year-old man with altered mental status. MR examination of the brain without contrast material reveals multi-focal axial FLAIR hyperintensity within the deep and subcortical white matter and the deep gray structures (*A–D*). Multiple voxel MR spectroscopy (*E*) is remarkable for decreased NAA, choline-to-creatine ratio of approximately unity, and no definite other abnormal peaks or ratios. See the text for expected clinical implications of these peaks. This constellation of findings is most consistent with acute disseminated encephalomyelitis, and the patient's symptoms and imaging abnormalities resolved with steroid treatment.

considered, and the MR spectroscopy is interpreted within the setting of the remaining conventional imaging and clinical scenario. Evaluation of NAA and lactate levels has been of interest in chronic liver failure and hypoxic encephalopathy, presumably related to glutamine metabolic derangements [22]. Nelson and colleagues have reported bilateral basis pontis decreased NAA and CRE with elevated CHO in Wilson disease [23].

Abscess

Differentiation between necrotic tumor and cerebral abscess may be difficult. MR spectroscopy may assist in this characterization by identifying peak combinations that are more consistent with one or the other diagnosis. For example, a necrotic tumor may have some residual NAA, whereas an abscess will typically not (unless adjacent brain is included in the voxel). Lactate may be visualized in either necrotic tumor or abscess. Amino acid peaks may be seen with abscess and are typically not seen with brain tumor.

Schizophrenia

Relative amounts of NAA may vary within particular portions of the brain in schizophrenia, perhaps representing neuronal and volume loss [14]. Ratios of metabolites appear to be of more utility than absolute metabolites in the brain MR imaging of patients with schizophrenia [14]. There is no consensus, however, regarding these implications, and further study is thus needed.

Neurodegenerative and dementia disorders

Abnormalities of NAA, choline, creatine, and ratios thereof, with evaluation related to anatomical localization, have been reported in many, different neurodegenerative disorders including Parkinson's disease, multiple system atrophy [24], Alzheimer's disease [7,25], acquired immune dementia syndrome dementia complex [26], autism, and attention-deficit/hyperactivity disorder [27]. As with schizophrenia, however, there is no consensus regarding these implications, and further study is thus needed.

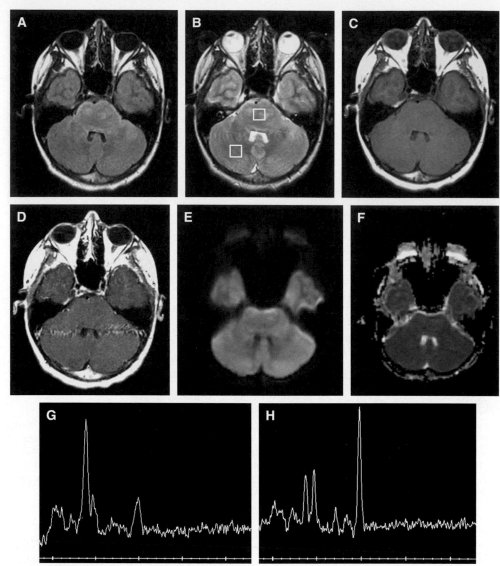

Fig. 4. 5-year-old boy with altered vision symptomatology cranial nerve dysfunction on physical examination. MR examination of the brain without and with contrast material reveals axial FLAIR (*A*) and axial T2-weighted imaging (*B*) hyperintensity within the pons, abnormality on axial T1-weighted imaging (*C*) that partially enhances on axial postcontrast T1-weighted imaging (*D*). There is some irregularity on axial diffusion-weighted imaging map (*E*) and apparent diffusion coefficient map (*F*) without definite restricted diffusion, and this appearance is most consistent with T2 shine-through effect. Single voxel MR spectroscopy (*G*) performed at the site of pontine abnormality is remarkable for markedly decreased NAA and markedly elevated choline:creatine ratio; please see the text for expected clinical implications of these peaks. An internal comparison single voxel spectroscopy image (*H*) performed within normal-appearing brain is overall normal. This constellation of findings is most consistent with high-grade brainstem glioma. This case remains presumptive in diagnosis, as no biopsy or postmortem examination has been performed; presumptive treatment in this context is not unusual.

Interpretation

Maps versus peaks

Traditionally, MR spectroscopy data are presented as a combination of a screen save showing the overlay of the voxel placement(s) on a conventional MR image combined with a separate image with the resultant one-dimensional spectra (that is, peaks).

Information may be extracted from that data to form maps based upon certain parameters. For example, NAA peak intensity may be forged into a color or gray scale map to indicate (relative) intensity overlaid on a conventional MR image. Other popular maps include choline and choline:creatine ratio, but theoretically any individual peak or ratio

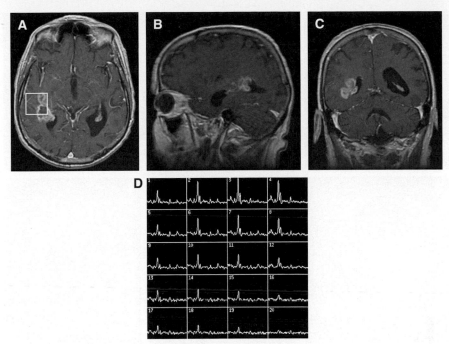

Fig. 5. 55-year-old man with headache. MR examination of the brain with contrast material reveals axial T1-weighted axial (*A*), sagittal (*B*), and coronal (*C*) predominant irregular ring enhancement centered at the atrium of the right lateral ventricle. Multiple voxel MR spectroscopy (*D*) is remarkable for markedly decreased NAA, markedly elevated choline:creatine ratio, and a small amount of lipid signal. See the text for expected clinical implications of these peaks. This constellation of findings is most consistent with high-grade glioma, and glioblastoma multiforme was obtained at surgery.

could be used. Some observers prefer the visual nature of the map, whereas others prefer the one-dimensional peak maps.

Peak heights, ratios, and area under the curve
Unless internal or external standards are used, the intensity yielded by MR spectroscopy cannot be used reliably to indicate a particular concentration of a substance within the area interrogated by MR spectroscopy. If standards are not used, the spectrum then becomes an indicator of the presence (or absence) of a sufficient enough amount of the substance to be identified (also assuming that it should show up on MR spectroscopy). Usually this is in the nanomolar concentration range. Technical problems and much higher concentrations of other compounds within the range of the spectrum evaluated may obscure identification of particular compounds. Once peaks are identified, they may be evaluated individually or in ratios. Clinical MR spectroscopy evaluation has adopted measurement of peak height (relative to the baseline) as an indicator of molecular amounts. In general, the area under the curve better represents the number of spins identified and should be used clinically; however, this involves computer calculations based upon best-fit approximations and thus requires extra

time, and usually, specialized software. Both of these theoretically contribute to increased cost. In most instances, the peak width is sufficiently narrow to make this approximation not egregious.

Correlation to so-called normal-appearing brain
Often, it is preferable to perform spectroscopy in an area of the brain or tissue being interrogated by MR spectroscopy that is unaffected by the primary disease process. In many cases, this involves the contralateral brain hemisphere [13]. This provides a seemingly normal side for comparison. There are several diseases, however, that may result in abnormal MRS in an area that appears normal on other, conventional MR sequences, and is thus likely abnormal [10]. It is important to remember this potential complication of internal comparison. The author prefers to look at this type of data as extra information, yielding identification of abnormal brain tissue elsewhere, not identified by conventional sequences and thus diffuse—also possibly of clinical interest. Additionally, MR spectroscopy results may not be bilaterally symmetrically equal [28], even at baseline, and this potentially could bias interpretation of MR spectroscopy without prior (baseline) examinations

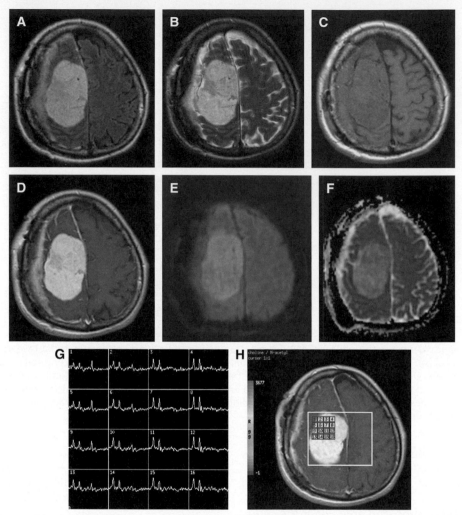

Fig. 6. 47-year-old woman for follow-up status after and before debulking surgery for meningioma. MR examination of the brain without and with contrast material reveals postoperative changes (including edema and an extra-axial collection) at the right convexity with a dominant extra-axial mass that exhibits axial FLAIR (*A*) and axial T2-weighted imaging (*B*) hyperintensity most consistent with vasogenic edema, abnormality on axial T1-weighted imaging (*C*) that is clarified as nearly solid, prompt enhancement on axial postcontrast T1-weighted imaging (*D*). There is lesional hyperintensity on axial diffusion-weighted imaging map (*E*) and mixed hypointensity on apparent diffusion coefficient map (*F*) most consistent with a highly cellular tumor. Multiple voxel MR spectroscopy (*G*) with screen save of the voxel locations (*H*) is remarkable for markedly decreased choline, creatine, and NAA, and myoinositol peak prominence. See the text for expected clinical implications of these peaks. This constellation of findings is most consistent with recurrent meningioma, which was confirmed at surgery.

available for comparison of interval change. The work of Nagae-Poetscher and colleagues provides some reference for absolute measurement of metabolites and ratios within different portions of the brain and suggests that most portions of the brain are indeed symmetric on MR spectroscopy excepting the thalamus and area of Wernicke [28]. Their work also suggests no gender effect [28]. Others, however, have pointed out more extensive regional differences and age-dependent changes [17].

MR spectroscopy performance literature

Does it really add anything to the workup?

This is a deceptively difficult question to address. Generally speaking, there is not incontrovertible proof (as is typically manifested by prospective, blinded, randomized human testing, and pathological proof) in the literature of an added benefit of MR spectroscopy in the imaging evaluation of any patient population. Moreover, such a study may not be forthcoming, as it may not be ethical. Thus, one is left to examine suboptimal results to determine whether MR spectroscopy is indicated and worth the time, money, and equipment that comes with it. Moreover, many disagree on whether MR spectroscopy adds anything to a particular patient's work-up, even anecdotally. Lin and colleagues addressed this topic for neurological diagnosis and neurotherapeutic decision making and came up with the following conclusions:

- **There is added value from MR spectroscopy where MR imaging is positive.**
- **There is unique decision-making information in MR spectroscopy when MR imaging is negative**
- **MR spectroscopy usually informs decision making in neurotherapeutics [7]**

The author feels that future optimized studies are indicated across the board to solidify the case for MR spectroscopy equipment installation, training, performance, billing, and reimbursement.

Potential pitfalls

Pediatrics

If the specific absorption rate (SAR) is considered safe, and the patient is MR compatible, MR spectroscopy generally may be performed on children without specific exclusions based upon age. It is important to remember that the normally maturing brain and CNS not only has variations in signal intensity on conventional imaging over time, but also that MR spectroscopy varies normally. This is of particular importance when evaluating a newborn, where small amounts of lactate may be visualized normally, as well as decreased NAA and increased choline; this constellation of findings in an adult is distinctly abnormal. To date, there does not exist a good reference tool for assessing normalcy of spectroscopy in the same manner that white matter evaluation has been documented. Nonetheless, there are some reference materials in the literature. When in doubt, consider consulting a pediatric neuroradiologist or spectroscopy expert.

Postcontrast imaging

As mentioned previously, there is a theoretical risk that the contrast material will modify the inherent MR spectroscopy results and that this may bias the results and thus the interpretation. There has been no convincing study to show that this should affect clinical results, and thus the decision to opt for the ease of performance of MR spectroscopy at the end of the examination has been adopted. Moreover, Smith and colleagues have studied this aspect and found that there should be no significant interpretive difference [29]. Performing MR spectroscopy before postcontrast images have been performed without reassessing whether additional MR spectroscopy locations should be interrogated may lead to MR spectroscopy not being performed at an area of interest.

Volume averaging, susceptibility and good shimming

In terms of MR spectroscopy, this expression is meant to describe a situation where a voxel includes more than the tissue to be interrogated. In other words, the voxel is contaminated by other tissues or substances (such as the air around the patient or metal hardware from prior surgery). In some instances, the inclusion of these contaminants may make the MR spectroscopy examination technically fail or may produce images that are not of diagnostic quality. In general, this is from the prominent susceptibility of the contaminants. In general, voxels placed near the outside of the patient, air-containing structures (including paranasal sinuses and mastoid air cells), or the skull base (eg, dental amalgam artifact, air outside the patient, and other issues) typically are degraded and may not work. In the author's experience, creative placement of the voxels may help; moreover, it is not completely predictable what MR spectroscopy examinations will work. Thus, as long as the patient is MR-compatible, the author tries to work with the MR technologist to get the voxels placed in such as way that the examination has its best chance of working and being clinically useful. Again, attention to detail is important, and, in the author's experience, good MR spectroscopy starts with good shimming.

A careful assessment of the tissues in the voxels is prudent, as this may affect the resultant MR spectroscopy spectrum and thus the diagnosis. For example, inclusion of the scalp may introduce fat signal. The most common pitfall here is when adjacent brain is included with a lesion; the brain signal may dilute and modify the resultant MR spectroscopy signal such that its interpretation may not be optimized. With single-voxel spectroscopy and lesions smaller than a single voxel, this is a frequent issue. Multiple-voxel spectroscopy provides smaller voxels and a survey of the area. A last word of caution is to remember what may or may not be on one's screensave of the voxel placement: what is not in the plane shown but is included in the voxels. Some vendors provide a triplanar visual representation of voxel placements, but most do not. Thus one must remember to think of what lies a slice or two above and below the slice shown, because these may be included in the area interrogated and manifested on its results.

Placement of voxel

Placement of voxels at the time of scanning and reliable pairing with spectra at the time of interpretation are paramount to effective MR spectroscopy contribution to diagnosis. In some cases, voxels may be standardized to include portions of the body that can be stereotyped and thus taught to the MR technologist so that radiologist participation in voxel placement in these cases is not necessary. The most common situation here is the metabolic protocol, where pictures showing voxels at the biparietal gray matter, centrum semiovale, and lentiform nucleus can be posted for the MR technologists to use. In most other cases, it is preferable to have a radiologist involved in placement of the voxels. This provides the best opportunity for MR spectroscopy to make a contribution to the examination and minimizes the need for callbacks. In some instances, the target is an enhancing lesion, whereas in others it is unenhancing abnormal T2/FLAIR signal. If there are comparison examinations, consider reviewing them to see where the voxels were placed previously and to decide if placing them at the same location is appropriate. If there is a new lesion, additional MR spectroscopy voxel placements may be indicated.

Interpretation in the setting of the remaining information

MR spectroscopy spectra should be interpreted in the setting of the remaining conventional MR images and any additional imaging results and clinical history that is available. MR spectroscopy results may confirm or refute findings and impressions of additional imaging or the clinical scenario. In the author's experience, their specificity improves dramatically if this is done routinely. The converse is also true. In instances where MR spectroscopy and other imaging conflict in their implications, further review of all available data is indicated to discern the clinical implications.

Future

MR spectroscopy future applications

Two-dimensional MR spectroscopy
One of the drawbacks of currently used one-dimensional MR spectroscopy is the noise of the baseline, and this may decrease the radiologist's ability to discern what relevant peaks are present. Certainly, better SNR would improve this determination but, hopefully, SNR has been optimized already (this should be a goal during each and every acquisition). Given this, the idea of spreading out the peaks onto two dimensions, where artifact versus real findings can be elucidated further is at least a potential laudable goal for clinical MR spectroscopy. Moreover, more information about the interaction of a spectrum's peaks may be discerned, and thus, more information may be characterized in

regards to a more specific diagnosis also. It is unclear when, if ever, this technology will be routinely used clinically for MR spectroscopy.

Heteronuclear MR spectroscopy
Most MR spectroscopy is performed using proton nuclei interrogation. Some phosphorous [6,9], very little nitrogen or carbon [3,6,22], and trace fluorine [3] clinical in vivo MR spectroscopy are being performed, even at highly academic research centers. In theory, these spectra could provide more physiologically interesting and potentially important clinical information about molecular states such as pH and energy levels (phosphorous) or nitric oxide and neuronal function in stroke (nitrogen). As with two-dimensional MR spectroscopy, it is unclear when, if ever, this technology will be routinely used clinically for MR spectroscopy.

Noncentral nervous system MR spectroscopy
This technique holds the most promise for the near future. There are articles in the radiology literature that discuss the use of non-CNS MR spectroscopy [6], especially as it pertains to the musculoskeletal (MSK) system [3], prostate tumors [2], and breast imaging [30]. Theoretically, the tissue examined by MR spectroscopy should be relatively immobile, and in terms of molecular signature, it is preferable that the disease processes are known to be quite different from normal, thus simplifying the interpretation. Optimally, the molecular signal also would be specific for a particular disease, but that takes time to acquire cases at a facility and also in the literature to determine what congeners are known to occur. In 2005, Meisamy and colleagues reported that "the addition of quantitative ^{1}H MR spectroscopy to the breast MR imaging examination resulted in higher sensitivity, specificity, accuracy, and interobserver agreement regarding patient treatment compared with the values achieved by using MR imaging alone" [30].

These types of examination are available at some centers, but they generally are thought to be relatively experimental. Local radiologists and MR staff may provide this service and not view it as experimental. The author recommends checking with local MR experts.

Outlook for the future

In the past few years, the length of time necessary to perform MR spectroscopy has decreased dramatically; this has made MR spectroscopy a viable addition to brain MR imaging examinations. Decreased time in the scanner decreases motion artifact and helps maintain patient throughput. The resultant images can be viewed as one-dimensional spectra,

CSI, and overlay maps. Many different molecular substances can be identified with MR spectroscopy, helping with more effective diagnosis. The author believes this trajectory remains quite steep, and he expects the contribution of MR spectroscopy in neuroimaging and other areas of imaging to continue to take increased prominence and importance. Certainly, continued study is indicated to ascertain how MR spectroscopy can contribute to a clinical imaging work-up. Further studies likely will help guide new engineering and clinical applications of MR spectroscopy, and these will help define the evidence base to support reimbursement for its performance.

Summary

Although MR spectroscopy remains somewhat controversial in terms of when and where to use it, many authors believe that it is quite useful. In particular, its use in neuroimaging is well-documented. MR spectroscopy is, by its very nature, molecular imaging, and as such, it should be considered as a continued active participant in the future of radiology.

References

[1] Sakellariou D, Meriles CA, Martin RW, et al. NMR in rotating magnetic fields: magic-angle field spinning. Magn Reson Imaging 2005;23: 295–9.

[2] Schick F. Whole-body MRI at high field: technical limits and clinical potential. Eur Radiol 2005;15: 946–59.

[3] Burt CT, Koutcher J, Roberts JT, et al. Magnetic resonance spectroscopy of the musculoskeletal system. Radiol Clin North Am 1986;24:321–31.

[4] Constantinidis I. MRS methodology. Adv Neurol 2000;83:235–46.

[5] Castillo M. Neuroimaging and cartography: mapping brain tumors. AJNR Am J Neuroradiol 2001; 22:597–8.

[6] Gillies RJ, Morse DL. In vivo magnetic resonance spectroscopy in cancer. Annu Rev Biomed Eng 2005;7:287–326.

[7] Lin A, Ross BD, Harris K, et al. Efficacy of proton magnetic resonance spectroscopy in neurological diagnosis and neurotherapeutic decision making. NeuroRx 2005;2:197–214.

[8] Rudkin TM, Arnold DL. Proton magnetic resonance spectroscopy for the diagnosis and management of cerebral disorders. Arch Neurol 1999;56: 919–26.

[9] Pirko I, Fricke ST, Johnson AJ, et al. Magnetic resonance imaging, microscopy, and spectroscopy of the central nervous system in experimental animals. NeuroRx 2005;2:250–64.

[10] De Stefano N, Bartolozzi ML, Guidi L, et al. Magnetic resonance spectroscopy as a measure of brain damage in multiple sclerosis. J Neurol Sci 2005;233:203–8.

[11] Butteriss DJ, Ismail A, Ellison DW, et al. Use of serial proton magnetic resonance spectroscopy to differentiate low grade glioma from tumefactive plaque in a patient with multiple sclerosis. Br J Radiol 2003;76:662–5.

[12] Castillo M, Smith JK, Kwock L. Correlation of myo-inositol levels and grading of cerebral astrocytomas. AJNR Am J Neuroradiol 2000;21: 1645–9.

[13] Croteau D, Scarpace L, Hearshen D, et al. Correlation between magnetic resonance spectroscopy imaging and image-guided biopsies: semiquantitative and qualitative histopathological analyses of patients with untreated glioma. Neurosurgery 2001;49:823–9.

[14] Tibbo P, Hanstock CC, Asghar S, et al. Proton magnetic resonance spectroscopy (1H-MRS) of the cerebellum in men with schizophrenia. J Psychiatry Neurosci 2000;25:509–12.

[15] Kwock L, Smith JK, Castillo M, et al. Clinical applications of proton MR spectroscopy in oncology. Technol Cancer Res Treat 2002;1:17–28.

[16] Smith JK, Castillo M, Kwock L. MR spectroscopy of brain tumors. Magn Reson Imaging Clin N Am 2003;11:415–29 [v–vi].

[17] Vuori K, Kankaanranta L, Hakkinen AM, et al. Low-grade gliomas and focal cortical developmental malformations: differentiation with proton MR spectroscopy. Radiology 2004;230: 703–8.

[18] Chang YW, Yoon HK, Shin HJ, et al. MR imaging of glioblastoma in children: usefulness of diffusion/perfusion-weighted MRI and MR spectroscopy. Pediatr Radiol 2003;33:836–42.

[19] Krieger MD, Panigrahy A, McComb JG, et al. Differentiation of choroid plexus tumors by advanced magnetic resonance spectroscopy. Neurosurg Focus 2005;18:E4.

[20] Castillo M, Smith JK, Kwock L. Proton MR spectroscopy in patients with acute temporal lobe seizures. AJNR Am J Neuroradiol 2001;22: 152–7.

[21] Weybright P, Sundgren PC, Maly P, et al. Differentiation between brain tumor recurrence and radiation injury using MR spectroscopy. AJR Am J Roentgenol 2005;185:1471–6.

[22] Zwingmann C, Butterworth R. An update on the role of brain glutamine synthesis and its relation to cell-specific energy metabolism in the hyperammonemic brain: further studies using NMR spectroscopy. Neurochem Int 2005;47: 19–30.

[23] Nelson JW, White ML, Zhang Y, et al. Proton magnetic resonance spectroscopy and diffusion-weighted imaging of central nervous system whipple disease. J Comput Assist Tomogr 2005; 29:320–2.

[24] Seppi K, Schocke MF. An update on conventional and advanced magnetic resonance imaging techniques in the differential diagnosis of

neurodegenerative parkinsonism. Curr Opin Neurol 2005;18:370–5.

[25] Cheng LL, Newell K, Mallory AE, et al. Quantification of neurons in Alzheimer and control brains with ex vivo high resolution magic angle spinning proton magnetic resonance spectroscopy and stereology. Magn Reson Imaging 2002;20:527–33.

[26] Yiannoutsos CT, Ernst T, Chang L, et al. Regional patterns of brain metabolites in AIDS dementia complex. Neuroimage 2004;23:928–35.

[27] Castillo M. Autism and ADHD: common disorders, elusive explanations. Acad Radiol 2005; 12:533–4.

[28] Nagae-Poetscher LM, Bonekamp D, Barker PB, et al. Asymmetry and gender effect in functionally lateralized cortical regions: a proton MRS imaging study. J Magn Reson Imaging 2004;19: 27–33.

[29] Smith JK, Kwock L, Castillo M. Effects of contrast material on single-volume proton MR spectroscopy. AJNR Am J Neuroradiol 2000;21: 1084–9.

[30] Meisamy S, Bolan PJ, Baker EH, et al. Adding in vivo quantitative 1H MR spectroscopy to improve diagnostic accuracy of breast MR imaging: preliminary results of observer performance study at 4.0 T. Radiology 2005;236:465–75.

NEUROIMAGING
CLINICS
OF NORTH AMERICA

Neuroimag Clin N Am 16 (2006) 619–632

Diffusion Imaging: Insight to Cell Status and Cytoarchitecture

Thomas L. Chenevert, PhD*, Pia C. Sundgren, MD, PhD,
Brian D. Ross, PhD

Molecular imaging is commonly defined as the ability to localize and measure biologic processes on the cellular and molecular level in the living organism. An imaging probe that essentially "switches on" based on a highly specific biologic event, such as the presence of a targeted gene expressed enzyme, certainly qualifies as a molecular imaging modality. Although diffusion-sensitive MR imaging techniques do not reach this level of biologic specificity, diffusion is often discussed within the context of molecular imaging objectives. Diffusion MR imaging is sensitive to molecular water interactions that occur at the cellular level, and human studies geared to address specific cellular status issues are well within the reach of diffusion MR imaging.

The central contrast mechanism in diffusion-based imaging is molecular mobility. With rare exception, water molecules are the signal source; therefore, water mobility is probed in diffusion-weighted imaging (DWI). In pure water, temperature is the only significant modulator of molecular mobility, and, in fact, diffusion MR imaging has been used to measure temperature noninvasively [1]. Fortunately, tissues are not comprised of pure water, and biologic factors on the cellular level have a strong impact on molecular mobility, which makes DWI a powerful diagnostic tool [2–5]. Indeed, DWI is used extensively in clinical practice owing to its exquisite sensitivity to cellular status, cytotoxic edema, cellular density, and cellular organization of tissues [6–10]. The objective of this article is provide a broad overview of basic methodologies and applications of diffusion MR imaging. Although DWI is commonly performed in routine brain screening examinations and has unique value in the detection of acute stroke, this article focuses on oncologic applications of DWI, which coincides with many of the objectives of other molecular imaging modalities.

This work was sponsored in part by NIH grant P01 CA 85878.
Thomas L. Chenevert and Brian D. Ross have intellectual property related to a portion of the underlying technology.
Department of Radiology, University of Michigan Health Systems, 1500 East Medical Center Drive, Ann Arbor, MI 48109, USA
* Corresponding author.
E-mail address: tlchenev@umich.edu (T.L. Chenevert).

Introduction of MR imaging into clinical practice has been among the most important advances in the radiologic diagnosis of patients, particularly within the neuroimaging arena. Excellent soft tissue differentiation, rapid technologic advancements, and widespread availability of clinical MR scanners have resulted in crucial roles performed by routine anatomic MR imaging. Moreover, by specific design of acquisition sequences, the imaging can be geared to reflect fundamental biophysical, physiologic, metabolic, or functional properties of tissues. A variety of MR techniques are sensitive to tissue perfusion [11,12], vascular permeability [13–16], tissue oxygenation [17–19], cellular status [4,5,9], cellular density [20,21], and microstructural organization [8,22–24], all of which are used in clinical and research studies. Diffusion-weighted sequences are specifically sensitive to cellular status, density, and microstructural organization. Molecular mobility may be exploited to help characterize lesion type, grade, and cellular alteration in response to intervention.

Imaging techniques

Diffusion-weighted imaging

Original diffusion-weighted MR imaging of in vivo systems was performed in the 1980s [2,10,25], and excellent reviews on the technical aspects of diffusion imaging are available from several sources [6,26,27]. A brief qualitative synopsis of diffusion principles is presented herein. Molecular diffusion refers to the thermally driven random translational motion of molecules in media. Diffusion is also referred to as brownian motion in which media viscosity, temperature, and the molecular mass are key elements that determine mobility. Unlike magnetization relaxation (ie, T1 and T2) that drives conventional MR imaging contrast, diffusion is not a magnetization-related process. Nevertheless, MR imaging is clearly the modality of choice to measure noninvasively the effect of diffusion in vivo. Gradient hardware essential to localize tissue signals in conventional imaging also serves to "encode" initial locations of constituents in an ensemble of water molecules in the medium. After a short interval (typically tens of milliseconds), the same gradient hardware "decodes" the molecular locations. If there is any displacement of ensemble constituents over the interval, decoding is incomplete, leading to spin dephasing or signal loss. Dephasing is more pronounced in proportion to the distance translated between encode/decode diffusion gradient pulses. Highly mobile molecules tend to loose signal, whereas immobile tissue environments yield relatively strong signal on diffusion-weighted sequences. Careful determination of the degree of signal loss at various diffusion gradient settings allows one to calculate molecular mobility in the medium, that is, the diffusion coefficient is precisely measurable in simple fluids. In more complex systems, such as tissues comprised of multiple intra- and extracellular compartments separated by semi-permeable membranes, the concept of a single diffusion coefficient is no longer valid. One easy remedy to this complex situation is simply to loosen terminology to measure an "apparent diffusion coefficient" (ADC) when performing diffusion-sensitive sequences on tissues [2,6]. Use of an ADC allows for a myriad of effects that impede molecular motions, such as cell membranes, high cellular packing, and interaction with macromolecules, as well as processes that enhance mobility via active transport, convective motion, and perfusion. Classic theory predicts the average displacement distance of molecules freely diffusing to be SQRT(6DT), where D is the diffusion coefficient and T is the time interval the molecules diffuse. In MR imaging, hardware and other factors typically set the measurement interval to around 50 to 100 ms. Pure water at body temperature has a diffusion coefficient of D $\approx 3 \times 10^{-3}$ mm^2/s; therefore, free water molecules normally migrate a displacement distance of 0.03 mm, or 30 µm, in 50 ms. Considering the fact that the size scale of neurons (ie, short axis) is on the order of a few microns to tens of microns, and that other entities such as membranes, organelles, myelin layers, and macromolecules span yet smaller dimensions, it is reasonable to assume that a given water molecule will encounter many interactions with cellular or subcellular entities over this measurement interval. Transient association of water with large slow-moving macromolecules as well as impediment by membranes and other structures effectively reduce water mobility to an ADC lower than free water diffusion. The greater the density of structures that impede water mobility, the lower the ADC. For this reason, ADC is considered a noninvasive indicator of cellularity or cell density. This is not to say that, between two tissues with different ADC values, the lower ADC tissue necessarily has the greater number of cells per unit volume. Other factors such as cell size, relative extra- versus intracellular volume, and membrane permeability also affect water mobility and ADC. Within a given tissue or cell type, ADC is useful as an indicator of the relative cellularity, such as in the evolution of tumor over time following therapy. Cellular alterations due to disease or intervention, as well as changes in cellular organization or integrity of cellular elements, are available for study by diffusion imaging.

It is truly remarkable that cellular distance scale motions are measurable amidst other much larger physiologic motions. The most widely used DWI acquisition method is single-shot echo-planar imaging (EPI) [28–30] because its speed allows the entire set of echoes for an image to be collected within one single acquisition period of 25 to 100 ms. This imaging method essentially freezes bulk tissue motion that would otherwise overwhelm measurement of molecular motion. The EPI technique is efficient and insensitive to bulk tissue motion, as well as readily available on most contemporary clinical MR imaging scanners. Although EPI virtually eliminates motion artifacts, the images are sensitive to other artifacts such as distortion and signal loss owing to magnetic susceptibility. These limitations aside, EPI is the most commonly used clinical sequence combined with diffusion-sensitization gradient pulses to perform DWI.

Despite underlying complexities related to tissue-water interaction and acquisition technique, measured ADC values of normal neurologic tissues are remarkably consistent across institutions, MR imaging hardware platforms, and operating field strengths as long as comparable acquisition techniques are used. The key acquisition parameter that describes the degree of sensitivity to diffusion is the b-value [2,6]. The b-value increases with gradient strength, duration, and the temporal separation of gradient pulses used to encode and decode molecular positions, and higher b-values yield higher diffusion weighting in the resultant MR image. Usually, two or more b-values are acquired to isolate diffusion effects from other MR imaging contrasts. For most neuroimaging applications, at least one low (b ≈ 0 s/mm²) and high (b ≈ 800–1000 s/mm²) setting are used. DWI acquired with the high b-value will exhibit high mobility

environments (eg, necrotic cyst and cerebrospinal fluid) as dark, whereas environments that impede molecular mobility, such as cellular-dense tissues, will appear bright. In most instances, the high b-value DWI will have contrast that appears reversed to that of the corresponding ADC map because ADC displays intensity in proportion to mobility. As illustrated in **Fig. 1**, highly mobile water in cerebrospinal fluid is rapidly attenuated as the b-value is increased.

Diffusion tensor imaging

The second crucial technical element in diffusion imaging relates to the fact that water mobility in tissues is often highly directional, that is, diffusion in tissue is anisotropic [8,22,31,32]. The greatest natural example of this is diffusion in white matter. Water mobility perpendicular to the long axis of white matter fibers is greatly impeded by the multiple layers of myelin encasing the neuron compared with relatively unimpeded movement of water along the fiber axis. In areas where the white matter tracks are highly organized and omnidirectional, such as in the corpus callosum, the measured diffusion value parallel to the fiber direction is several-fold greater than diffusion perpendicular to the fiber axis. To account for the eventuality of anisotropic diffusion, DWIs along multiple gradient directions are acquired. To interpret DWI and ADC properly in clinical practice, one needs to eliminate anisotropy effects; otherwise, suspiciously high-intensity regions on DWI may simply be artifact related to the relative orientation of normal white matter pathways and the diffusion gradient direction. Fortunately, it is not difficult to acquire and display DWI (and ADC) representing an average molecular mobility without confounding anisotropy effects. The minimum effort to accomplish this is to acquire three high b-value

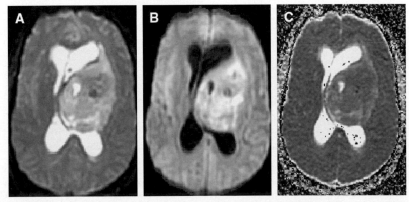

Fig. 1. DWI performed on a 29-year-old man with a high-grade glioma. (*A*) DWI at low diffusion sensitivity b-value ≈ 0 and (*B*) high b-value = 1000 s/mm² show this tumor as hyperintense, suggesting dense tissue. The calculated ADC map (*C*) also indicates water mobility is low in this tumor, consistent with high cellularity.

DWIs along orthogonal directions and one b≈0 image. By proper mathematical combination, rotationally invariant DWI and ADC are generated free of anisotropy effects.

Alternatively, anisotropy may be the specific objective of the diffusion examination, because the presence of anisotropy provides unique insight into microstructural and cytoarchitectural tissue properties. By proper extension in the number of directions probed by the diffusion-sensitization gradient pulses and choice of an appropriate mathematical model, one can generate maps representing the degree of anisotropy in tissue. The diffusion "tensor" is a mathematical construct to describe more fully the mobility of the molecules in anisotropic systems [6,27,33–35]. Because the tensor is symmetric and represented by a 3×3 matrix, at least six unique elements are required to characterize it fully [35,36]. The tensor can be reorganized mathematically or "diagonalized" such that only three non-zero elements ($\lambda1$, $\lambda2$, and $\lambda3$) remain along the diagonal. These elements are known as the eigenvalues and represent the diffusivities along directions of greatest structural anisotropy established by cytoarchitecture. Each eigenvalue is associated with an eigenvector ($\varepsilon1$, $\varepsilon2$, and $\varepsilon3$), where the largest of the three eigenvalues ($\lambda1$) corresponds to the eigenvector $\varepsilon1$ and describes the principal direction of the diffusion at that point, that is, the direction along which molecules move most freely. The concepts of mean diffusivity (ie, ADC) and directional mobility are often represented by a "diffusion ellipsoid," where eigenvalues and eigenvectors provide the size and direction of the principle axes of an ellipsoid as illustrated in Fig. 2.

Diffusion tensor imaging (DTI) yields a rich data set because six independent values are derived for each voxel in the imaged object. Unfortunately, display of an array of ellipsoids as an image is difficult to interpret and is not commonly performed for clinical applications. A common way to summarize diffusion measurements in DTI is the calculation of a parameter for the overall diffusivity and another parameter that reflects anisotropy. The ADC serves for overall diffusivity and is derived from the diffusion tensor by the simple average of eigenvalues (Fig. 2). Anisotropy is usually represented by the fractional anisotropy (FA) or, alternatively, the relative anisotropy (RA) [24,31,33,35]. The FA is a measure of the portion of the magnitude of the diffusion tensor owing to anisotropy, and the RA is derived from a ratio between the anisotropic and isotropic portions of the diffusion tensor. The mathematical definition of the most commonly used anisotropy index, FA, is provided in Fig. 2,

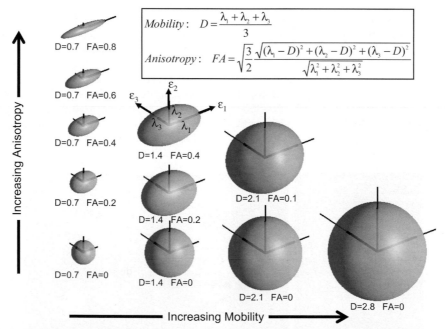

$$Mobility: \quad D = \frac{\lambda_1 + \lambda_2 + \lambda_3}{3}$$

$$Anisotropy: \quad FA = \sqrt{\frac{3}{2}} \frac{\sqrt{(\lambda_1 - D)^2 + (\lambda_2 - D)^2 + (\lambda_3 - D)^2}}{\sqrt{\lambda_1^2 + \lambda_2^2 + \lambda_3^2}}$$

Increasing Anisotropy

D=0.7 FA=0.8
D=0.7 FA=0.6
D=0.7 FA=0.4
D=0.7 FA=0.2
D=0.7 FA=0

D=1.4 FA=0.4
D=1.4 FA=0.2
D=1.4 FA=0

D=2.1 FA=0.1
D=2.1 FA=0

D=2.8 FA=0

Increasing Mobility

Fig. 2. Diffusion ellipsoid representation of anisotropic water mobility in tissues. Mean diffusivity, D (in units of $\times 10^{-3}$ mm^2/s), is given by the average of eigenvalues $\lambda1$, $\lambda2$, and $\lambda3$, which represent the mobility along each of the ellipsoid principle axes denoted by eigenvectors $\varepsilon1$, $\varepsilon2$, and $\varepsilon3$. The direction of greatest mobility is given by $\varepsilon1$ and is often associated with the long axis of neurons in white matter. Fractional anisotropy (FA) (unitless) is commonly used to quantify the degree of anisotropy. Theoretically, FA values can range from 0 to 1, although maximal FA in tissue is approximately 0.8 (eg, in genu of corpus callosum, D = 0.7×10^{-3} mm^2/s, FA = 0.8).

which also serves to illustrate the range of FA values measured in tissues. Typical acquisition techniques on clinical DTI scans yield maximal FA values in highly anisotropic omnidirectional tissue of around 0.8, although maximal FA values typically decrease as ADC increases, as indicated in Fig. 2. From previous work it is known that the water ADC and the diffusion anisotropy differ markedly between pediatric brain and adult brain, and that both parameters vary with increasing age as well as in different regions of the brain [37,38]. The FA and RA are 0.0 for a purely isotropic medium. For a highly idealized anisotropic medium, the FA tends toward 1, whereas the RA tends toward $\sqrt{2}$. Both FA and RA maps can be presented as gray-scale images for the purpose of visual evaluation of patterns of tissue structural order. FA and RA represent intravoxel anisotropy, whereas the lattice anisotropy index measures the intervoxel anisotropy. The lattice measures of diffusion anisotropy allow neighboring voxels to be considered together in a region of interest without losing anisotropy effects that result from different fiber orientations across voxels [24,31].

DTI requires at least six non-collinear diffusion gradient directions plus the obligatory b = 0 image to determine diffusion tensor elements, although, often, many more directions are sampled to improve tensor calculations. High anisotropy values (eg, FA ≥ 0.4) suggest a more omnidirectional microstructural organization. The effective "grain" direction of the microstructure is provided by the principle eigenvector. Maps of anisotropy indices (eg, FA, RA) allow one to inspect the degree of anisotropy but do not indicate directional aspects of the anisotropy; therefore, newer and more sophisticated methods to demonstrate diffusion directions such as directional color coding and fiber tracking as have been proposed [39–43]. By choosing the eigenvector associated with the largest eigenvalue, the principal diffusion direction of the brain structure to be examined can be encoded with color, resulting in directionally encoded (DEC) FA maps. In these color-encoded maps, the white matter tracts are given different colors depending on their different diffusion directions (red = right↔left, green = anterior↔posterior, and blue = superior↔inferior) [40]. Fig. 3 illustrates a high-grade glioma depicted by contrast-enhanced T1 (Fig. 3A), as well as the ADC derived from the trace of the diffusion tensor (Fig. 3B) and FA (Fig. 3C). The DEC FA map in Fig. 3D

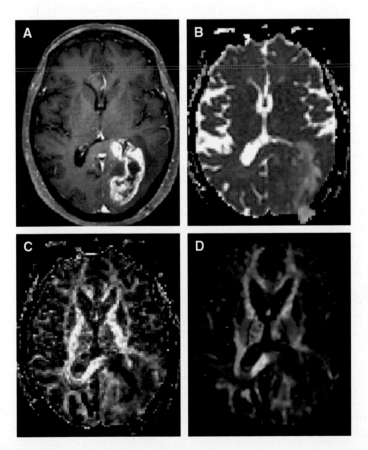

Fig. 3. MR imaging performed on a 62-year-old woman with biopsy proven glioblastoma in the left occipital lobe. (*A*) Post contrast-enhanced axial T1-weighted images demonstrate a large heterogenous contrast enhancing mass in the left occipital lobe with involvement of the splenium of the corpus callosum. (*B*) Moderately low ADC indicates a cellular tumor. (*C*) Low FA indicates random cellular order typical for tumor. Low FA also suggests the tumor has infiltrated white matter of the splenium and destroyed the normally high directional order there. (*D*) Color-encoded FA maps show directionality of remaining white matter tracts (red = right/left, green = anterior/posterior direction, and blue = superior/inferior direction).

contains directional information of the white matter fiber pathways. FA and DEC FA maps facilitate visualization of redirected or infiltrated normal white matter pathways by tumor. FA and DEC FA maps clearly show infiltration and destruction of normal white matter tract pathways in the splenium adjacent to this glioblastoma.

Because FA and eigenvalues are measured at all points in the imaged object, fiber tracking algorithms have been devised to estimate continuity and trajectory of the fibers. These synthetic fibers are then displayed in three dimensions and are often superimposed on anatomic images. Fiber tracking techniques have high potential for applications in neurosurgical planning, neurodevelopment studies, and assessing tumor and lesion invasion of white matter pathways.

Applications of diffusion imaging

Diffusion imaging in tissue characterization

One of the earliest successful applications of DWI and ADC mapping was in the detection and characterization of stroke. As demonstrated by many investigators, DWI offers unique sensitivity to early ischemic damage in the brain [4,5,9]. Moreover, the DWI/ADC response is time dependent such that acute and old ischemic stroke can be distinguished. Acute ischemic stroke exhibits a hyperintensity on DWI (ie, low ADC). One prevalent theory is that acute ischemia leads to cytotoxic edema because cell energetics hinder normal homeostasis, preferentially shifting water to the lower mobility intracellular compartment. Alternatively, active transport within the cell may cease owing to damaged cell energetics, leading to reduction of intracellular ADC. In addition, swollen cells increase the tortuosity of mobility paths in the extracellular space. The state of lower water mobility in acute stroke is quantifiable via the ADC. In normal adult brain, the ADC is $\approx 0.7 \times 10^{-3}$ mm^2/s, whereas in acute ischemic damage in brain, the ADC is reduced by 30% to 40%. As the ischemic tissue ages over days to weeks, vasogenic edema and cytolysis liberate water to yield ADC values greater than in normal brain and may eventually evolve to frank acellular necrosis or cyst with an ADC of 2.5 to 3.5×10^{-3} mm^2/s, consistent with the diffusion coefficient of body temperature water.

In terms of tumors, ADC maps generated from DWI or DTI data have proved helpful in defining solid enhancing tumor, non–contrast enhancing lesion, peritumoral edema, and necrotic or cystic regions from normal surrounding brain tissue. It has been suggested in several studies that ADC values can be helpful to discriminate edema from tumor [44,45], but there are also several examples of the contrary [46–48]. Because of the continuum and overlap in water environments that exist between tumor and edema, it appears unlikely that ADC values alone can differentiate with certainty between peritumoral edema and non–contrast enhancing neoplasm in individual patients [49]. Nevertheless, the observation of progressively increasing ADC from dense cellular tumor to necrotic cyst has been widely observed and is consistent with known histologic properties of tumor. The ADCs for exceptionally cellular dense tumors are 0.6×10^{-3} mm^2/s [50] and 0.78×10^{-3} mm^2/s [47] for medulloblastoma and meningioma, respectively, whereas the ADCs for solid enhancing high-grade glioma span a range from a low of 0.8×10^{-3} mm^2/s (see Fig. 1) to 1.3×10^{-3} mm^2/s [32,47,45]. Edematous brain has an intermediate ADC of 1.3 to 1.4×10^{-3} mm^2/s [32,45,47], and the necrotic core of gliomas typically has an ADC of 1.8 to 2.4×10^{-3} mm^2/s [32,45].

Necrotic regions have the highest ADC values [32,45], whereas contrast enhancing parts of the tumor have lower ADC values, presumably due to the presence of tumor cell elements impeding mobility [51]. Diffusion has also been valuable to distinguish extra-axial cysts from epidermoid tumor, which otherwise have similar contrast properties on non-diffusion MR imaging sequences [52]. A significant increase in mean diffusivity and a significant decrease in FA have been demonstrated in the peritumoral region of gliomas and metastatic tumors when compared with normal appearing white matter [53]. Furthermore, the mean diffusivity of peritumoral metastatic lesions is significantly greater than that of gliomas, whereas the FA values show no discrepancy between tumor and metastasis, suggesting that the FA changes surrounding gliomas can be attributed to increased water content and tumor infiltration [53].

Diffusion imaging in tumor grading

The possibility of differentiating the type and grade of a tumor has also been explored using DWI and DTI in adult as well as pediatric populations. Several studies have shown that low-grade astrocytoma has high ADC values, whereas high-grade malignant glioma has low ADC values, findings reflecting more restricted diffusion with increasing tumor cellularity [20,46,54,55].

It remains uncertain whether anisotropy indices will be able to differentiate tumor type and grade. Tumor cytoarchitecture is predominantly random; therefore, anisotropy tends to be low in tumor. In addition, the large variation in normal tissue anisotropy depends heavily on its location in the brain [31,56], which implies that the contrast of tumor to normal background, as depicted by anisotropy, will be dependent on lesion location. There is justifiable optimism that anisotropy will be valuable in assessing the effect of tumor on normally omnidirectional white matter structures. Mass effect that displaces and compresses white matter tracks as well as destruction of track organization by tumor infiltration have been documented by anisotropy-based diffusion imaging, suggesting that this technology will have a role in presurgical planning [32,41,57,58].

Diffusion imaging to assess tumor cellularity and therapy response

Both intra- and extracellular spaces and their exchange contribute to the measured ADC. Normally the extracellular space is considered to have higher mobility relative to intracellular water; therefore, relatively small changes in the extracellular space have a disproportionately strong influence on ADC. As cellular density increases, the added tortuosity to extracellular mobility paths also reduces water mobility. The inverse relationship between ADC and cellular density has been noted by several groups [20,21,57]. The gradation of increasing diffusion from solid, cellular, viable tumor to the acellular necrotic tumor suggests that the temporal evolution from viable tumor to treatment-induced necrotic tumor may also be measurable by diffusion. Moreover, because molecular and cellular changes precede macroscopic changes in tumor size, it is reasonable to expect that the diffusion assay may be an early response indicator in clinical cancer therapeutics and preclinical drug trials. Indeed, over the past 10 years, many investigators have explored diffusion MR imaging as an indicator of anti-tumor therapeutic efficacy in animal models [20,21,57,59,60,61–64]. Initial studies using diffusion MR imaging to detect changes in water diffusion in animal tumor models following high-dose chemotherapy were found to be promising. As hoped, changes in ADC values were observed to precede changes in tumor volume regression, supporting the potential of this approach to be an early predictor of therapy response. In addition, several clinical studies have shown a correlation between an early change in the ADC and a delayed clinical response to therapy [62,65–68]. Evaluation of the clinical potential of diffusion MR imaging for the detection of early therapeutic-induced changes in tissue structure is ongoing. It is hoped that the use of diffusion MR imaging will provide early evidence of treatment efficacy in individual patients before completion of a given regimen, offering a rational basis to continue effective or discontinue ineffective treatment.

Initial human studies further suggest that diffusion imaging may be a sensitive tool in the evaluation of tumor response to therapy [66,67] and helpful in predicting the chemosensitivity of glial tumors [69] as well as overall survival [70]. These data are supported by other studies demonstrating a significant difference in the mean ADC between responders and nonresponders to therapy, as well as a linear correlation between the relative change in ADC and the normalized change in tumor volume [67]. Early increasing ADC values during therapy are hypothesized to relate to therapy-induced cellular necrosis. The subsequent drop in ADC values within the tumor to pretreatment levels is thought to be an indicator of tumor regrowth. This theory is supported by observations of lower ADC values in contrast enhancing portions of recurrent high-grade gliomas when compared with those obtained in patients with radiation injury and necrosis [71]. The combination of ADC maps and relative cerebral blood volume measurements has been used to evaluate chemosensitivity. Areas of the tumor with the lowest ADC values and highest cerebral blood volume demonstrated a significant volume reduction during treatment, whereas other components of the tumor demonstrated no change in volume [69]. An increase in tumor ADC upon apoptotic cell death has also been noted in animal studies [61,72,73], suggesting this signature ADC change following effective anticancer therapy is reasonably general.

A rapid diffusion change due to cytolysis and possibly vasogenic edema in animal tumor models given single-dose chemotherapy is consistent across many studies. Translation of diffusion indices to monitor treatment of human brain tumors is hampered by the fact that the efficacy of available treatments is generally poor, and human treatments tend to be fractionated over long intervals. Protracted administration of marginally effective treatment may cause overlap in periods of therapy-induced cellular necrosis, excess water and debris clearance, and cellular repopulation by disease progression. To address these issues, some investigations of brain tumor therapy assessment in humans have involved additional methodologic procedures. Pretreatment ADC tumor values alone may predict response to radiotherapy [74]. In a study by Mardor and coworkers, lower ADC tumors were more responsive to radiation than initially high ADC tumors. These same investigators showed that a more detailed analysis of multi-exponential ADC behavior may provide additional diffusion parameters predictive of eventual clinical outcome. At the expense of long scan times, signal attenuation in tumor over many b-values demonstrated that tissue and tumor have multi-valued diffusion components. Often, this behavior is interpreted as a superposition of intra- (low mobility) and extracellular (high mobility) domains. These same investigators showed that the ratio of the high ADC value to the volume fraction of the low ADC domain was a predictor of clinical response [67].

Not surprisingly, tumor heterogeneity is a major confounding factor in assigning a single indicator to patient or tumor response. A given lesion often contains wide gradations of viable cellularity and necrosis, and the response of tumor subregions to treatment is nonuniform and dependent on many factors. Diffusion properties in subregions of the tumor are measurable on ADC maps, but the criteria used to select representative regions become an issue. Histogram analysis of ADC values throughout the tumor is one means to address heterogeneity. Population shifts in voxels stratified by mobility as opposed to location may prove valuable to detect subtle therapy effects.

Cellular changes in tumor after therapy may involve a combination of cell swelling owing to loss of cellular water homeostasis and subsequent necrosis or apoptotic cell shrinkage and death. In addition, there may be a redistribution or resorption of excess water from edema and cysts. The balance of these effects can yield transient and spatially focal reductions and increases in diffusion values. The magnitude of these regional changes may be underestimated by whole-tumor averages. An alternative potential remedy to heterogeneity is proposed in a method referred to as "functional diffusion mapping" (fDM) [75]. A key element of fDM is spatial registration of all three-dimensional image sets into a common geometrical framework. In this way, diffusion changes are measurable on a voxel-by-voxel basis from spatially aligned pretreatment, during treatment, and posttreatment image sets. In recent fDM studies, all images were registered to the initial pretreatment T2-weighted images using an automated mutual information algorithm and affine transformation [70,75]. After image registration, brain tumors were manually contoured, and only voxels identified as "tumor" on pretreatment and 3 weeks after the start of therapy were quantitatively compared. The tumor was further segmented into three different categories representing (1) voxels for which ADC increased by a specified threshold, (2) voxels for which ADC decreased by the same magnitude, and (3) voxels that did not change outside this threshold range (voxelwise scatterplot of ADC pretreatment versus at 3 weeks of treatment as illustrated in Fig. 4B). The specified threshold in these studies was $\pm 55 \times 10^{-5}$ mm^2/s, where the basis for this threshold was empirically determined to be the 95% confidence intervals calculated from normal contralateral brain tissues, including white matter,

gray matter, and cerebrospinal fluid. The fractional volume of tumor in these three categories was then calculated. These fDM-derived volumes represent the relative volume of tumor that exhibits a significant increase in ADC, a decrease in ADC, and no change in ADC, respectively. A key finding of these early studies was that tumors exhibiting a significant change in fDM volumes measured at 3 weeks into treatment were predictive of the radiographic response measured at 10 weeks [70,75]. Moreover, tumor assessment by fDM at 3 weeks into treatment provided an early indicator of the eventual clinical responses of disease time to progression and overall survival in patients with malignant glioma [70]. As exemplified in the case in Fig. 4, fDM also provides a visual indication of regions of the tumor that appear to be responsive to treatment as well as regions unaltered and possibly resistant to treatment. The patient in Fig. 4 was treated for a primitive neuroectodermal tumor by chemotherapy. Signs of heterogeneous response in this patient are the red overlay areas indicating necrosing tumor after treatment, the blue overlay areas indicating decreasing mobility, and the green areas that did not change significantly after 3 weeks of treatment.

Although diffusion processes are independent of MR imaging field strength, the quality of diffusion imaging improves from the signal-to-noise gain at higher magnetic fields. This improvement, in turn, affords efficient exploration at yet greater diffusion sensitivities. Fig. 5 illustrates a patient with a grade 3 anaplastic glioma scanned on a 3-T MR imaging unit with diffusion sensitivity increased to b = 4000 s/mm^2 (Fig. 5A), which is roughly fourfold higher than the sensitivity typically used in most clinical studies. The slope in log (Signal) versus b-value provides a graphical measure of ADC as implicitly performed in standard two-point calculations (usually, b = 0 and 1000 s/mm^2). Inspection of Fig. 5B illustrates that this slope becomes more shallow in tissue at higher b-values. To further illustrate multi-exponential diffusion properties, ADC maps were calculated using b-value pairs of b = 0 and 1000 (ie, "standard" ADC1000) and b = 2000 and 4000 (to yield ADC4000) as shown in Fig. 5C. Although contrast and brightness of the ADC maps were adjusted independently to better show tissue features, the ADC values for normal appearing white matter were ADC1000 = $(0.76 \pm 0.05) \times 10^{-3}$ mm^2/s and ADC4000 = $(0.28 \pm 0.05) \times 10^{-3}$ mm^2/s. These findings suggest that higher b-values may provide yet greater sensitivity to the more solid or cellular elements of the tissue (ie, low ADC) and their subtle alteration owing to therapy, because the signals from cystic necrosis and highly edematous tissues are essentially erased at high b-values. After spatial registration of images,

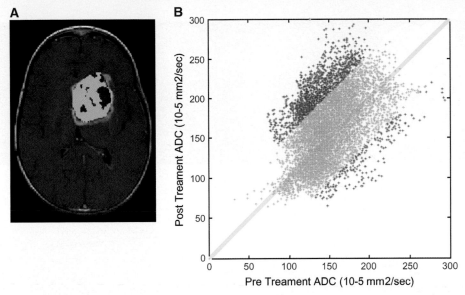

Fig. 4. fDM of a patient treated for a primitive neuroectodermal tumor. (*A*) Pretreatment gadolinium contrast-enhanced axial T1-weighted image with change in ADC values measured 3 weeks from the start of chemotherapy superimposed in color. Voxels that increased ADC by at least 55×10^{-5} mm^2/s are coded in red; voxels that decreased by at least 55×10^{-5} mm^2/s are coded in blue and voxels that did not change outside of this threshold are coded green. (*B*) Scatterplot of ADC pretreatment versus 3 weeks into chemotherapy performed on a voxel-by-voxel basis provides a whole-tumor overview of ADC change. The relative volume of tumor that increased ADC (ie, red voxels) was 17%; the volume of tumor that decreased ADC was 2% (blue voxels); and the volume of unchanged ADC (green voxels) was 81%, which suggests a partial response to stable disease in this patient. The regions shown in red on the anatomic image correspond to tissue that evolved toward necrosis during therapy, indicating tumor zones more responsive to treatment.

the differences in mobility are displayed as color maps in Fig. 5D representing the percent change in ADC1000 and ADC4000 after 3 weeks of chemo-radiation therapy. The region of decreasing ADC in the genu of the corpus callosum is best seen on the change in ADC4000. FLAIR images (pretreatment and at 3 weeks of treatment) indicate significant disease progression in the genu, and DEC FA and fiber track images in Fig. 5E and 5F indicate complete loss of tissue microstructural organization in the genu and tumor compared with contralateral tissues. This technology has the potential to provide rational guidance of spatially directed therapies such as intensity modulated radiation therapy (IMRT) and intratumoral injection of agents [76]. Further evaluation of this technique is warranted to determine whether it is useful for more timely individualization of treatment in clinical protocols.

Diffusion imaging in differentiation of recurrent tumor from radiation injury

Delayed effects of treatment with chemo- and radiotherapy for brain tumors can result in white matter injury. A recent study showed that the mean FA value decreased and the average mean isotropic ADC value increased significantly in normal

appearing white matter in patients treated with radiation when compared with the values found in normal white matter in control subjects [77]. Long-term reduction in anisotropy in normal appearing white matter has also been demonstrated in children treated with combination therapy for medulloblastoma [78]. Although these and other studies suggest that diffusion anisotropy is highly sensitive to microstructural changes that might not be seen on conventional imaging, the pathologic specificity is relatively low. More sophisticated approaches will be required for tissue characterization using DTI.

Newly enhancing lesions that arise on routine follow-up brain MR imaging at the site of a previously treated primary brain neoplasm present a significant diagnostic dilemma. Many lesions do not have specific imaging characteristics that enable the neuroradiologist to discriminate tumor recurrence from the inflammatory or necrotic changes that result from treatment with radiation or chemotherapy. Recurrent tumors and treatment-related changes (ie, necrosis) typically demonstrate enhancement with gadolinium and are commonly surrounded by an area of increased T2 signal. Recent reports have suggested that diffusion

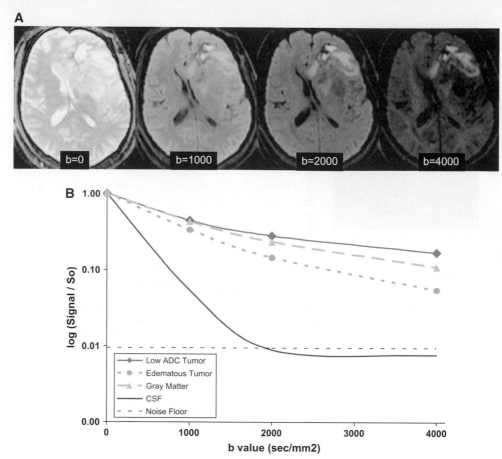

Fig. 5. ADC mapping at high b-values to monitor therapy response in a patient treated for an anaplastic glioma. All images are spatially registered to a common geometric frame. (*A*) DWI acquired on 3 T MR imaging with b-values increasing from 0 to 4000 s/mm² where cellular dense tumor is seen as hyperintense particularly at high b-values. (*B*) Graph of log (Signal/So) illustrates multi-exponential signal loss with increasing b-value and greater relative contrast of low and intermediate ADC tissues. (*C*) Pretreatment FLAIR MR imaging and ADC maps. ADC1000 is calculated from 0 to1000 b-value range and ADC4000 from b-value range 2000 to 4000, which is more heavily weighted to lower water mobility elements of tissue. (*D*) FLAIR MR imaging at 3 weeks of chemoradiation treatment and percent change in ADC1000 and ADC4000 on ± 50% scale (positive values indicate an increase in ADC at week 3 of treatment). The tumor exhibits significant growth over this interval, particularly through the genu of the corpus callosum, which is easily seen as a strong negative change on the ADC4000 map, suggesting a drop in mobility owing to an increase in cellular density. "Zero" ADC values in ventricles and necrosis on the ADC4000 maps result when the signal-to-noise ratio drops below acceptable threshold levels at high diffusion weighting. Zero pixel values are artifactual on ADC maps and are ignored by analysis routines. (*E*) Directional encoded color FA map and (*F*) fiber tracts superimposed on FLAIR image illustrate loss of anisotropy due to tumor infiltration in white matter, particularly in genu of the corpus callosum, which typically has high anisotropy (see DEC FA in **Fig. 3**).

measurements can potentially provide important diagnostic information regarding newly enhancing lesions as well as surrounding areas of signal abnormality that may appear months to years after therapy [71]. In a recent study of 19 patients who presented with new contrast enhancing lesions at or nearby the site of previous treatment, ADC values were significantly higher in patients with tumor recurrence (mean, 1.23×10^{-3} mm²/s) than in

those with treatment-related changes (mean, 1.07×10^{-3} mm²/s) [79]. Contradictions exist in the literature regarding whether an increased or decreased ADC is to be expected in tumor or radiation injury and necrosis. In one study, recurrent tumor showed statistically lower mean ADC values (1.18×10^{-3} mm²/s) when compared with the mean ADC value for treatment-induced necrosis (1.40×10^{-3} mm²/s) [71]; however, other studies

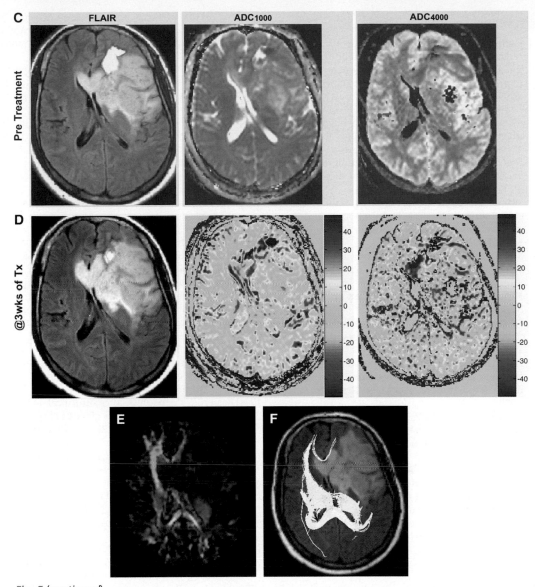

Fig. 5 (continued)

have demonstrated higher ADC in recurrent tumors relative to radiation-injured tissue [7,80,81].

Summary

MR imaging methods such as DWI and DTI based on tissue biophysical properties are rapidly being incorporated in routine brain imaging protocols to improve the diagnosis, characterization, and management of patients with brain tumors. In the future, these methods combined with other physiology-based methods, such as MR perfusion and MRS metabolite mapping, as well as excellent anatomic images are anticipated to improve brain tumor diagnosis, biopsy guidance, pretreatment and presurgical planning, and the assessment of therapeutic efficacy in individuals. In their current form, DWI and DTI yield remarkable insight into tissue and tumor cellularity and organization in a totally noninvasive fashion. In the future, more sophisticated forms of diffusion-based image acquisition and analysis may increase the specificity of these approaches. Existing studies demonstrate that DWI and DTI are indicators of tumor cell density and microstructural organization. Further research is needed to determine how to best use diffusion information to impact positively patient management.

References

[1] Gellermann J, Wlodarczyk W, Feussner A, et al. Methods and potentials of magnetic resonance imaging for monitoring radiofrequency hyperthermia in a hybrid system. Int J Hyperthermia 2005;21:497–513.

[2] Le Bihan D, Breton E, Lallemand D, et al. Separation of diffusion and perfusion in intravoxel incoherent motion MR imaging. Radiology 1988;168:497–505.

[3] Szafer A, Zhong J, Gore JC. Theoretical model for water diffusion in tissues. Magn Reson Med 1995;33:697–712.

[4] Warach S, Gaa J, Siewert B, et al. Acute human stroke studied by whole brain echo planar diffusion-weighted magnetic resonance imaging. Ann Neurol 1995;37:231–41.

[5] Sorensen AG, Buonanno FS, Gonzalez RG, et al. Hyperacute stroke: evaluation with combined multisection diffusion-weighted and hemodynamically weighted echo-planar MR imaging. Radiology 1996;199:391–401.

[6] Le Bihan D. Molecular diffusion nuclear magnetic resonance imaging. Magn Reson Q 1991; 7:1–30.

[7] Le Bihan D, Douek P, Argyropoulou M, et al. Diffusion and perfusion magnetic resonance imaging in brain tumors. Top Magn Reson Imaging 1993;5:25–31.

[8] Moseley ME, Cohen Y, Kucharczyk J, et al. Diffusion-weighted MR imaging of anisotropic water diffusion in cat central nervous system. Radiology 1990;176:439–45.

[9] Moseley ME, Kucharczyk J, Mintorovitch J, et al. Diffusion-weighted MR imaging of acute stroke: correlation with T2-weighted and magnetic susceptibility-enhanced MR imaging in cats. AJNR Am J Neuroradiol 1990;11:423–9.

[10] Thomsen C, Henriksen O, Ring P. In vivo measurement of water self-diffusion in the human brain by magnetic resonance imaging. Acta Radiol 1987;28:353–61.

[11] Wong JC, Provenzale JM, Petrella JR. Perfusion MR imaging of brain neoplasms. AJR Am J Roentgenol 2000;174:1147–57.

[12] Rosen BR, Belliveau JW, Vevea JM, et al. Perfusion imaging with NMR contrast agents. Magn Reson Med 1990;14:249–65.

[13] Schwickert HC, Stiskal M, Roberts TP, et al. Contrast-enhanced MR imaging assessment of tumor capillary permeability: effect of irradiation on delivery of chemotherapy. Radiology 1996;198: 893–8.

[14] Tofts PS, Kermode AG. Measurement of the blood-brain barrier permeability and leakage space using dynamic MR imaging. 1. Fundamental concepts. Magn Reson Med 1991;17:357–67.

[15] Larsson HB, Tofts PS. Measurement of blood-brain barrier permeability using dynamic Gd-DTPA scanning: a comparison of methods. Magn Reson Med 1992;24:174–6.

[16] Weisskoff R, Boxerman JL, Sorenson AG, et al. Simultaneous blood volume and permeability mapping using a single Gd-based contrast injection. ISMRM 1994,1994;279.

[17] Fujita N, Matsumoto K, Tanaka H, et al. Quantitative study of changes in oxidative metabolism during visual stimulation using absolute relaxation rates. NMR Biomed 2006;19:60–8.

[18] Rodrigues LM, Howe FA, Griffiths JR, et al. Tumor R2* is a prognostic indicator of acute radiotherapeutic response in rodent tumors. J Magn Reson Imaging 2004;19:482–8.

[19] Su FC, Chu TC, Wai YY, et al. Temporal resolving power of perfusion- and BOLD-based event-related functional MRI. Med Phys 2004;31: 154–60.

[20] Guo AC, Cummings TJ, Dash RC, et al. Lymphomas and high-grade astrocytomas: comparison of water diffusibility and histologic characteristics. Radiology 2002;224:177–83.

[21] Lyng H, Haraldseth O, Rofstad EK. Measurement of cell density and necrotic fraction in human melanoma xenografts by diffusion weighted magnetic resonance imaging. Magn Reson Med 2000;43:828–36.

[22] Chenevert TL, Brunberg JA, Pipe JG. Anisotropic diffusion in human white matter: demonstration with MR techniques in vivo. Radiology 1990; 177:401–5.

[23] Basser PJ, Pierpaoli C. Microstructural and physiological features of tissues elucidated by quantitative-diffusion-tensor MRI. J Magn Reson B 1996;111:209–19.

[24] Pierpaoli C, Basser PJ. Toward a quantitative assessment of diffusion anisotropy. Magn Reson Med 1996;36:893–906.

[25] Merboldt KD, Bruhn H, Frahm J, et al. MRI of "diffusion" in the human brain: new results using a modified CE-FAST sequence. Magn Reson Med 1989;9:423–9.

[26] Conturo TE, McKinstry RC, Aronovitz JA, et al. Diffusion MRI: precision, accuracy and flow effects. NMR Biomed 1995;8:307–32.

[27] Bammer R. Basic principles of diffusion-weighted imaging. Eur J Radiol 2003;45:169–84.

[28] Mansfield P. Real-time echo-planar imaging by NMR. Br Med Bull 1984;40:187–90.

[29] Turner R, Le Bihan D, Maier J, et al. Echo-planar imaging of intravoxel incoherent motion. Radiology 1990;177:407–14.

[30] Edelman RR, Wielopolski P, Schmitt F. Echo-planar MR imaging. Radiology 1994;192: 600–12.

[31] Pierpaoli C, Jezzard P, Basser PJ, et al. Diffusion tensor MR imaging of the human brain. Radiology 1996;201:637–48.

[32] Brunberg JA, Chenevert TL, McKeever PE, et al. In vivo MR determination of water diffusion coefficients and diffusion anisotropy: correlation with structural alteration in gliomas of the cerebral hemispheres. AJNR Am J Neuroradiol 1995; 16:361–71.

[33] Basser PJ, Mattiello J, LeBihan D. MR diffusion tensor spectroscopy and imaging. Biophys J 1994;66:259–67.

[34] Basser PJ, Mattiello J, LeBihan D. Estimation of the effective self-diffusion tensor from the NMR spin echo. J Magn Reson B 1994;103: 247–54.

[35] Le Bihan D, Mangin JF, Poupon C, et al. Diffusion tensor imaging: concepts and applications. J Magn Reson Imaging 2001;13:534–46.

[36] Basser PJ, Jones DK. Diffusion-tensor MRI: theory, experimental design and data analysis—a technical review. NMR Biomed 2002;15:456–67.

[37] Mukherjee P, Miller JH, Shimony JS, et al. Normal brain maturation during childhood: developmental trends characterized with diffusion-tensor MR imaging. Radiology 2001;221: 349–58.

[38] Pfefferbaum A, Sullivan EV, Hedehus M, et al. Age-related decline in brain white matter anisotropy measured with spatially corrected echo-planar diffusion tensor imaging. Magn Reson Med 2000;44:259–68.

[39] Lori NF, Akbudak E, Shimony JS, et al. Diffusion tensor fiber tracking of human brain connectivity: acquisition methods, reliability analysis and biological results. NMR Biomed 2002;15: 494–515.

[40] Pajevic S, Pierpaoli C. Color schemes to represent the orientation of anisotropic tissues from diffusion tensor data: application to white matter fiber tract mapping in the human brain. Magn Reson Med 1999;42:526–40.

[41] Mori S, Frederiksen K, van Zijl PC, et al. Brain white matter anatomy of tumor patients evaluated with diffusion tensor imaging. Ann Neurol 2002;51:377–80.

[42] Mori S, van Zijl PC. Fiber tracking: principles and strategies—a technical review. NMR Biomed 2002;15:468–80.

[43] Basser PJ, Pajevic S, Pierpaoli C, et al. In vivo fiber tractography using DT-MRI data. Magn Reson Med 2000;44:625–32.

[44] Bastin ME, Sinha S, Whittle IR, et al. Measurements of water diffusion and T1 values in peritumoural oedematous brain. Neuroreport 2002; 13:1335–40.

[45] Sinha S, Bastin ME, Whittle IR, et al. Diffusion tensor MR imaging of high-grade cerebral gliomas. AJNR Am J Neuroradiol 2002;23:520–7.

[46] Castillo M, Smith JK, Kwock L, et al. Apparent diffusion coefficients in the evaluation of high-grade cerebral gliomas. AJNR Am J Neuroradiol 2001;22:60–4.

[47] Provenzale JM, McGraw P, Mhatre P, et al. Peritumoral brain regions in gliomas and meningiomas: investigation with isotropic diffusion-weighted MR imaging and diffusion-tensor MR imaging. Radiology 2004;232:451–60.

[48] Stadnik TW, Chaskis C, Michotte A, et al. Diffusion-weighted MR imaging of intracerebral masses: comparison with conventional MR imaging and histologic findings. AJNR Am J Neuroradiol 2001;22:969–76.

[49] Field AS, Alexander AL. Diffusion tensor imaging in cerebral tumor diagnosis and therapy. Top Magn Reson Imaging 2004;15:315–24.

[50] Rodallec M, Colombat M, Krainik A, et al. Diffusion-weighted MR imaging and pathologic findings in adult cerebellar medulloblastoma. J Neuroradiol 2004;31:234–7.

[51] Krabbe K, Gideon P, Wagn P, et al. MR diffusion imaging of human intracranial tumours. Neuroradiology 1997;39:483–9.

[52] Nguyen JB, Ahktar N, Delgado PN, et al. Magnetic resonance imaging and proton magnetic resonance spectroscopy of intracranial epidermoid tumors. Crit Rev Comput Tomogr 2004; 45:389–427.

[53] Lu S, Ahn D, Johnson G, et al. Peritumoral diffusion tensor imaging of high-grade gliomas and metastatic brain tumors. AJNR Am J Neuroradiol 2003;24:937–41.

[54] Bulakbasi N, Guvenc I, Onguru O, et al. The added value of the apparent diffusion coefficient calculation to magnetic resonance imaging in the differentiation and grading of malignant brain tumors. J Comput Assist Tomogr 2004; 28:735–46.

[55] Kono K, Inoue Y, Nakayama K, et al. The role of diffusion-weighted imaging in patients with brain tumors. AJNR Am J Neuroradiol 2001;22: 1081–8.

[56] Shimony JS, McKinstry RC, Akbudak E, et al. Quantitative diffusion-tensor anisotropy brain MR imaging: normative human data and anatomic analysis. Radiology 1999;212:770–84.

[57] Chenevert TL, McKeever PE, Ross BD. Monitoring early response of experimental brain tumors to therapy using diffusion magnetic resonance imaging. Clin Cancer Res 1997;3:1457–66.

[58] Wieshmann UC, Symms MR, Parker GJ, et al. Diffusion tensor imaging demonstrates deviation of fibres in normal appearing white matter adjacent to a brain tumour. J Neurol Neurosurg Psychiatry 2000;68:501–3.

[59] Galons JP, Altbach MI, Paine-Murrieta GD, et al. Early increases in breast tumor xenograft water mobility in response to paclitaxel therapy detected by non-invasive diffusion magnetic resonance imaging. Neoplasia 1999;1:113–7.

[60] Hakumaki JM, Poptani H, Puumalainen AM, et al. Quantitative 1H nuclear magnetic resonance diffusion spectroscopy of BT4C rat glioma during thymidine kinase-mediated gene therapy in vivo: identification of apoptotic response. Cancer Res 1998;58:3791–9.

[61] Poptani H, Puumalainen AM, Grohn OH, et al. Monitoring thymidine kinase and ganciclovir-induced changes in rat malignant glioma in vivo by nuclear magnetic resonance imaging. Cancer Gene Ther 1998;5:101–9.

[62] Ross BD, Moffat BA, Lawrence TS, et al. Evaluation of cancer therapy using diffusion magnetic

resonance imaging. Mol Cancer Ther 2003;2: 581–7.

[63] Stegman LD, Rehemtulla A, Hamstra DA, et al. Diffusion MRI detects early events in the response of a glioma model to the yeast cytosine deaminase gene therapy strategy. Gene Ther 2000;7:1005–10.

[64] Zhao M, Pipe JG, Bonnett J, et al. Early detection of treatment response by diffusion-weighted 1H-NMR spectroscopy in a murine tumour in vivo. Br J Cancer 1996;73:61–4.

[65] Chenevert TL, Meyer CR, Moffat BA, et al. Diffusion MRI: a new strategy for assessment of cancer therapeutic efficacy. Mol Imaging 2002;1:336–43.

[66] Chenevert TL, Stegman LD, Taylor JM, et al. Diffusion magnetic resonance imaging: an early surrogate marker of therapeutic efficacy in brain tumors. J Natl Cancer Inst 2000;92:2029–36.

[67] Mardor Y, Pfeffer R, Spiegelmann R, et al. Early detection of response to radiation therapy in patients with brain malignancies using conventional and high b-value diffusion-weighted magnetic resonance imaging. J Clin Oncol 2003;21:1094–100.

[68] Mardor Y, Roth Y, Lidar Z, et al. Monitoring response to convection-enhanced taxol delivery in brain tumor patients using diffusion-weighted magnetic resonance imaging. Cancer Res 2001; 61:4971–3.

[69] Jager HR, Waldman AD, Benton C, et al. Differential chemosensitivity of tumor components in a malignant oligodendroglioma: assessment with diffusion-weighted, perfusion-weighted, and serial volumetric MR imaging. AJNR Am J Neuroradiol 2005;26:274–8.

[70] Hamstra DA, Chenevert TL, Moffat BA, et al. Evaluation of the functional diffusion map as an early biomarker of time-to-progression and overall survival in high-grade glioma. Proc Natl Acad Sci USA 2005;102:16759–64.

[71] Hein PA, Eskey CJ, Dunn JF, et al. Diffusion-weighted imaging in the follow-up of treated high-grade gliomas: tumor recurrence versus radiation injury. AJNR Am J Neuroradiol 2004; 25:201–9.

[72] Kauppinen RA. Monitoring cytotoxic tumour treatment response by diffusion magnetic resonance imaging and proton spectroscopy. NMR Biomed 2002;15:6–17.

[73] Valonen PK, Lehtimaki KK, Vaisanen TH, et al. Water diffusion in a rat glioma during ganciclovir-thymidine kinase gene therapy-induced programmed cell death in vivo: correlation with cell density. J Magn Reson Imaging 2004;19: 389–96.

[74] Mardor Y, Roth Y, Ochershvilli A, et al. Pretreatment prediction of brain tumors' response to radiation therapy using high b-value diffusion-weighted MRI. Neoplasia 2004;6:136–42.

[75] Moffat BA, Chenevert TL, Lawrence TS, et al. Functional diffusion map: a noninvasive MRI biomarker for early stratification of clinical brain tumor response. Proc Natl Acad Sci USA 2005; 102:5524–9.

[76] Pietronigro D, Drnovsky F, Cravioto H, et al. DTI-015 produces cures in T9 gliosarcoma. Neoplasia 2003;5:17–22.

[77] Kitahara S, Nakasu S, Murata K, et al. Evaluation of treatment-induced cerebral white matter injury by using diffusion-tensor MR imaging: initial experience. AJNR Am J Neuroradiol 2005; 26:2200–6.

[78] Khong PL, Kwong DL, Chan GC, et al. Diffusion-tensor imaging for the detection and quantification of treatment-induced white matter injury in children with medulloblastoma: a pilot study. AJNR Am J Neuroradiol 2003; 24:734–40.

[79] Dong Q, Sundgren PC, Weybright P, et al. Differentiation of tumor recurrence from radiation-induced necrosis using diffusion tensor imaging. Proc Int Soc MagReson Med 2004;12:2076.

[80] Biousse V, Newman NJ, Hunter SB, et al. Diffusion weighted imaging in radiation necrosis. J Neurol Neurosurg Psychiatry 2003;74:382–4.

[81] Tung GA, Evangelista P, Rogg JM, et al. Diffusion-weighted MR imaging of rim-enhancing brain masses: is markedly decreased water diffusion specific for brain abscess? AJR Am J Roentgenol 2001;177:709–12.

NEUROIMAGING
CLINICS
OF NORTH AMERICA

Neuroimag Clin N Am 16 (2006) 633–654

Molecular Imaging Using Visible Light to Reveal Biological Changes in the Brain

Christopher H. Contag

As biomedical research moves from reductionist approaches to systems approaches, imaging modalities that reveal cellular and molecular changes comprise a key set of technologies to evaluate biology within the context of the living body. The high-density screening methods and large-scale sequencing projects began the process of moving biological investigation from evaluating single genes or single proteins to the next level, were multiple single genes or proteins are analyzed. Approaches to assemble the multi-parameter data sets into coherent patterns of multiple single elements can point to regulatory networks that control given biological processes. The next step in the analysis of the wealth of information generated by multi-parametric analyses performed on excised tissues is to study biological processes using integrated approaches, where the biological context is retained, and the

identified genes, proteins, or mutations can be analyzed in the living body. Spatiotemporal interrogation of cellular and molecular events in the context of the living body is the ultimate form of systems biology, and this is the primary aim in the emerging field of molecular imaging. The emergence of this field marks another transition phase in the era of integrated biomedical research, or systems biology.

Application of molecular imaging to animal models of human biology and disease can provide more predictive information about a biological process than can be obtained in cell culture or using biochemical assays on excised tissues. Before the development of imaging tools for small animals, many animal studies were performed by serially sacrificing subjects at predetermined time points and performing assays on predetermined tissues. The sampling bias inherent in these types of

Departments of Pediatrics, Microbiology & Immunology and Radiology, E150 Clark Center, MC 5427, Stanford University School of Medicine, Stanford, CA 94305, USA
E-mail address: ccontag@stanford.edu

doi:10.1016/j.nic.2006.08.002

experiments includes the times and tissues that are selected based on preconceived notions of the process being studied. To obviate these biases, data need to be obtained in real time using dynamic measures of biological functions that can interrogate all tissues in the body. This is the basis of preclinical molecular imaging. Imaging approaches also can eliminate the variability inherent in studies where each time point is represented by a different group of animals, and this reduces the statistical variation in the data. Because there is a range of established animal models that have been characterized, imaging strategies that can be superimposed on existing animal models will offer advantages over those that require significant modifications to, or redevelopment of, an animal model. The use of visible light and relevant reporter molecules can be used with existing animal models to refine and accelerate their study.

Real-time access to cellular and molecular information in intact tissues and organs of animal models enables the researcher to observe mechanisms of action or cascading events within the animal that otherwise would not be detected using conventional methods. These imaging approaches have been based on imaging modalities that already are used clinically; however, numerous tools have been developed specifically for the study of small animal models of human biology and disease [1–5]. The major advances in small animal imaging have been based largely on the use of visible light, which offers the advantages of rapid and high throughput measures of biological function using relatively low-cost instrumentation with tremendous sensitivity. Because of their ease of use, the optical imaging methods have had and will continue to have an impact on drug studies where it is necessary to evaluate disease process in models with intact biological pathways that interact with the potential therapies. The complexity of the regulatory networks in disease processes needs to be studied in the context of intact organs and living tissues and cannot be modeled readily in culture.

The emerging optical imaging techniques have the potential to reveal steps in biological pathways in mouse models of human biology and disease. Optical imaging of intact animals has been applied to the study of infectious processes, host response to infection, hematopoietic reconstitution, tumor vascularization, response to chemotherapy, antitumor immune responses to therapy, and tissue regeneration [3,4,6,7]. This article describes the basis of the optical imaging methods, describes those that have been applied to small animal studies, and discusses potential applications for optical imaging in the clinic.

Cellular and molecular biology as a basis for in vivo optical imaging

Large-scale sequencing efforts and tremendous advances in high-density screens and gene expression studies have identified many key elements in physiology and disease [8]. Understanding these elements in biology or in the context of the disease processes requires integrative approaches where the context of living cells and tissues are preserved. This has been the driving force behind the development of methods for studying biology in live cells and thick tissues [9–12], and more recently for the emerging field of molecular imaging, in which tools are being developed to reveal cellular and molecular changes in the living body. Complex biological responses consist of coordinated expression of multiple interrelated genes, proteins, and biological pathways, where expression of a gene and its protein product may depend on a regulatory cascade involving multiple cell types, some of which are recruited into the site, and some of which are resident in the tissue. The true spatiotemporal patterns of expression for a specific gene in this dynamic environment may, therefore, only be understood through imaging where the organs, tissue structure and circulation remain intact. Reconstructing the pathways and networks that are comprised of multiple single elements will require technological advances and a systems approach to biology beyond the capabilities of today. It likely will involve a linkage between multiplexed ex vivo and in vivo assays. Imaging approaches that can be used to monitor biochemical events in living cells is emerging as an integral part of systems biology, and optically based imaging methods will be at the forefront of these developments, given their ease of use, amenability to multiplexing, and their availability for biologists. The transition to clinical imaging is more limited for optical imaging tools because of the attenuation of visible light by mammalian tissues, but the insights gained from animal models will be invaluable for clinical advances.

Cell biology has consisted largely of assays on cell lysates and tissue extracts and live cell assays using vital dyes and reporters with microscopy. This has formed the foundation of in vivo optical imaging, where instruments are used to detect the signals from reporter genes and vital dyes from outside of the animal's body. Important temporal changes and patterns of activity have been revealed in live animals using these approaches. In vivo studies of biological processes, however, typically have used only single markers, and although the influences on these reporters are multi-fold, the readout has remained largely singular.

Correlative cell culture assays

Ready-made validation assays exist for the new imaging approaches because of the shared roots in molecular and cell biology. These consist of correlative cell culture assays, where the probes and dyes used in vivo can be evaluated in cells in culture as a means of developing an imaging strategy before in vivo use of the imaging approach, and also after imaging for validation. Preimaging cell culture correlates can be used to design probes and test their validity, and then postimaging validation can be performed using biochemical assays on tissue lysates using well-established measures of enzyme activity, mRNA, and protein levels [13,14]. The data obtained in vivo have tremendous utility for selecting the times, and tissues for analyses can be selected based on the image data or cell numbers. This image guidance can be used to improve the data set by confining the study to the relevant times and tissues. The new advances in imaging are based on advances in cellular and molecular biology, and the tools of these fields are essential components of the field of molecular imaging.

Imaging of small animal models has gone through transitions that are similar to those that have occurred in the field of cell biology. Initially, tools like radiograph imaging were developed to see dense structures such as bone, and then contrast-enhanced CT, MR imaging, and ultrasound (US) were developed to obtain soft tissue contrast. Such structural analyses have proven extraordinarily useful in the clinic, and development of CT, MR imaging, and US instruments for small animal imaging have enabled preclinical studies of organ and tissue structure similar to those in the clinic. But more importantly, however, the availability of these tools in small animal imaging laboratories is leading to development of new molecular contrast agents [15] for some of these modalities that will have an impact on clinical imaging. In addition, use of these instruments for small animal imaging is leading to the development of multi-modality instruments that combine optical measures of function with structural analyses. Combination instruments will enrich and improve data sets through attenuation correction and improved localization of signals.

Imaging modalities

Numerous imaging modalities have been applied to the study of biology in animal models, including MR imaging, positron emission tomography (PET), and single-photon emission CT (SPECT). Each of these also is used clinically for diagnostic applications and to assess treatment outcomes.

MR imaging uses magnetic fields and radio frequency pulses to induce and measure signals from hydrogen atoms in the body. The image resolution is excellent in animal and human subjects, but sensitivity to molecular changes is less than that of other modalities. MR imaging is largely an anatomic imaging modality, as approaches for molecular contrast are relatively new, and the sensitivity with existing contrast agents is less than what is needed for detecting relevant biological changes in the body. PET imaging is based on the simultaneous emission of two gamma rays upon annihilation of positrons emitted from radioactive tracers injected into the subject. The tracers can be designed into many different compounds and drugs. Thus PET offers a tremendous opportunity for biochemical analyses in vivo. Resolution in PET is less than that which can be achieved by MR imaging, but the cross-sectional information and three-dimensional reconstruction capability offers significant information. SPECT is based on detection of gamma emission directly from the spontaneous decay of radioisotopes. The resolution and sensitivity of SPECT are similar to that of PET, but the isotopes used in SPECT generally have longer half-lives then those used in PET. Thus SPECT can be a more accessible modality. To use PET imaging effectively, a cyclotron needs to be located nearby because the short half-lives of the isotopes used. Additionally, onsite chemistry is necessary to generate the appropriate radioactive compounds for injection into research subjects. For routines using radioactive fluoro-deoxyglucose, the compounds can be purchased from off site locations, but any custom probes require radiochemistry expertise on site. Both PET and SPECT, as they relate to routine small animal imaging, are somewhat limited by the special handling required for the use of radioisotopes. There is increasing availability of specialized MR imaging, PET and SPECT scanners, however, for small animal imaging, and this has led to development of new reagents and approaches for assessing molecular changes in vivo. The improved performance and capabilities of the instrumentation are leading to increased use in animal models. Development of these tools likely will lead to powerful technologies with potential for translation to the clinic.

Optical imaging

The relative opacity of tissue permits limited transmission of visible light through the body, and although largely attenuated by both absorption and scattering, light in the visible and near infrared (nir) region of the spectrum has been used successfully for imaging of biological process in living subjects [16,17]. Optical imaging is not comprised simply of one modality, but the field consists of numerous approaches that use light in the visible region of the spectrum to sense and image in the living body. Some of these use the inherent optical properties of the tissue and are based on reflected light, intrinsic absorptive properties, or autofluorescence [18–23]. Many of these are well-developed, and the molecular changes that are associated with differences between normal and disease tissues and give rise to unique signatures are being resolved, such that information about the biology can be inferred from the image or the spectra of the tissues. One example of these tools is diffuse optical tomography (DOT), which is being tested clinically as a means of detecting recurrence of breast cancer following therapy [24]. This method measures changes in the tissue optical properties several centimeters into the tissues, and it is sensitive to changes in blood oxygenation, water, fat, and other tissue components [17]. The data in DOT are usually a spectrum and not an image; however, images based on these tissue changes can be made. Optical coherence tomography (OCT), is an optical method analogous to US that provides high-resolution images [25,26] with small fields of view and shallow tissue penetration (less than 1 mm). This modality is finding utility in ophthalmology and is being tested for use in endoscopy and intravascular imaging. Neither DOT nor OCT use exogenous contrast, although efforts are being made to either adapt the modality to novel contrast agents (OCT) or to use new contrast agents that provide a useful signal (DOT). In contrast to these optical modalities being developed for largely for clinical applications, in vivo bioluminescence (BLI) and fluorescence imaging (FLI) may have their greatest application in the study of small animal models. Their development has been largely for preclinical imaging.

Optical imaging using bioluminescence and fluorescence

Whole-body imaging using BLI and fluorescence can refine small animal models of human physiology and disease and accelerate their evaluation. In general, imaging using these two approaches is rapid and can be exquisitely sensitive. Molecular markers can be delivered as exogenous dyes or genetically engineered into cells or animal subjects. Each of these two modalities is versatile and has been applied broadly across many disciplines. BLI and FLI, in their most common forms, produce planar projection data using pseudocolored images to represent signal intensity, and these images are localized over grayscale reference images of the subjects. Recent developments in three-dimensional

reconstruction are leading to instruments that generate three-dimensional data sets from either multiple images from several views, or from temporal [27] or spectral data [28,29]. Optimal detection of bioluminescent or fluorescent signals requires the use of imaging systems that are sensitive to the weak signals that escape the scattering and absorbing environment of the mammalian body. These systems typically are based on CCD detectors and lenses and filters that operate in the visible to near infrared regions of the spectrum. These devices tend to be less expensive than those of other imaging modalities. Anatomic resolution is relatively poor in whole-body images, but when necessary, a high-magnification lens can be directed at sites in the body where labeled cells have been localized by whole-body imaging to produce high-resolution images that complement the lower resolution images taken noninvasively of the whole animal. The use of a high-magnification lens in living animals, intravital microscopy, has been published for numerous cell trafficking studies, and tremendous insights have been gained in this manner [30–35]. The extreme attenuation of light in the visible and nir regions of the spectrum by human tissues will limit the translation of optical imaging modalities to specialized niches in the clinic. Because radioactivity is not required, however, and because the instruments are relatively lower in cost, optical modalities may be more accessible and available for studying small animal models.

Bioluminescence imaging

The use of light-emitting enzymes, luciferases, and external imaging of the light transmitted through mammalian tissue first was demonstrated using bacteria labeled through the expression a bacterial reporter gene [3]. The versatility of this method has led to rapid adaptation to revealing tumor growth and response to therapy (Fig. 1) [6], stem cell engraftment and proliferation (Figs. 2, 3) [36], gene expression (Fig. 4) [4], and protein–protein interactions [37–41]. Application of BLI to these areas of biology has grown rapidly, and there are numerous papers and reviews [7,42–44] describing the use of this approach to study mammalian biology. The bases of this method are light-emitting enzymes, luciferases, and their substrates. Probably the most significant advantage to this method is an extraordinary signal-to-noise ratio. This is because of the absence of noise in that there is very little light generated by mammalian tissues. Because neither the enzyme nor the substrate produce signal alone, there is a switch that occurs when the two come together, and unlike fluorescence, it does not require an excitation light source. In fluorescent imaging, the excitation light also will excite naturally

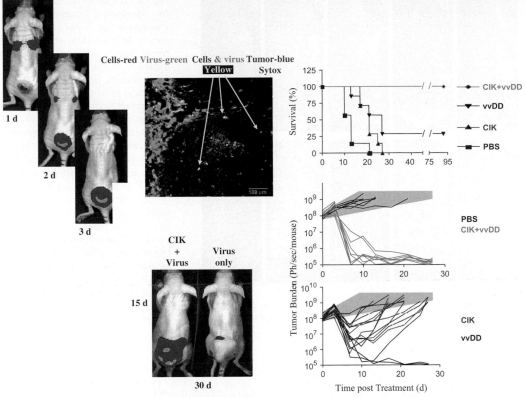

Fig. 1. Optimizing therapies using optically based molecular imaging tools. Optimization of combination therapies is challenging because of the numerous different possible treatment times and dosing schemes. Imaging serves to reduce the number of animal groups required to obtain a specific answer and thus can reduce and refine the preclinical phase of development. Here an immune cell population was used to deliver an ocolytic vaccinia virus, and imaging was used to localize immune cells and sites of virus replication and to assess tumor growth. The images on the left reveal the temporal patterns of viral replication, and the micrograph demonstrates that the virally infected immune cells are present deep in the tumor. Animal survival (*top right*) and tumor burden (*middle and bottom right*) indicate that the combination therapy is more effective than either one alone. (*Reprinted from* Thorne SH, Negrin RS, Contag CH. Synergistic antitumor effects of immune cell viral biotherapy. Science 2006;311:1780–4; with permission. © Copyright 2006 AAAS.)

occurring fluors in the tissue (autofluorescence) in addition to the fluorescent tag. This is the source of noise in FLI, and it can be significant, especially at shorter wavelengths of light (300 to 600 nm). At longer wavelengths of light (greater than 600 nm), absorbance and autofluorescence decrease dramatically, and the scatter also decreases. The new fluorescent probes for in vivo applications are being developed largely in the near infrared region of the spectrum (600 to 900 nm) given the significantly lower background signals and greater tissue penetration that occurs at the shorter wavelengths.

Attempts also have been made to increase the wavelength of emission of the luciferases for BLI, but there have been only modest red shifts in the emission spectra reported to date with the longest emitting luciferase at 615 nm, which has been achieved for the click beetle and firefly luciferases [45–47]. All luciferases have broad emission spectra, and for enzymes with spectra that peak above 600 nm, approximately 60% of the light output is above 600 nm [48]. The most commonly used luciferase is that from the North American firefly, and this luciferase red shifts at 37°C, making it among the longest emitting luciferases at mammalian body temperatures [48]. Despite its reported emission peak of 560 nm (collected at 22°C), its emission at 37°C is 612 nm [48]. Other luciferases appear to be temperature stable [48]. The advances in instrumentation for detection of weak bioluminescent signals in the body take advantage of the broad emission spectra, and methods that use the differential transmission of light at different wavelengths to obtain depth information are being developed. Spectrally resolved imaging of luciferase emission also enables localizing emitters of two different wavelengths in the body [49]. All of the advances in instrumentation for BLI are based on

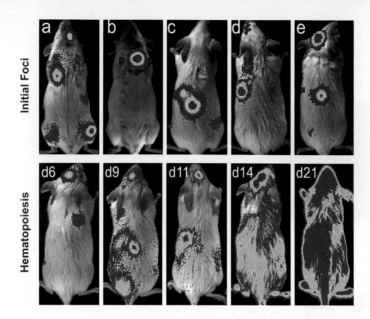

Initial Foci

a   b   c   d   e

Hematopoiesis

d6   d9   d11   d14   d21

Fig. 2. Location of bioluminescent foci following transplantation of transgenic luc + HSC. Foci were apparent in individual animals at anatomic sites corresponding to the location of the spleen, skull, vertebrae, femurs, and sternum (*A–E*) at 6 to 9 days after transfer. The patterns of engraftment were dynamic, with formation and expansion or formation and loss of the bioluminescent foci. One recipient of 250 HSC was monitored over time (*second row*). In this animal, two initial foci were apparent on day 6. By day 9, one was no longer detectable, and another remained at nearly the same intensity as on day 6. New foci were apparent on day 9, and then the intensity at these sites weakened or disappeared by day 11. Pseudo-colored images reflecting optical signal intensity are overlaid upon a grayscale reference image of the animal. (*From* Cao YA, Wagers AJ, Beilhack A, et al. Shifting foci of hematopoiesis during reconstitution from single stem cells. Proc Natl Acad Sci USA 2004;101:221–6; with permission. © Copyright 2004 National Academy of the Sciences USA.)

the same basic design, which includes an imaging chamber that excludes ambient light and a sensitive CCD as a detector [16].

Despite the simple design, there are numerous instrumentation advances for detecting bioluminescent signals in the body. Most of these advances have been for the purpose of obtaining data that would permit the reconstruction of three-dimensional data sets. These designs include a ring of detectors for obtaining multiple views, a stage for moving the animal coupled with a rotating mirror for obtaining multiple views, and improved spectral imaging using filters [28,50]. Many of these advances are relatively new, and many have been made by the instrument vendors. For these reasons, there have not been many publications on these new designs.

Fluorescence imaging

Recent advances in the detection of fluorescent signals in vivo are based on the versatility of dyes and reporters that fluoresce and the approaches of separating signal to noise in the living body [51–57]. The wavelengths of light that are needed to excite many of the fluors that have been developed for use in microscopy and cytometry are in the blue and green region of the visible spectrum. Light of these wavelengths has limited penetration through mammalian tissues because of absorption, which is, in large part, caused by hemoglobin [17,58]. These shorter wavelengths provide high-resolution

images (see Fig. 1), and modulation of the excitation wavelength [54] offers control over signal intensity. For these reasons, fluorescent techniques have tremendous utility in the study cells in culture, excised tissues, small transparent organisms, or biological processes that occur at superficial tissue sites in mammals. Fluorescence, however, can be detected through relatively thick mammalian tissue, and development of nir dyes [59–61] and reporters that are red shifted [62–64] have led to increased signal-to-noise ratios and improvement in in vivo imaging. The advances in this area of investigation have led to the development of fluors that may have clinical utility [65]. Indocyanin green (ICG [66,67]) has been approved for clinical use and is being investigated for clinical imaging and in animal models [51,54,55,68–73]. The basic problem of limited penetration of visible light through tissues can be overcome by placing the detector inside of the body, and two advances that will bring this type of approach into widespread clinical use will be coupled macro- and microscopic imaging devices that provide a choice of a wide field of view or high-resolution imaging, and miniaturization of microscopes that will enable either implantation and use in endoscopy [74–79]. Multi-photon systems greatly improve detection of fluorescent signals, as the excitation is accomplished with longer wavelengths, yielding deeper tissue penetration [74]. Advances in microendoscopy are taking advantage of this phenomenon.

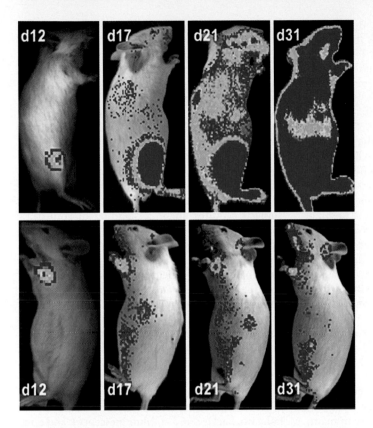

Fig. 3. Temporal analyses of hematopoiesis following single-cell transplants. These mice demonstrate the variability in contribution to reconstitution that was observed following the establishment of initial foci of hematopoietic engraftment after transplantation of a single transgenic luc + HSC. Pseudo-colored images reflecting optical signal intensity are overlaid upon a grayscale reference image of the animal. (*From* Cao YA, Wagers AJ, Beilhack A, et al. Shifting foci of hematopoiesis during reconstitution from single stem cells. Proc Natl Acad Sci U S A 2004;101:221–6; with permission. © Copyright 2004 National Academy of the Sciences USA.)

Genetic labels and dyes

The various optical reporters and dyes available for optical imaging have contributed tremendous versatility to BLI and FLI, and significant advances in in vivo optical imaging will be made in the area of probe development and advances in molecular contrast agents. By analogy to light microscopy, dyes can be used to stain tissues in the body. Unlike staining a tissue section for microscopy, however, the inability to wash off unbound dye in vivo is

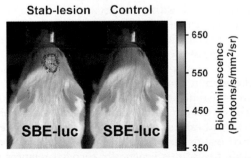

Stab-lesion   Control

SBE-luc   SBE-luc

650
550
450
350

Bioluminescence
(Photons/s/mm²/sr)

Fig. 4. Activation of Smad expression after traumatic brain injury. Transgenic mice reveal gene activation using BLI. (*Reprinted from* Lin AH, et al. Global analysis of Smad2/3-dependent TGF-beta signaling in living mice reveals prominent tissue-specific responses to injury. J Immunol 2005;175:547–54; with permission.)

a significant limitation. Therefore dyes often are used to label cells outside the body before transfer into an animal model and imaging macroscopically or microscopically [80–82]. Fluorescent dyes can have a relatively intense signal. As the labeled cells divide, however, the progeny cells have half as much dye, and the optical signals eventually drop below background fluorescence. Compounds that contain a fluor and a quencher where the fluor can be dequenched (activated) in vivo by separation the two components is one method for obviating the problem of noise from the fluorescent dye at sites that are off target [83]. In these strategies, the signal from the dye is not detectable until it encounters its molecular target. This eliminates the problem of not being able to wash out the dye that has not encountered its target, and there should, in principle, be essentially no background signal. The best examples of these types of agents are protease substrates, in which a fluor and a quencher are joined by a peptide sequence that is cleaved by an extracellular protease [52]. This approach has been used for various proteases in the study of cancer, inflammation, and autoimmunity [53,84,85].

In animal models, reporter genes that express proteins with intrinsic optical properties may be used for obtaining specificity and reducing background signals, but most importantly for genetically linking an optical signal to a biological process where the two are not readily dissociated. These reporter genes function as labels that can be traced noninvasively over time (see Figs. 1–3). They typically encode proteins that interact with reporter probes, applied substrates (bioluminescence), or exogenous excitation light sources (fluorescence) to generate a signal that initially can be localized from outside the body. Then these data can serve as a guide for selecting the appropriate tissues and times where sampling will be most meaningful. Many of these reporter genes initially were developed for use in cell-based assays or for detection in excised tissues. Therefore, after imaging in live subjects and use of the image data to guide tissue sampling, measurements of the reporter activity also can be made on excised tissue using the same optical signal that generated in the in vivo image. This serves to link the in vivo and ex vivo assays to the correlative cell culture assays such that the animal model can be studied more effectively and more data generated per study. Effective use of optical imaging, therefore, results in studies of animal models that are more informative and predictive than studies that only use conventional assays on excised tissues. Genetically encoded reporters, where the molecular specificity can be engineered into the cell and detected from outside the body, have been modified for more effective use in mammalian subjects [3,4]. The specificity and signal to noise inherent in these types of agents contrast sharply those of agents that report blood pool and compounds that produce contrast through nonspecific accumulation. For measurements of tumor burden or for assessing cell trafficking patterns, it is necessary to use genes that are integrated into the genome and whose expression is constitutive such that the detectable signal is linked inextricably to the metabolic activity of the target cell population. This will circumvent problems of loss of signal because of dilution, and the confounding detection of signals that have dissociated from the viable target cell population. Additional development in the area of optical reporter genes will be motivated by the need for greater sensitivity and specificity.

The advances in understanding gene expression and the ability to assess expression levels of 30,000 genes simultaneously provide the information on how to regulate the expression of reporter genes and which genes to target in which disease state or developmental process. The molecular targeting of reporter genes can be at the level of transcription, where the cells are labeled by targeting specific genetic regulatory elements (ie, promoters) and linking them to sequences that encode reporter genes (see Fig. 4). Because this approach has been used in cell biology for decades, there is a significant background for rapidly translating the cell biology assays to in vivo assays using this strategy [86]. With imaging instrumentation specifically designed for small animals, the transition from cell-based assays to in vivo assays has been demonstrated for cancer, mammalian development, host response to infection, and other disease states. Alternatively, reporter genes have been developed that are constitutively expressed but lack an optical signal until another specific molecular event occurs. In this case, the activation of the reporter is post-translational [37–41,44,87,88].

The use of optical reporter genes in living animal subjects requires an understanding of control of gene expression, tissue optics, and detector technologies [89]. Optimal reporter genes for in vivo studies have several characteristics. They should encode well-characterized gene products, proteins that can result in generation or accumulation of deeply penetrating light emission with the potential for a high signal-to-noise ratio. The signal-to-noise ratio depends on levels and location of reporter gene expression, and also on the optical properties of mammalian tissues [16]. Noise in fluorescent imaging arises from the autofluorescence of tissue (this is not the case with reporter genes that encode bioluminescent proteins, because there is little, or essentially no, background autoluminescence), and once a reporter gene is expressed, the signal depends on the absorbing and scattering properties of the tissue, which are greater with shorter wavelengths of light [89–91]. Long wavelength emitters (greater than 600 nm) are desirable, and those that do not require an excitation wavelength offer the greatest signal-to-noise ratios (Table 1). Optimal detection of the optical signal requires sensitive detectors and elimination of ambient light. Although optical signals from inside the body can be detected without the exclusion of ambient light [92,93], detection with maximum sensitivity likely is not accomplished without collection of the data in complete darkness. Devices with excellent light collection capability are accessible and versatile for studying reporter gene expression in vivo.

Fluorescent proteins

After the initial report of using GFP as a reporter of gene expression in the worm *Caenorhabditis elegans* [94], and extensive use of GFP as a marker in excised mammalian tissues [95–106], attempts were made to use this genetically encoded reporter in live mammalian subjects [56]. This first green fluorescent protein was obtained from the jellyfish *Aequorea victoria*, and since the initial studies of gene expression performed in *C elegans*, numerous variants of GPF have been described and fluorescent homologs from anthozoa corals [62,107–114].

Table 1: Characteristics of luciferases used in vivo

Luciferase	Species of origin	[a]Peak emission	Substrate utilized	Protein size	Subcellular localization of enzyme	Energy source	Cofactors	Citations
Fluc	*Photinus pyralis* (firefly beetle)	612 nm[b]	Luciferin	61 kd[c]	Cytoplasmic	ATP	O_2[d] Mg^{++}	48
CBRed	*Pyrophorus plagiophthalamus* (click beetle)	615 nm	Luciferin	61 kd	Cytoplasmic	ATP	O_2	48, 121
CBGr68	*Pyrophorus plagiophthalamus* (click beetle)	543 nm	Luciferin	61 kd	Cytoplasmic	ATP	O_2	48, 121
Rluc	*Renilla reniformins*	480 nm	Coelenterazine	36 kd	Cytoplasmic	Substate	O_2	48
Rluc-mod	*Renilla reniformins*		Coelenterazine	36 kd	Cytoplasmic	Substate	O_2	
Gluc	*Gaussia princeps*		Coelenterazine	19.9 kd	Extracellular	Substate	O_2	127, 171, 172
Lux	*Photorhabdus luminescence* (bacteria)	490 nm	Decanal	77 kd[e]	Intracellular	FMN	O_2	173

[a] Emission peak (I_{max}) measured at 37° C.
[b] Nanometers.
[c] This is size of the protein in kilodaltons (kd).
[d] All luciferases characterized to date are oxygenases; however some require co-factors such as magnesium ions or calcium ions.
[e] The heterodimeric luciferase is on two genes (Lux A and Lux B) which encode 37 and 40 kd proteins. The lux genes are encoded on five gene operon.

These have been broadly used in cell biology. They also are being used in vivo, and are being modified for improved function and greater versatility [64].

There is significant spectral and chromophore diversity among this family of proteins of which there are now about 100 cloned and partially characterized members. The fluorescent proteins that have been characterized share common structural, biochemical, and photophysical features and have been derived from marine organisms. Modifications to all of these proteins have been made to alter excitation and emission light or to change other functions. There remain proteins that are better suited for one application over another [115]. The monomeric red and dimeric far red fluorescent proteins derived from the GFP-like proteins from anthozoa and their derivatives may hold the greatest potential for in vivo applications because of their longer wavelengths of excitation and emission and their monomeric nature Although the anthozoa GFP-like proteins provide this and other advantages over GFP, understanding the nature of these proteins is essential for use in vivo. Many of these proteins require oligomerization, and many show slow or incomplete fluorescence maturation, which may have utility in some applications [116]. They may hinder others. For in vivo studies, using reporters of the appropriate wavelength and stability for the application is essential for meaningful data and successful studies.

Luciferase and related proteins

Luciferase enzymes have been found in a range of organisms from several different genera, but there are essentially three basic biochemistries among the characterized enzymes [117]. Each of the biochemistries uses different substrates and conditions. Members of the three classes of luciferases have been cloned and their chemistries characterized to a point where they can be used routinely in the laboratory and in in vivo studies. These include the luciferases from beetles (coleoptera), jellyfish, and sea pansies (cnidaria), and bacteria (*Vibrio* species and *Photorhabdus luminescens*). All luciferases are oxygenases and require energy and a specific substrate (commonly known as luciferin), for light production, often in the presence of cofactors.

The luciferases from fireflies and related insects are a single polypeptides related to the CoA ligase family of proteins [118,119]. They use a benzothiazole luciferin substrate (commonly called luciferin) to generate light in the presence of ATP and oxygen. The gene encoding firefly luciferase (Fluc) is the most commonly used bioluminescent reporter, and it has been codon optimized for expression in mammalian cells. Other beetle luciferases also

have been codon optimized, including those from the click beetle [46,120,121]. These proteins offer the advantages of broad-spectrum emission and a sufficient red component of the spectrum. Both characteristics improve detection of small numbers of cells. Luciferases from the sea pansy (*Renilla reniformis*) [122–124], the jellyfish (*Aequorea aequorea*) [41,125,126], and marine copepod *Gaussia princeps* [127] also have been cloned, characterized, and used as in vivo reporter genes. All of the enzymes from marine organisms that have been described use coelenterazine as their substrate, but they all differ in some aspects. Selection of the appropriate reporter requires some understanding of their biochemistries and capabilities. Unfortunately, the greatest diversity is in the enzymes derived from marine organisms, and all of these are blue emitters and use the less desirable in vivo substrate, coelenterazine. The blue emission is absorbed largely by hemoglobin, and coelenterazine is less desirable because it has a relatively short circulation time in vivo with some autoluminescence [48,128]. The enzyme from the hydrozoan *Aequorea* (aequorin) requires a calcium ion for light production, and it has been used as a calcium sensor in cultured cells. Codon-optimized versions of the *Renilla* enzyme have been developed for use in vivo with a slight red shift and greater stability in vivo. This enzyme has served as a light source for self-illuminating quantum dots [129]. The luciferase from *Renilla* does not require cofactors that need to be provided by the host cell for other enzymes (ATP and magnesium), and this opens up the possibility of monitoring extracellular events. The differences in emission spectra and biochemistries of the luciferases offer the potential for multiplexing the cell culture and in vivo assays such that two, and possibly more, biological processes can be studied simultaneously [80,130]. Combining bioluminescence with other enzyme activities offers another layer for in vivo bioassay development.

Lac Z and activation of modified luciferins

Beta-galactosidase (beta-gal) has been used widely as a transgenic reporter enzyme in cell biology, and there were several early attempts to extend the use of this enzyme to in vivo imaging studies [54,131]. Several different fluorescent substrates are available for its detection, and these have been used for flow cytometry. Extension of this reporter into in vivo studies would offer a significant tool for biological research. Conjugates of the beta-galactoside substrates and 7-hydroxy-9H-(1,3-dichloro-9,9-dimethylacridin-2-one) (DDAO), are both chromogenic and red fluorescent [54], and activation events are used to increase the signal-to-noise ratios with a 50 nm red shift upon cleavage. This activation step enabled specific detection despite the presence of intact probe in the background tissues. In this study, 9L gliomas expressing beta-gal were detected using in vivo fluorescence imaging [54]. This enzyme also has been the focus of work aimed at creating MR imaging contrast agents, where gadolidium is caged and released upon catalysis by beta-gal [132–134]. Additional developments in the optical regime include the description of a sequential reporter enzyme luminescence strategy that is based on beta-gal activity. This approach uses cleavable substrates developed by Promega Corporation (Madison Wisconsin) [135]. The substrate for this reaction is a caged D-luciferin-galactoside conjugate that is cleaved by beta-gal to release D-luciferin that can be used as a substrate for the coleoptera luciferases such as that from the firefly and click beetles. This has enabled the visualization of beta-gal activity in vivo as an additional tool for molecular imaging. These reporter gene strategies have been used alone, and a trend in the field is to make combinations of reporters. Some of the new strategies will offer strengths in the development of combination or multi-functional reporters.

Substrate biodistribution

The biodistribution of the substrate will determine the signal intensity at different tissue sites, and thus the pharmacokinetics of luciferin and coelenterazine are important to consider in imaging studies involving these biochemical reactions. To obtain quantitative information from BLI data, the substrate must not be limiting; otherwise the images will reflect substrate levels and not reporter gene expression patterns. Proper imaging of luciferase reporters requires imaging at the time of peak substrate availability. The optimal time from administration to data acquisition depends upon the route of administration and the rate of clearance of the substrate in the body. The substrate for Fluc and CBRluc, D-luciferin, is relatively stable in the body and has a relatively long circulation time [4]. In contrast, the substrate for Rluc, coelenterazine, is cleared from the body rapidly and binds to serum proteins [128]. Coelenterazine, therefore, only can be administered intravenously, and data acquisition must be complete within a few seconds to a minute after injection. D-luciferin can be injected intraperitoneally or intravenously [128]. The biodistribution of D-luciferin, after i.p. injection, peaks at 15 to 20 min, and the bioluminescence signal stays relatively stable for another 15 to 20 min before degrading because of substrate clearance. After intravenous injection of D-luciferin, the peak of emission occurs at about 1 min and decreases rapidly.

Multi-functional reporter genes

Multi-modality imaging approaches have been described for the purpose of providing additional data to a study in the form of validation. These often will offer structural and function information, and the ease of linking genes through genetic tools has led to the development of numerous of these reporters [13,72,136]. Multi-reporter gene fusions first were described using luciferase and GFP for use in cells and flies [137], and similar fusions have been used as a means of connecting in vivo measurements in mice, using luciferase, to ex vivo assays such as flow cytometry, and fluorescence microscopy using GFP and related fluorescent proteins [13]. Triple gene fusions have been used to link optical imaging and ex vivo assays to PET imaging [72,136]. These multi-function reporter genes can increase the flexibility of a reporter for in vivo assays and perhaps even more importantly offer validation measures that are not possible using a single-function reporter [13,138,139].

A limitation to the use of reporter genes is the transfer of these genes to cells with stable integration and reliable expression. Selection of tumor cells in vivo is generally straightforward, although at times trying, but labeling primary cells and organs has remained a challenge despite advances in nonviral- and viral-mediated gene transfer methods. Therefore, transgenic mice have been developed that express the dual-function reporter genes, and these animals serve as universal donors to provide cells and tissue transplantation and cell trafficking studies (see **Figs. 2, 3**) [36]. Hematopoietic stem cells and immune cells from this transgenic donor have been transplanted and analyzed in vivo [36,140]. By crossing these transgenic mice with transgenic lines of mice that have been engineered to spontaneously develop malignancy, new insights into oncogenesis have been gleaned [141]. Because the reporter genes are integrated into the mouse genome, the signals are not lost through development or over time, and the labeled cells can be followed throughout the life of the animal or during the different phases of oncogenesis. Studies using labeled tumors generated through breeding a reporter transgenic line with a line that spontaneously develops tumors have revealed a persistent low-level signal after inactivation of the oncogene that supported the initial tumor growth [141]. The cells that persist in these animals have a normal appearance by all measures, but they can serve as a source of relapse. As such, they may constitute a cancer stem cell. Such studies would not be possible without the use of imaging, as other methods would not have allowed following animals through the entire disease course. Using transgenic animals that express multi-functional reporter genes has been a useful tool for developing new therapeutic strategies, because this method enables tracking any cell population of interest over time and links in vivo and ex vivo assays (see Fig. 1).

Other dyes and reagents

Quantum dots

Fluorescent proteins and even dyes are limited in the number of available colors. This is especially true in the region of the spectrum that is suited for in vivo imaging. One alternative to this shortfall is to use semiconductor quantum dots [142]. Quantum dots of different sizes and surface coatings can fluoresce at different colors over a broad region of the spectrum, and the emission is very narrow, lending this reagent to multiplexed assays, especially for cells in culture. The quantum dots that have been tested in vivo include amphiphilic poly(acrylic acid), short-chain (750 Da) methoxy-PEG and long-chain (3400 Da) carboxy-PEG quantum dots, which had fairly short circulating half lives (less than 12 min), and long-chain (5000 Da) methoxy-PEG quantum dots, which had long circulating half lives of about 70 min [143]. In the in vivo studies, localization of labeled quantum dots was assessed by fluorescence imaging of living animals. This was followed by analyses at necropsy using frozen tissue sections for optical microscopy, and by electron microscopy [143]. The versatility of this approach, from live animals to nanometer resolution images of excised tissues, suggests that this may be an ideal means of linking in vivo and ex vivo assays. The localization of these labels varied with surface coatings, and although not fully evaluated, localization also may be variable with size. Quantum dots initially were developed for use in biochemical and cell culture-based assays, but development for use in vivo may offer novel reagents for preclinical imaging and perhaps limited clinical application.

Self-illuminating quantum dots

A significant advantage of quantum dots is that particles of different sizes fluoresce at different wavelengths using a common excitation wavelength. The excitation light for quantum dots, however, is generally of short wavelengths, those largely absorbed by mammalian tissues. Development of quantum dots that contain their own light source would be valuable as in vivo agent, because the distance that the excitation light would have to travel would be significantly less than what would be needed for external excitation. A description of quantum dot conjugates that autoluminesce has been reported [129]. These conjugates use bioluminescence resonance energy transfer (BRET, also

known as chemiluminescent resonant energy transfer and luminescence resonance energy transfer) [144–147] to produce signals without external excitation. Carboxylate-presenting quantum dots were conjugated to a mutant form of the luciferase from R reniformis, and the blue emission from this enzyme was used to excite the quantum dot. The long wavelength of emission and the colocalization of the excitation source with the fluorescence resulted in improved sensitivity in small animal imaging and a high signal-to-noise ratio compared with quantum dots requiring an external excitation source.

Combination approaches

Combinations of instruments that provide structural information and functional data represent the most robust imaging approaches, and instruments that have this capability are being developed for radioactive and optical imaging strategies. The goal of molecular imaging is to develop contrast agents that are so specific that only the targeted biological process will be apparent in the image. Therefore, by providing structural, or anatomic, information, a multi-modality instrument can provide a reference image for localization of the molecular signal to a specific anatomic site. In addition, the structural information can be used for attenuation correction and can improve the functional image. This will be particularly useful for optical imaging, where attenuation can be severe. Many clinical imaging modalities are available in combined instruments, (eg, PET-CT and SPECT-CT systems). Because optical imaging largely has been used in the study of laboratory animals, however, similar multimodality instruments do not yet exist.

An underappreciated aspect of optical imaging is that optical detectors are generally sensitive to a range of energies in the visible to nir regions of the spectrum, and there are a range of emitters that can be used. Therefore, each wavelength, or energy, within the visible range can be used to multiplex optically based systems and create multi-modality optical imaging devices. This is essentially the basis for 12-color flow cytometry and multiplexed fluorescent-based cell imaging. Extension of this concept to in vivo assays is limited primarily by the more confined region of the spectrum with deep tissue penetration in mammalian subjects. The window for optics is between 600 and 1300 nm, where absorption of the signal is minimal, and optical signals are as affected scatter. As probes and dyes that operate in this region of the spectrum are developed, one is likely to see multiplexed and multi-modality optical imaging that will enrich the data obtained from animal models and possibly from human subjects.

Applications

The CNS has been the subject of numerous studies using optics to interrogate biology and disease. The skull represents a barrier to these studies, but because bone is a scattering material and not particularly absorbing, relative to other mammalian tissues, it presents a challenge for obtaining resolution but not sensitivity in the optical regime. Numerous studies have aimed at using optics to reveal CNS function based on intrinsic optical properties. Because of the resolution issue, these studies have aimed at sensing changes and not necessarily at obtaining an image [90,148–151]. Because intrinsic optical properties are being used in these studies, injection of contrast is not necessary, and thus clinical studies are uncomplicated. Numerous studies have been reported [90]. In animal models, both FLI and BLI have been used to reveal biological changes in the brain, including gene expression patterns, distribution of infectious agents, and extent of tumor growth. Coupled with other imaging modalities for localization, the use of light to assess function comprises a powerful set of tools for brain imaging of animal models to clinical studies. Several selected examples of molecular imaging of the brain are described.

Gene expression in the central nervous system

The TGF-β superfamily of proteins, including TGF-βs, activins, and bone morphogenic proteins (BMPs), controls cellular processes ranging from patterning and differentiation to proliferation and apoptosis. The proteins have been implicated in tumorigenesis, fibrosis, inflammation, and neurodegeneration, and imaging the expression patterns of these genes could have a tremendous impact on our understanding of developmental processes and oncogenesis. Smad2 and Smad3 (Smad2/3) proteins are key signaling molecules that influence the expression of TGF-β. Study of the temporal and spatial patterns of Smad2/3-dependent signaling was accomplished by generating transgenic mice, where the transgene consisted of Smad-responsive luciferase reporter construct (SBE-luc mice), and the patterns of gene expression were evaluated in normal and pathological conditions in the brain in living animals and in excised tissues [18]. Whole-body imaging revealed that luciferase activity was highest in brain, intestine, heart, and skin, and the image data correlated with biochemical measurements of luciferase activity. In this study, traumatic brain injury caused by a needle stab resulted in a several fold increase in bioluminescence in living mice and correlated local activation

of Smad2/3-dependent genes (see **Fig. 4**). These data further indicated that luciferin crosses the blood–brain barrier and that gene expression in the CNS can be studied noninvasively over time.

RNA-containing viruses

Imaging of infectious agents, their interaction with host cells and the host response is possible using optical methods in small animal models and a number of agents have been studied in this manner. In addition, as infectious agents are being converted to biotherapies for gene transfer or oncolysis, their efficacy has been studied using optical imaging (see **Fig. 1**). Many of these studies assess only the infectious agent or only the tissue response. It is possible to monitor both in the same animal, and an example of moving toward multiplexed assays is described.

Viral encephalitis caused by small RNA-containing viruses are presenting an ever increasing health problem, as viruses like West Nile virus and other encephalitic viruses are carried to new parts of the globe. Sindbis virus infection of mice serves as a model for these diseases of humans, and identification of viral determinants of virulence and host determinants of susceptibility can be evaluated using this model. Some strains of Sindbis virus cause encephalomyelitis in some genetic backgrounds of mice, and thus this model of encephalitis offers an excellent opportunity for revealing viral and host factors of susceptibility. In murine models of viral encephalitis, BLI was used to monitor the extent and location of Sindbis virus replication over time [152]. In this study, the authors demonstrated that there was a direct correlation between the amount of light detected from the labeled virus and the amount of infectious virus in the brain. In addition to revealing what was known for the various strains of virus in susceptible and nonsusceptible hosts, the study suggested that virus entry into the nervous system could occur by retrograde axonal transport, either from neurons innervating the initial site of replication or from the olfactory epithelium after viremic spread. Integration of reporter genes into other viruses and into genetic loci of the host has the potential of revealing the biology host pathogen interaction with a temporal resolution that was not previously possible, as such the intricate interaction between the host and the virus will be revealed.

DNA-containing viruses

Mouse models of herpes simplex virus type 1 (HSV-1) infection have been developed to reveal aspects of host pathogen interaction, and optical imaging is being used to reveal the viral and host genes that regulate pathogenesis [153]. BLI can be used to determine the full extent of viral spread, replication, and cellular responses by expressing luciferases from various viral or host promoter sequences. In the study by Luker and colleagues, labeled HSV was introduced into mice by means of injection into the footpad, peritoneal cavity, brain, and eyes, and the infectious process followed over time [153]. Luciferase assays performed on excised tissues validated the in vivo images, indicating that the input titers were reflected in the images. In this manner, response to antiviral therapy was assessed, and the BLI data correlated well with the drug response. In this study, both luciferases from the firefly and *Renilla* were used to label and study the virus, and the problem of substrate delivery [128] was evident when using viruses labeled with the *Renilla* luciferase. To visualize *Renilla*-labeled viruses, it was necessary to inject the substrate locally, whereas the enzyme from the firefly enabled systemic delivery and whole-body imaging. This study emphasizes the need to select the appropriate reporter for the questions being addressed. If understanding viral spread to the CNS following peripheral inoculation is the objective of the study, incorporation of a reporter that uses a substrate with effective systemic delivery is essential. Dual-function reporters that either provide good in vivo and histological markers, or the ability to monitor infection by multiple modalities can enhance the study significantly [154,155].

Because HSV can infect neurons, HSV-based vectors have been developed for carrying genetic payloads into the brain. Understanding the distribution of the delivered vector [156] and the delivery of therapeutic genes can be accomplished with optical imaging, where one of the transferred genes is an optical reporter [155,157,158]. These vectors have been used for cancer therapy and for gene replacement studies [155,157]. Unfortunately, the state of the art is still at the level of demonstration and validation [157], and imaging studies that reveal new information about viral-mediated gene delivery to the brain have not been reported. In contrast, new information about agents that infect other parts of the body has been demonstrated [159,160]. The obvious questions pertaining to HSV-mediated gene transfer that could be addressed using imaging include, "What is the duration of corrective expression of therapeutic transgenes?" and "Can restoration of function be revealed using imaging, and are there clinical applications?" The outstanding questions are significant, and emerging molecular imaging technologies have tremendous potential for revealing answers to basic questions in gene transfer studies and the nuance and subtlety about viral vectors and gene delivery that may advance the field.

In a study of vaccinia virus infection, the role that interferons play in the distribution and temporal progression of vaccinia infection was revealed by BLI [161]. In this study, vaccinia viruses were labeled with reporter genes encoding firefly luciferase or a monomeric orange fluorescent protein. The validation studies revealed that the reporter genes served as reliable markers of vaccinia infection and supported the major finding of the study that replication of vaccinia was significantly greater in mice where the genes encoding the receptors for type I interferons (IFN I R$-/-$) had been deleted, relative to wild-type mice. Both wild-type and knock-out animals developed focal infections in the lungs and brain after intranasal inoculation. The extent of infection was greater in the absence of interferon receptors. The use of vaccinia virus as an oncolytic therapy and the ability to deliver this virus to the tumor site were revealed using optical imaging [80]. In the study by Luker and colleagues, the protective effects of interferons were shown to occur primarily through parenchymal cells rather than hematopoietic cells, and this may play a role in immune cell-mediated delivery of oncolytic agents.

DNA-containing viruses have been used for cancer gene therapy, where prodrug-converting enzymes are inserted into the viral genome in attempts to reduce toxicity of chemotherapy and increase its specificity. Noninvasive assessment of the therapeutic response and correlating the location, magnitude, and duration of transgene expression can be assessed in vivo using optical measures, and such data would enhance the development of these approaches to treating cancers of the brain greatly. Adenoviral vectors containing therapeutic transgenes and reporter genes have been developed and tested in vivo using imaging. In one study, the yeast cytosine deaminase (yCD), along with luciferase, was inserted into an adenoviral vector and used in an intratumoral injection model to treat experimental gliomas [162]. Both optical imaging and MIR were used to monitor the processes of gene delivery and therapeutic efficacy. The MR images revealed significant reduction in tumor growth rates after therapy using yCD and its nontoxic prodrug substrate 5-fluorocytosine (5FC). BLI could predict the level of viral gene transfer. Combination therapies and approaches such as the one described in this study are complicated by having many moving parts. The level of viral replication, gene expression, and prodrug conversion are all variables that can affect therapeutic outcome. Knowing the optimal times of prodrug delivery relative to virus replication, for example, will be critical for developing these therapeutic strategies, and imaging is the only means by which these data can be obtained with the efficiency and temporal resolution necessary for effective preclinical and clinical evaluation. This is an excellent example of how imaging can accelerate preclinical studies, provide information not previously available, and refine animal models of disease.

Glial fibrillary acidic protein transgenic reporter mouse and bacterial meningitis

The level of the host response to infection relative to the replication levels of an infecting agent typically is related. That is as the agent is cleared, the host response subsides. In a model of bacterial meningitis, however, imaging revealed a disconnect between the host response and the presence and absence *Streptococcus pneumoniae* [163]. Here, the pathogen was labeled through the expression of a bacterial luciferase (lux) [3] and used to infect a transgenic reporter mouse where the promoter from glial fibrillary acidic protein (GFAP) was used to express the firefly luciferase gene. The two luciferases are spectrally and biochemically distinct, and the spectral differences were used to image bacterial infection and GFAP expression levels. The level of neuronal damage and recovery following antibiotic treatment was found to depend on the time of treatment, and the GFAP expression levels were found to persist after clearance of the infection. These data suggest that long-term damage to the CNS following infection has a significant host component that is initiated by the infection but sustained independent of the agent. The multi-parameter imaging in this study revealed aspects of infection and host response not otherwise resolved and serves as a basis for further development of multi-parameter optical imaging.

Similar to the study of interferon knock-out mice and vaccinia infection, toll-like receptor 2 (TLR2) function has been investigated in a murine model of *S pneumoniae* meningitis [164]. Here the pathogen was labeled, and the extent and location of infection were used as a guide for selecting the times and tissues for sampling. The host response was assessed on excised tissues. Wild-type and TLR2-deficient mice were evaluated. Plasma interleukin-6 levels and bacterial numbers in blood and peripheral organs were found to be similar for both strains of mice. Three hours after infection, TLR2($-/-$) mice had higher bacterial loads in the brain than wild-type mice, and tumor necrosis factor (TNF) activity was higher in cerebrospinal fluid of infected knock-out mice that wild-type. Absence of TLR2 was associated with earlier death from meningitis linked to reduced clearance of bacteria in the brain. This study demonstrates the strength of image guidance for tissue sampling, in that the numbers of animals required to access these data without imaging would have precluded this study.

Tracking and monitoring of neuronal stem cells

Imaging of stem cells poses new challenges to established imaging technologies in that the aspects of their biology that are so valuable for tissue regeneration, including extensive proliferation and differentiation through numerous cell types with different physiologies, result in dilution of dyes and differential regulation of promoter sequences that may be used to control reporter gene expression. Transgenic reporter mouse lines that use strong, constitutive, ubiquitous, synthetic promoters to express reporter genes can be used as a source of labeled stem cells [36,140]. Use of specific promoters in the generation of transgenic mice can provide stage-specific expression and be used to assess stem cell function [165]. Hematopoietic stem cells from these mice are sufficiently bright that foci arising from individual cells can be detected early after transplantation. The promoters are not regulated significantly through development so that cells at different developmental stages can be visualized after transplantation (see **Figs. 2, 3**). For established stem cell lines, it is necessary to transfect or transduce the reporter genes into these cells [166,167]. Often times, this approach also is used for cells isolated from animals [168]. Although necessary in some situations, labeling by viral transduction results in each cell having a unique integration site, each with its own influence on gene expression and the potential for disrupting genes that are needed for tissue regeneration. Imaging has been used to look at hematopoiesis from single hematopoietic stem cells, stem cell survival in damaged cardiac tissue, and in the participation of stem cells in regeneration of neuronal tissues.

Neural progenitor cells (NPCs) are essential for developing the CNS in embryonic development. Additionally, they play a role in the ongoing processes of neurogenesis in specialized regions of the adult brain, and they may be manipulated to regenerate or repair tissue damage after injury. The characteristics of these cells linked to their potential in tissue regeneration include the potential for multi-lineage differentiation, recruitment into sites of tissue damage, and a capacity for self-renewal. Although not fully realized, efficiency of using NPCs for treatment of Parkinson's disease, multiple sclerosis, brain ischemia, and traumatic injury of CNS has been reported [169]. In a model of spinal cord injury, NSPC survival and location were assessed using BLI, and expression of GFP enabled microscopic analyses of the tissues after macroscopic localization using BLI. The primary cultured

NSPCs were labeled with firefly luciferase and a variant of GFP and the cells transferred into mice with spinal cord injuries. The image data demonstrated stability of signals from NPCs that were transplanted into the lesion, and the cells remained at that site for the entire study period. The signal from the cells appeared to remain at the site of transplantation with a reduction in intensity over time. The data suggested an 80% loss of NSPCs within the first 4 days after transplantation, while signal from the remaining cells persisted for 6 weeks. Histological examination of the injury site revealed t a morphology of the survival cells that were different depending on the time of transplant relative to the injury, which suggested that imaging would be an essential tool for developing cell-based therapies and serve as a guide for tissue selection and microscopic examination. Recovery of function was also different for the animal receiving cells at different times relative to time of injury.

Neural precursor cells also have been use for treating glioma, and in one study the ability to traffic to malignant cells was used as a means to deliver therapeutic molecules [170]. Murine neural precursor cells were engineered to express TNF-related apoptosis-inducing ligand (S-TRAIL) and firefly luciferase and used to treat *Renilla*-expressing gliomas. The implanted neural precursor cell-FL-sTRAIL migrated to the tumor site, and using *Renilla* expression, antitumor effects could be visualized. The dual luciferase imaging, based on previous work [130], was useful for maximizing the data obtained from groups of animals and provided a dynamic picture of cell-mediated delivery of antitumor therapies. Additional data could have been obtained using intravital microscopy and assessing the cell migration and antitumor effects at a cellular level.

Studies of stem cell and tumor cell migration have been performed in murine bone marrow [34]. These studies used in vivo confocal imaging to reveal cell migration to unique anatomic regions in the skull that the authors could define by specialized endothelial markers. The vasculature at these tissue sites expressed the adhesion molecule E-selectin and the chemoattractant stromal-cell-derived factor 1 (SDF-1). The expression patterns appeared in clearly defined regions that attracted metastatic cancer cells and bone marrow cells. These studies revealed that there are distinct cellular microdomains that attract cells and that these regions are defined by specialized vascular structures. Linking macroscopic and microscopic imaging modalities will offer the most data from these preclinical studies by providing a global picture and cellular interaction patterns in the same animals. As the field progresses, integrated studies of mammalian biology and disease will be based on image data that can be linked to multiplexed molecular assays to reveal disease patterns and potential molecular targets for intervention.

Summary and future outlook

The future of the imaging sciences is the development of multi-modality instrumentation, and multi-functional contrast reagents that are designed to sense cellular events and display the data in the context of ultra fine structural information, and linking these approaches to the tools being developed as part of the omics revolution. The field of molecular imaging is in its infancy. Yet the advances already have been significant, and the potential of these tools is appreciated. The convergence of cell biology, chemistry, physics, engineering, and imaging will lead to a range of tools for probing biology in vivo and as a basis for imaging molecular changes in the human body. Optical imaging will have a significant role in preclinical studies and find its strength in unique niches of clinical imaging. The low-cost instrumentation and ability to monitor patients frequently will have great utility in screening high-risk patients who have been identified through genetic screens as having a predisposition, or who have been treated and need to be monitored for relapse and disease progression. The exploitation of these techniques will accelerate and refine studies of biology and improve analyses of new therapeutic approaches through refinement of animal models. With the advent of many small animal imaging systems, it is possible to more rapidly test new imaging approaches and refine these applications such that in translation to the clinic, one will have a greater understanding of the properties of imaging agents and the utility for making outcome measures in the clinic.

References

[1] Germano G, Chen BC, Huang SC, et al. Use of the abdominal aorta for arterial input function determination in hepatic and renal PET studies. J Nucl Med 1992;33:613–20.

[2] Choi Y, Hawkins RA, Huang SC, et al. Parametric images of myocardial metabolic rate of glucose generated from dynamic cardiac PET and 2-[18F]fluoro-2-deoxy-d-glucose studies. J Nucl Med 1991;32:733–8.

[3] Contag CH, Contag PR, Mullins JI, et al. Photonic detection of bacterial pathogens in living hosts. Mol Microbiol 1995;18:593–603.

[4] Contag CH, Spilman SD, Contag PR, et al. Visualizing gene expression in living mammals using a bioluminescent reporter. Photochem Photobiol 1997;66:523–31.

[5] Tjuvajev JG, Stockhammer G, Desai R, et al. Imaging the expression of transfected genes in vivo. Cancer Res 1995;55:6126–32.

[6] Sweeney TJ, Mailander V, Tucker AA, et al. Visualizing the kinetics of tumor-cell clearance in living animals. Proc Natl Acad Sci U S A 1999; 96:12044–9.

[7] Contag CH, Bachmann MH. Advances in in vivo bioluminescence imaging of gene expression. Annu Rev Biomed Eng 2002;4:235–60.

[8] Nielsen TO, West RB, Linn SC, et al. Molecular characterisation of soft tissue tumours: a gene expression study. Lancet 2002;359:1301–7.

[9] Krogsgaard M, Huppa JB, Purbhoo MA, et al. Linking molecular and cellular events in T cell activation and synapse formation. Semin Immunol 2003;15:307–15.

[10] Davis MM, Krogsgaard M, Huppa JB, et al. Dynamics of cell surface molecules during T cell recognition. Annu Rev Biochem 2003;72:717–42.

[11] Huppa JB, Gleimer M, Sumen C, et al. Continuous T cell receptor signaling required for synapse maintenance and full effector potential. Nat Immunol 2003;4:749–55.

[12] Stephens DJ, Allan VJ. Light microscopy techniques for live cell imaging. Science 2003;300: 82–6.

[13] Edinger M, Cao YA, Verneris MR, et al. Revealing lymphoma growth and the efficacy of immune cell therapies using in vivo bioluminescence imaging. Blood 2003;101:640–8.

[14] Lipshutz GS, Gruber CA, Cao Y, et al. In utero delivery of adeno-associated viral vectors: intraperitoneal gene transfer produces long-term expression. Mol Ther 2001;3:284–92.

[15] Weber SM, Peterson KA, Durkee B, et al. Imaging of murine liver tumor using microCT with a hepatocyte-selective contrast agent: accuracy is dependent on adequate contrast enhancement. J Surg Res 2004;119:41–5.

[16] Rice BW, Cable MD, Nelson MB. In vivo imaging of light-emitting probes. J Biomed Opt 2001;6:432–40.

[17] Tromberg BJ, Shah N, Lanning R, et al. Noninvasive in vivo characterization of breast tumors using photon migration spectroscopy. Neoplasia 2000;2:26–40.

[18] Lin AH, Luo J, Mondshein LH, et al. Global analysis of Smad2/3-dependent TGF-beta signaling in living mice reveals prominent tissue-specific responses to injury. J Immunol 2005; 175:547–54.

[19] DaCosta RS, Andersson H, Cirocco M, et al. Autofluorescence characterisation of isolated whole crypts and primary cultured human epithelial cells from normal, hyperplastic, and adenomatous colonic mucosa. J Clin Pathol 2005; 58:766–74.

[20] DaCosta RS, Wilson BC, Marcon NE. Optical techniques for the endoscopic detection of dysplastic colonic lesions. Curr Opin Gastroenterol 2005;21:70–9.

[21] Chwirot BW, Kowalska M, Plociennik N, et al. Variability of spectra of laser-induced fluorescence of colonic mucosa: its significance for fluorescence detection of colonic neoplasia. Indian J Exp Biol 2003;41:500–10.

[22] Haringsma J, Tytgat GN, Yano H, et al. Autofluorescence endoscopy: feasibility of detection of GI neoplasms unapparent to white light endoscopy with an evolving technology. Gastrointest Endosc 2001;53:642–50.

[23] Wang CY, Lin JK, Chen BF, et al. Autofluorescence spectroscopic differentiation between normal and cancerous colorectal tissues by means of a two-peak ratio algorithm. J Formos Med Assoc 1999;98:837–43.

[24] Tromberg BJ, Cerussi A, Shah N, et al. Imaging in breast cancer: diffuse optics in breast cancer: detecting tumors in pre-menopausal women and monitoring neoadjuvant chemotherapy. Breast Cancer Res 2005;7:279–85.

[25] Fujimoto JG. Optical coherence tomography for ultrahigh resolution in vivo imaging. Nat Biotechnol 2003;21:1361–7.

[26] Fujimoto JG, Pitris C, Boppart SA, et al. Optical coherence tomography: an emerging technology for biomedical imaging and optical biopsy. Neoplasia 2000;2:9–25.

[27] Bloch S, Lesage F, McIntosh L, et al. Whole-body fluorescence lifetime imaging of a tumor-targeted near-infrared molecular probe in mice. J Biomed Opt 2005;10:054003.

[28] Chaudhari AJ, Darvas F, Bading JR, et al. Hyperspectral and multispectral bioluminescence optical tomography for small animal imaging. Phys Med Biol 2005;50:5421–41.

[29] Ntziachristos V, Ripoll J, Wang LV, et al. Looking and listening to light: the evolution of whole-body photonic imaging. Nat Biotechnol 2005;23:313–20.

[30] von Andrian UH, Berger EM, Ramezani L, et al. In vivo behavior of neutrophils from two patients with distinct inherited leukocyte adhesion deficiency syndromes. J Clin Invest 1993;91:2893–7.

[31] Mazo IB, Gutierrez-Ramos JC, Frenette PS, et al. Hematopoietic progenitor cell rolling in bone marrow microvessels: parallel contributions by endothelial selectins and vascular cell adhesion molecule 1. J Exp Med 1998;188:465–74.

[32] Dewhirst MW, Shan S, Cao Y, et al. Intravital fluorescence facilitates measurement of multiple physiologic functions and gene expression in tumors of live animals. Dis Markers 2002; 18:293–311.

[33] Sumen C, Mempel TR, Mazo IB, et al. Intravital microscopy: visualizing immunity in context. Immunity 2004;21:315–29.

[34] Sipkins DA, Wei X, Wu JW, et al. In vivo imaging of specialized bone marrow endothelial microdomains for tumour engraftment. Nature 2005;435:969–73.

[35] Germain RN, Castellino F, Chieppa M, et al. An extended vision for dynamic high-resolution

intravital immune imaging. Semin Immunol 2005;17:431–41.

[36] Cao YA, Wagers AJ, Beilhack A, et al. Shifting foci of hematopoiesis during reconstitution from single stem cells. Proc Natl Acad Sci U S A 2004;101:221–6.

[37] Paulmurugan R, Umezawa Y, Gambhir SS. Noninvasive imaging of protein-protein interactions in living subjects by using reporter protein complementation and reconstitution strategies. Proc Natl Acad Sci U S A 2002;99: 15608–13.

[38] Ray P, Pimenta H, Paulmurugan R, et al. Noninvasive quantitative imaging of protein–protein interactions in living subjects. Proc Natl Acad Sci U S A 2002;99:3105–10.

[39] Paulmurugan R, Gambhir SS. Monitoring protein–protein interactions using split synthetic *Renilla* luciferase protein fragment-assisted complementation. Anal Chem 2003;75: 1584–9.

[40] Luker KE, Piwnica-Worms D. Optimizing luciferase protein fragment complementation for bioluminescent imaging of protein–protein interactions in live cells and animals. Methods Enzymol 2004;385:349–60.

[41] Wang Y, Wang G, O'Kane DJ, et al. A study of protein-protein interactions in living cells using luminescence resonance energy transfer (LRET) from *Renilla* luciferase to aequorea GFP. Mol Gen Genet 2001;264:578–87.

[42] Sadikot RT, Blackwell TS. Bioluminescence imaging. Proc Am Thorac Soc 2005;2:511–40.

[43] McCaffrey A, Kay MA, Contag CH. Advancing molecular therapies through in vivo bioluminescent imaging. Mol Imaging 2003;2:75–86.

[44] Contag CH, Ross BD. It's not just about anatomy: in vivo bioluminescence imaging as an eyepiece into biology. J Magn Reson Imaging 2002;16:378–87.

[45] Doyle TC, Burns SM, Contag CH. In vivo bioluminescence imaging for integrated studies of infection. Cell Microbiol 2004;6:303–17.

[46] Stolz U, Velez S, Wood KV, et al. Darwinian natural selection for orange bioluminescent color in a Jamaican click beetle. Proc Natl Acad Sci U S A 2003;100:14955–9.

[47] Wood KV. Luc genes: introduction of colour into bioluminescence assays. J Biolumin Chemilumin 1990;5:107–14.

[48] Zhao H, Doyle TC, Coquoz O, et al. Emission spectra of bioluminescent reporters and interaction with mammalian tissue determine the sensitivity of detection in vivo. J Biomed Opt 2005; 10:41210.

[49] Kadurugamuwa JL, Modi K, Coquoz O, et al. Reduction of astrogliosis by early treatment of pneumococcal meningitis measured by simultaneous imaging, in vivo, of the pathogen and host response. Infect Immun 2005;73:7836–43.

[50] Tonary AM, Pezacki JP. Simultaneous quantitative measurement of luciferase reporter activity and cell number in two- and three-dimensional cultures of hepatitis C virus replicons. Anal Biochem 2006;350:239–48.

[51] Ntziachristos V, Tung CH, Bremer C, et al. Fluorescence molecular tomography resolves protease activity in vivo. Nat Med 2002;8:757–60.

[52] Weissleder R, Tung CH, Mahmood U, et al. In vivo imaging of tumors with protease-activated near-infrared fluorescent probes. Nat Biotechnol 1999;17:375–8.

[53] Chen J, Tung CH, Mahmood U, et al. In vivo imaging of proteolytic activity in atherosclerosis. Circulation 2002;105:2766–71.

[54] Tung CH, Zeng Q, Shah K, et al. In vivo imaging of beta-galactosidase activity using far red fluorescent switch. Cancer Res 2004;64: 1579–83.

[55] Kircher MF, Weissleder R, Josephson L. A dual fluorochrome probe for imaging proteases. Bioconjug Chem 2004;15:242–8.

[56] Yang M, Baranov E, Jiang P, et al. Whole-body optical imaging of green fluorescent protein-expressing tumors and metastases. Proc Natl Acad Sci U S A 2000;97:1206–11.

[57] Hoffman R. Green fluorescent protein imaging of tumour growth, metastasis, and angiogenesis in mouse models. Lancet Oncol 2002;3:546–56.

[58] Nighswander-Rempel SP, Kupriyanov VV, Shaw RA. Relative contributions of hemoglobin and myoglobin to near-infrared spectroscopic images of cardiac tissue. Appl Spectrosc 2005; 59:190–3.

[59] Ye Y, Bloch S, Xu B, et al. Design, synthesis, and evaluation of near infrared fluorescent multimeric RGD peptides for targeting tumors. J Med Chem 2006;49:2268–75.

[60] Ntziachristos V, Bremer C, Weissleder R. Fluorescence imaging with near-infrared light: new technological advances that enable in vivo molecular imaging. Eur Radiol 2003;13:195–208.

[61] Lin Y, Weissleder R, Tung CH. Novel near-infrared cyanine fluorochromes: synthesis, properties, and bioconjugation. Bioconjug Chem 2002;13:605–10.

[62] Zacharias DA, Tsien RY. Molecular biology and mutation of green fluorescent protein. Methods Biochem Anal 2006;47:83–120.

[63] Shaner NC, Steinbach PA, Tsien RY. A guide to choosing fluorescent proteins. Nat Methods 2005;2:905–9.

[64] Giepmans BN, Adams SR, Ellisman MH, et al. The fluorescent toolbox for assessing protein location and function. Science 2006;312:217–24.

[65] Hsu ER, Anslyn EV, Dharmawardhane S, et al. A far-red fluorescent contrast agent to image epidermal growth factor receptor expression. Photochem Photobiol 2004;79:272–9.

[66] Sakatani K, Kashiwasake-Jibu M, Taka Y, et al. Noninvasive optical imaging of the subarachnoid space and cerebrospinal fluid pathways based on near-infrared fluorescence. J Neurosurg 1997;87:738–45.

[67] Reynolds JS, Troy TL, Mayer RH, et al. Imaging of spontaneous canine mammary tumors using fluorescent contrast agents. Photochem Photobiol 1999;70:87–94.

[68] Zheng G, Li H, Yang K, et al. Tricarbocyanine cholesteryl laurates labeled LDL: new near infrared fluorescent probes (NIRFs) for monitoring tumors and gene therapy of familial hypercholesterolemia. Bioorg Med Chem Lett 2002;12:1485–8.

[69] Becker A, Hessenius C, Licha K, et al. Receptor-targeted optical imaging of tumors with near-infrared fluorescent ligands. Nat Biotechnol 2001;19:327–31.

[70] Becker A, Riefke B, Ebert B, et al. Macromolecular contrast agents for optical imaging of tumors: comparison of indotricarbocyanine-labeled human serum albumin and transferrin. Photochem Photobiol 2000;72:234–41.

[71] Shah K, Tung CH, Chang CH, et al. In vivo imaging of HIV protease activity in amplicon vector-transduced gliomas. Cancer Res 2004;64:273–8.

[72] Ponomarev V, Doubrovin M, Serganova I, et al. A novel triple-modality reporter gene for whole-body fluorescent, bioluminescent, and nuclear noninvasive imaging. Eur J Nucl Med Mol Imaging 2004;31:740–51.

[73] Doubrovin M, Ponomarev V, Serganova I, et al. Development of a new reporter gene system—dsRed/xanthine phosphoribosyltransferase-xanthine for molecular imaging of processes behind the intact blood–brain barrier. Mol Imaging 2003;2:93–112.

[74] Flusberg BA, Cocker ED, Piyawattanametha W, et al. Fiber-optic fluorescence imaging. Nat Methods 2005;2:941–50.

[75] Funovics MA, Alencar H, Su HS, et al. Miniaturized multichannel near infrared endoscope for mouse imaging. Mol Imaging 2003;2:350–7.

[76] Wang TD, Mandella MJ, Contag CH, et al. Dual-axis confocal microscope for high-resolution in vivo imaging. Opt Lett 2003;28:414–6.

[77] Sokolov K, Sung KB, Collier T, et al. Endoscopic microscopy. Dis Markers 2002;18:269–91.

[78] Sokolov K, Aaron J, Hsu B, et al. Optical systems for in vivo molecular imaging of cancer. Technol Cancer Res Treat 2003;2:491–504.

[79] Drezek RA, Richards-Kortum R, Brewer MA, et al. Optical imaging of the cervix. Cancer 2003;98:2015–27.

[80] Thorne SH, Negrin RS, Contag CH. Synergistic antitumor effects of immune cell viral biotherapy. Science 2006;311:1780–4.

[81] Halin C, Rodrigo Mora J, Sumen C, et al. In vivo imaging of lymphocyte trafficking. Annu Rev Cell Dev Biol 2005;21:581–603.

[82] Sosnovik D, Weissleder R. Magnetic resonance and fluorescence based molecular imaging technologies. Prog Drug Res 2005;62:83–115.

[83] Graves EE, Weissleder R, Ntziachristos V. Fluorescence molecular imaging of small animal tumor models. Curr Mol Med 2004;4:419–30.

[84] Figueiredo JL, Alencar H, Weissleder R, et al. Near infrared thoracoscopy of tumoral protease activity for improved detection of peripheral lung cancer. Int J Cancer 2006;118:2672–7.

[85] Bremer C, Ntziachristos V, Weitkamp B, et al. Optical imaging of spontaneous breast tumors using protease sensing 'smart' optical probes. Invest Radiol 2005;40:321–7.

[86] Safran M, Kim WY, O'Connell F, et al. Mouse model for noninvasive imaging of HIF prolyl hydroxylase activity: assessment of an oral agent that stimulates erythropoietin production. Proc Natl Acad Sci U S A 2006;103: 105–10.

[87] Zhang GJ, Kaelin WG Jr. Bioluminescent imaging of ubiquitin ligase activity: measuring Cdk2 activity in vivo through changes in p27 turnover. Methods Enzymol 2005;399: 530–49.

[88] Laxman B, Hall DE, Bhojani MS, et al. Noninvasive real-time imaging of apoptosis. Proc Natl Acad Sci U S A 2002;99:16551–5.

[89] Troy T, Jekic-McMullen D, Sambucetti L, et al. Quantitative comparison of the sensitivity of detection of fluorescent and bioluminescent reporters in animal models. Mol Imaging 2004;3: 9–23.

[90] Benaron DA, Cheong WF, Stevenson DK. Tissue optics. Science 1997;276:2002–3.

[91] Jobsis FF. Noninvasive, infrared monitoring of cerebral and myocardial oxygen sufficiency and circulatory parameters. Science 1977;198: 1264–7.

[92] Yang M, Luiken G, Baranov E, et al. Facile whole-body imaging of internal fluorescent tumors in mice with an LED flashlight. Biotechniques 2005;39:170–2.

[93] Yang M, Reynoso J, Jiang P, et al. Transgenic nude mouse with ubiquitous green fluorescent protein expression as a host for human tumors. Cancer Res 2004;64:8651–6.

[94] Chalfie M, Tu Y, Euskirchen G, et al. Green fluorescent protein as a marker for gene expression. Science 1994;263:802–5.

[95] Yang M, Jiang P, Sun FX, et al. A fluorescent orthotopic bone metastasis model of human prostate cancer. Cancer Res 1999;59:781–6.

[96] Yang M, Jiang P, An Z, et al. Genetically fluorescent melanoma bone and organ metastasis models. Clin Cancer Res 1999;5:3549–59.

[97] Yang M, Chishima T, Wang X, et al. Multi-organ metastatic capability of Chinese hamster ovary cells revealed by green fluorescent protein (GFP) expression. Clin Exp Metastasis 1999; 17:417–22.

[98] Naumov GN, Wilson SM, MacDonald IC, et al. Cellular expression of green fluorescent protein, coupled with high-resolution in vivo videomicroscopy, to monitor steps in tumor metastasis. J Cell Sci 1999;112(Pt 12):1835–42.

[99] Yang M, Hasegawa S, Jiang P, et al. Widespread skeletal metastatic potential of human lung

cancer revealed by green fluorescent protein expression. Cancer Res 1998;58:4217–21.

[100] Hoffman RM. Orthotopic transplant mouse models with green fluorescent protein-expressing cancer cells to visualize metastasis and angiogenesis. Cancer Metastasis Rev 1998;17:271–7.

[101] Chishima T, Yang M, Miyagi Y, et al. Governing step of metastasis visualized in vitro. Proc Natl Acad Sci U S A 1997;94:11573–6.

[102] Chishima T, Miyagi Y, Wang X, et al. Cancer invasion and micrometastasis visualized in live tissue by green fluorescent protein expression. Cancer Res 1997;57:2042–7.

[103] Chishima T, Miyagi Y, Wang X, et al. Visualization of the metastatic process by green fluorescent protein expression. Anticancer Res 1997; 17:2377–84.

[104] Chishima T, Miyagi Y, Wang X, et al. Metastatic patterns of lung cancer visualized live and in process by green fluorescence protein expression. Clin Exp Metastasis 1997;15:547–52.

[105] Chishima T, Miyagi Y, Li L, et al. Use of histoculture and green fluorescent protein to visualize tumor cell host interaction. In Vitro Cell Dev Biol Anim 1997;33:745–7.

[106] Ropp JD, Donahue CJ, Wolfgang-Kimball D, et al. Aequorea green fluorescent protein analysis by flow cytometry. Cytometry 1995;21: 309–17.

[107] Zaccolo M, De Giorgi F, Cho CY, et al. A genetically encoded, fluorescent indicator for cyclic AMP in living cells. Nat Cell Biol 2000;2:25–9.

[108] Campbell RE, Tour O, Palmer AE, et al. A monomeric red fluorescent protein. Proc Natl Acad Sci U S A 2002;99:7877–82.

[109] Patterson GH. A new harvest of fluorescent proteins. Nat Biotechnol 2004;22:1524–5.

[110] Shaner NC, Campbell RE, Steinbach PA, et al. Improved monomeric red, orange and yellow fluorescent proteins derived from Discosoma sp. red fluorescent protein. Nat Biotechnol 2004;22:1567–72.

[111] Miyawaki A. Green fluorescent protein-like proteins in reef Anthozoa animals. Cell Struct Funct 2002;27:343–7.

[112] Fradkov AF, Verkhusha VV, Staroverov DB, et al. Far-red fluorescent tag for protein labeling. Biochem J 2002;368:17–21.

[113] Gurskaya NG, Savitsky AP, Yanushevich YG, et al. Color transitions in coral's fluorescent proteins by site-directed mutagenesis. BMC Biochem 2001;2:6.

[114] Matz MV, Fradkov AF, Labas YA, et al. Fluorescent proteins from nonbioluminescent Anthozoa species. Nat Biotechnol 1999;17:969–73.

[115] Liu ZM, Chen GG, Ng EK, et al. Upregulation of heme oxygenase-1 and p21 confers resistance to apoptosis in human gastric cancer cells. Oncogene 2004;23:503–13.

[116] Terskikh A, Fradkov A, Ermakova G, et al. Fluorescent timer: protein that changes color with time. Science 2000;290:1585–8.

[117] Hastings JW. Chemistries and colors of bioluminescent reactions: a review. Gene 1996;173: 5–11.

[118] Franks NP, Jenkins A, Conti E, et al. Structural basis for the inhibition of firefly luciferase by a general anesthetic. Biophys J 1998;75:2205–11.

[119] Conti E, Franks NP, Brick P. Crystal structure of firefly luciferase throws light on a superfamily of adenylate-forming enzymes. Structure 1996; 4:287–98.

[120] Wood KV, Lam YA, McElroy WD, et al. Bioluminescent click beetles revisited. J Biolumin Chemilumin 1989;4:31–9.

[121] Wood KV, Lam YA, Seliger HH, et al. Complementary DNA coding click beetle luciferases can elicit bioluminescence of different colors. Science 1989;244:700–2.

[122] Karkhanis YD, Cormier MJ. Isolation and properties of Renilla reniformis luciferase, a low molecular weight energy conversion enzyme. Biochemistry 1971;10:317–26.

[123] Matthews JC, Hori K, Cormier MJ. Purification and properties of Renilla reniformis luciferase. Biochemistry 1977;16:85–91.

[124] Srikantha T, Klapach A, Lorenz WW, et al. The sea pansy Renilla reniformis luciferase serves as a sensitive bioluminescent reporter for differential gene expression in Candida albicans. J Bacteriol 1996;178:121–9.

[125] Shimomura O, Johnson FH. Chemical nature of bioluminescence systems in coelenterates. Proc Natl Acad Sci U S A 1975;72:1546–9.

[126] Greer LF III, Szalay AA. Imaging of light emission from the expression of luciferases in living cells and organisms: a review. Luminescence 2002;17:43–74.

[127] Tannous BA, Kim DE, Fernandez JL, et al. Codon-optimized gaussia luciferase cDNA for mammalian gene expression in culture and in vivo. Mol Ther 2005;11:435–43.

[128] Zhao H, Doyle TC, Wong RJ, et al. Characterization of coelenterazine analogs for measurements of Renilla luciferase activity in live cells and living animals. Mol Imaging 2004;3:43–54.

[129] So MK, Xu C, Loening AM, et al. Self-illuminating quantum dot conjugates for in vivo imaging. Nat Biotechnol 2006;24:339–43.

[130] Bhaumik S, Gambhir SS. Optical imaging of Renilla luciferase reporter gene expression in living mice. Proc Natl Acad Sci U S A 2002; 99:377–82.

[131] Alam J, Cook JL. Reporter genes: application to the study of mammalian gene transcription. Anal Biochem 1990;188:245–54.

[132] Modo M, Cash D, Mellodew K, et al. Tracking transplanted stem cell migration using bifunctional, contrast agent-enhanced, magnetic resonance imaging. Neuroimage 2002;17:803–11.

[133] Louie AY, Huber MM, Ahrens ET, et al. In vivo visualization of gene expression using magnetic resonance imaging. Nat Biotechnol 2000;18: 321–5.

[134] Jacobs RE, Ahrens ET, Meade TJ, et al. Looking deeper into vertebrate development. Trends Cell Biol 1999;9:73–6.

[135] Wehrman TS, von Degenfeld G, Krutzik PO, et al. Luminescent imaging of beta-galactosidase activity in living subjects using sequential reporter-enzyme luminescence. Nat Methods 2006;3:295–301.

[136] Ray P, De A, Min JJ, et al. Imaging trifusion multimodality reporter gene expression in living subjects. Cancer Res 2004;64:1323–30.

[137] Day RN, Kawecki M, Berry D. Dual-function reporter protein for analysis of gene expression in living cells. Biotechniques 1998;25:844–56.

[138] Edinger M, Hoffmann P, Contag CH, et al. Evaluation of effector cell fate and function by in vivo bioluminescence imaging. Methods 2003; 31:172–9.

[139] Mandl S, Mari C, Edinger M, et al. In vivo dynamics of tumor cell death: multi-modality imaging identifies key imaging times for assessing response to chemotherapy using an orthotopic mouse model of lymphoma. 2003.

[140] Cao YA, Bachmann MH, Beilhack A, et al. Molecular imaging using labeled donor tissues reveals patterns of engraftment, rejection, and survival in transplantation. Transplantation 2005;80:134–9.

[141] Shachaf CM, Kopelman AM, Arvanitis C, et al. MYC inactivation uncovers pluripotent differentiation and tumour dormancy in hepatocellular cancer. Nature 2004;431:1112–7.

[142] Mattheakis LC, Dias JM, Choi YJ, et al. Optical coding of mammalian cells using semiconductor quantum dots. Anal Biochem 2004;327: 200–8.

[143] Swenson DL, Warfield KL, Kuehl K, et al. Generation of Marburg virus-like particles by co-expression of glycoprotein and matrix protein. FEMS Immunol Med Microbiol 2004;40: 27–31.

[144] Arai R, Nakagawa H, Kitayama A, et al. Detection of protein-protein interaction by bioluminescence resonance energy transfer from firefly luciferase to red fluorescent protein. J Biosci Bioeng 2002;94:362–4.

[145] Issad T, Boute N, Pernet K. The activity of the insulin receptor assessed by bioluminescence resonance energy transfer. Ann N Y Acad Sci 2002;973:120–3.

[146] Boute N, Jockers R, Issad T. The use of resonance energy transfer in high-throughput screening: BRET versus FRET. Trends Pharmacol Sci 2002;23:351–4.

[147] Xu Y, Piston DW, Johnson CH. A bioluminescence resonance energy transfer (BRET) system: application to interacting circadian clock proteins. Proc Natl Acad Sci U S A 1999; 96:151–6.

[148] Platek SM, Fonteyn LC, Izzetoglu M, et al. Functional near infrared spectroscopy reveals differences in self-other processing as a function of schizotypal personality traits. Schizophr Res 2005;73:125–7.

[149] Chen Y, Intes X, Tailor DR, et al. Probing rat brain oxygenation with near-infrared spectroscopy (NIRS) and magnetic resonance imaging (MRI). Adv Exp Med Biol 2003;510: 199–204.

[150] Shiino A, Haida M, Beauvoit B, et al. Three-dimensional redox image of the normal gerbil brain. Neuroscience 1999;91:1581–5.

[151] Benaron DA, Stevenson DK. Optical time-of-flight and absorbance imaging of biologic media. Science 1993;259:1463–6.

[152] Cook SH, Griffin DE. Luciferase imaging of a neurotropic viral infection in intact animals. J Virol 2003;77:5333–8.

[153] Luker GD, Bardill JP, Prior JL, et al. Noninvasive bioluminescence imaging of herpes simplex virus type 1 infection and therapy in living mice. J Virol 2002;76:12149–61.

[154] Scheffold C, Kornacker M, Scheffold YC, et al. Visualization of effective tumor targeting by CD8 + natural killer T cells redirected with bispecific antibody F(ab')(2)HER2xCD3. Cancer Res 2002;62:5785–91.

[155] Soling A, Theiss C, Jungmichel S, et al. A dual function fusion protein of herpes simplex virus type 1 thymidine kinase and firefly luciferase for noninvasive in vivo imaging of gene therapy in malignant glioma. Genet Vaccines Ther 2004;2:7.

[156] Schellingerhout D, Rainov NG, Breakefield XO, et al. Quantitation of HSV mass distribution in a rodent brain tumor model. Gene Ther 2000; 7:1648–55.

[157] Pike L, Petravicz J, Wang S. Bioluminescence imaging after HSV amplicon vector delivery into brain. J Gene Med 2006.

[158] Kaplitt MG, Tjuvajev JG, Leib DA, et al. Mutant herpes simplex virus induced regression of tumors growing in immunocompetent rats. J Neurooncol 1994;19:137–47.

[159] Hardy J, Francis KP, DeBoer M, et al. Extracellular replication of Listeria monocytogenes in the murine gall bladder. Science 2004;303:851–3.

[160] Hardy J, Margolis JJ, Contag CH. Induced biliary excretion of Listeria monocytogenes. Infect Immun 2006;74:1819–27.

[161] Luker KE, Hutchens M, Schultz T, et al. Bioluminescence imaging of vaccinia virus: effects of interferon on viral replication and spread. Virology 2005;341:284–300.

[162] Rehemtulla A, Hall DE, Stegman LD, et al. Molecular imaging of gene expression and efficacy following adenoviral-mediated brain tumor gene therapy. Mol Imaging 2002;1:43–55.

[163] Zhu L, Ramboz S, Hewitt D, et al. Noninvasive imaging of GFAP expression after neuronal damage in mice. Neurosci Lett 2004;367:210–2.

[164] Echchannaoui H, Frei K, Schnell C, et al. Toll-like receptor 2-deficient mice are highly susceptible to *Streptococcus pneumoniae* meningitis

because of reduced bacterial clearing and enhanced inflammation. J Infect Dis 2002;186: 798–806.

[165] Bauer SM, Goldstein LJ, Bauer RJ, et al. The bone marrow-derived endothelial progenitor cell response is impaired in delayed wound healing from ischemia. J Vasc Surg 2006;43: 134–41.

[166] Cao F, Lin S, Xie X, et al. In vivo visualization of embryonic stem cell survival, proliferation, and migration after cardiac delivery. Circulation 2006;113:1005–14.

[167] Takamatsu S, Furukawa T, Mori T, et al. Noninvasive imaging of transplanted living functional cells transfected with a reporter estrogen receptor gene. Nucl Med Biol 2005;32:821–9.

[168] Okada S, Ishii K, Yamane J, et al. In vivo imaging of engrafted neural stem cells: its application in evaluating the optimal timing of transplantation for spinal cord injury. FASEB J 2005;19:1839–41.

[169] Lindvall O, Kokaia Z, Martinez-Serrano A. Stem cell therapy for human neurodegenerative disorders-how to make it work. Nat Med 2004; 10:S42–50.

[170] Shah K, Bureau E, Kim DE, et al. Glioma therapy and real-time imaging of neural precursor cell migration and tumor regression. Ann Neurol 2005;57:34–41.

[171] Wiles S, Ferguson K, Stefanidou M, et al. Alternative luciferase for monitoring bacterial cells under adverse conditions. Appl Environ Microbiol 2005;71:3427–32.

[172] Verhaegent M, Christopoulos TK. Recombinant gaussia luciferase. Overexpression, purification, and analytical application of a bioluminescent reporter for DNA hybridization. Anal Chem 2002;74:4378–85.

[173] Fisher AJ, Thompson TB, Thoden JB, et al. The 1.5-A resolution crystal structure of bacterial luciferase in low salt conditions. J Biol Chem 1996;271:21956–68.

NEUROIMAGING
CLINICS
OF NORTH AMERICA

Neuroimag Clin N Am 16 (2006) 655–679

Molecular Imaging of Novel Cell- and Viral-Based Therapies

Dawid Schellingerhout, MD

- ■ The fundamentals: technologies for cell- and viral-based tracking
- ■ Cell loading
- ■ Cell gene modification
  Treatment versus disease modeling in gene modification strategies
- ■ Viral loading
- ■ Viral gene modification
- ■ Dual/multiple imaging strategies
- ■ Human applications of cell- and viral-based imaging
- ■ Summary
- ■ Acknowledgements
- ■ References

Drugs, surgery, and radiation are the traditional modalities of therapy in medicine. To these are being added new therapies based on cells and viruses or their derivatives. In these novel therapies, a cell or viral vector acts as a "drug" in its own right, altering the host or a disease process to bring about healing. Most of these advances originate from the significant recent advances in molecular medicine, but some of them have been around for quite some time. Blood transfusions and cowpox vaccinations are part of the history of medicine, but, nevertheless, are examples of cell- and viral-based therapies. This review focuses on the modern molecular incarnations of these therapies and, specifically, on how imaging is used to track and guide these novel agents.

Cell-based therapies typically are based on stem cells, but immunocytes are another favorite cell-based therapy . Even non-mammalian cells, in the form of bacteria, have been used as therapeutic agents. Viral agents typically are used in gene therapy, to alter the genetic composition of host or disease tissue. They are either modified viruses such as

herpes simplex virus (HSV), adenovirus (AV), or they can be artificial virus-like vectors not based on naturally occurring viruses.

The number of diseases potentially treatable by these new therapeutics is limited only by human ingenuity. The National Institutes of Health (NIH) list 1130 clinical trials involving stem cells and 617 gene therapy trials. This represents a massive investment by industry and government in these new therapies. These trials deal with various diseases such as cancer (415 stem cell trials, 197 gene therapy trials), heart disease (77 stem cell trials, 45 gene therapy trials), stroke (five stem cell trials, 12 gene therapy trials), and spinal cord injury (13 stem cell trials, five gene therapy trials).

With the huge increase in sophistication and therapeutic potential of these new modes of therapy is born the need for advanced imaging that is similarly sophisticated. Imaging, in the clinical context, is needed to: assess the need for these therapies, track and guide the administration of these agents, and assess treatment outcomes. Traditional anatomic imaging cannot perform all of these

Neuroradiology Section, Department of Radiology and Experimental Diagnostic Imaging, Division of Diagnostic Imaging, M D Anderson Cancer Center, 1515 Holcombe Boulevard, Houston, TX 77030, USA
E-mail address: dawid.schellingerhout@di.mdacc.tmc.edu

doi:10.1016/j.nic.2006.06.006

functions, and new molecular imaging technologies are being invented to fill this need. This article reviews several of the imaging modalities used to image these new therapies.

These therapies are reviewed from an imaging perspective, and the article attempts to provide a structured overview of the literature on this topic, ranging from experimental systems to the first human applications. This should be seen as a survey of the field, lightly touching many aspects, and serving as an entry point for the reader to learn more about the field.

The fundamentals: technologies for cell- and viral-based tracking

There are two very different approaches to tracking a cell or viral therapy: loading technologies or gene modification technologies (Table 1). Loading technologies usually are performed in vitro, and involve the administration of an exogenous label to a purified cell or viral preparation. The label must: be nontoxic, leave the cell/virus fully functional, have a stable association with the cell/virus, and be imagable by a suitable technology once injected in vivo.

The main benefit of the loading (or prelabeling) approach is that, ideally, there is no background imaging signal to deal with. The only label in the body after injection is that associated with the loaded or prelabeled cell or viral particle. The main drawbacks of loading strategies are:

- **Labeling is often chemically harsh to cells/ viruses and may have a deleterious effect on the therapy.**
- **Labeling cannot be repeated; once the therapy is injected, the amount of label is fixed and nonrenewable.**
- **Imaging is therefore transient, as the label inevitably will be diluted, decayed or be broken down and excreted.**
- **Many biological processes, such as gene expression, are not amenable to imaging by this approach.**

Genetic modification technologies involve the manipulation of the cell/viral genome to insert a marker gene; that is a gene that has as its product a protein that can be imaged by some means. Genetic modification requires that:

- **The cell/ virus be genetically manipulated to insert the marker gene**
- **The marker gene be stably integrated in the genome**
- **The gene product be expressed reliably**
- **The gene product must be imagable**

The main benefit of gene modification is that the cell/virus becomes permanently imagable, and at future dates after administration even the cell/viral progeny (if proliferating) may be imaged without dilution. Gene modification is maintained by the same biological mechanisms that maintain normal genes in living tissues, and thus constantly is renewed. The main drawback of successful genetic modifications is:

- **They are permanent.**
- **They involve the genome and hence are considered with suspicion, as many diseases (cancer, viral infections) share these attributes.**
- **The full consequences of these manipulations may not be immediately apparent.**

On the other hand, some cells/viruses are difficult to modify genetically, or can be modified only transiently with loss of gene expression over time.

Table 1 shows the main organization of the literature in this article. All literature reviewed can be classified by asking two questions: What is labeled? And, how is it labeled? What is labeled can either be a cellular or a viral therapy. How it is labeled can be a loading technology or a genetic modification. Thus one creates a matrix with four quadrants: cell loading, viral loading, cell gene modification and viral gene modification. Each of these is considered separately. This simple classification breaks down for some of the more sophisticated multi-label studies, which are considered separately, but the guiding principle remains as a useful device for the reader who wishes to interpret the complex literature of this field.

Cell loading

A survey of available cell loading technologies is listed in Table 2. The basis of all these techniques

Table 1: Tracking of cellular and viral Therapies, overview of technologies

		Material labeled	
		Cells	*Virus*
Labeling method	Load	Table 2	Table 5
	Gene modification	Table 3	Table 6

Table 2: Cellular Loading technologies

Labeling Method	Material	Material labeled				
		Cells				Other
		Stem cells	Immunocytes	Bacteria	Cancer cells	
Iron Oxides	MION	[31,32]	[1]		[1]	
	MION–Tat	[16,17,21–28]	[32,258,254]		[32]	[29,30]
	SPIO	[17,34–39]	[2–6]			
	SPIO–transfection agent	[43,44]	[36,37,40]		[36,37,41,42]	[36,37]
	SPIO–protamine					
	SPIO–Tat peptide					
	SPIO–conjugate	[12,16,45–50]	[33]		[41,47,53]	[55–57]
	Dendromer	[11–13]	[48,51–54]		[41]	[265]
	Larger sized iron oxides	[7–9]	[8,9]		[8,9]	
	Magnetite complexes		[14]			
	Colloids	[15]				
	Liposomes	[16–18]	[19]			
	SPIO viral envelopes	[20]				
	Electro-poresis					
	Magneto-poresis	[58]				
	Non colloid iron particles	[10]	[40]			
	"Gene gun" iron oxide	[59–61]				
T1-agents	Gd(3+)	[62–64]				
	Gd-polymer				[65,66]	[68]
	Gd-peptide	[69]			[67]	
	Gd-transfection agent	[70]				
	Gd–HPDO3A an Eu–HPDO3A	[16]				
	Gd–liposome	[71]				
	Gadophrin					
	Manganese		[72]			
	Other lanthanides (Tb, Eur)					[73]
Nuclear	^{64}Cu–PTSM				[74]	
	^{18}FDG				[74]	
	^{111}Indium–"EGadMe"				[266]	
	Radiolabeled transferring	[268]				
	^{18}F–FEAU				[75]	
	^{111}Indium–oxine	[27,76]	[2,77]			
	^{99m}Tc–HMPAO		[77]			
Optical	PKH dye	[82]				[83]
	Quantum dots					[81]
	CM–DiI dye					[84]
	DiI dye	[23]				
	Rhodamine	[63,64]				
	Other fluorophore	[7,15,38]				

is the loading of cells of interest with a substance that is imagable. MR imaging contrast agents such as the iron oxides are a favorite for imaging based on T2-weighted contrast, with many variations in the type of iron oxide and the methodology used to achieve labeling. Iron oxides used range from the very small, typified by monocrystalline iron oxide nanoparticle (MION) [1], through midsize preparations typified by the various superparamagnetic iron oxides (SPIO) [2–6], to large-sized iron oxide [7–9] or even magnetic particles [10]. The most typical iron oxides used (MION and SPIO) are crystalline forms of iron oxide covered with dextran to render them soluble and biocompatible. Other formulations, however, have been used, including dendrimers [11–13], magnetite complexes [14], colloidal preparations [15], liposomes [16–19], and viral envelopes as covering material [20]. A large part of the effort in this area was driven by the difficulties of getting sufficient quantities of iron oxide loaded into the cells to be able to image the cells successfully. Many investigators used long incubations of cells with iron oxides in the media, trusting to fluid-phase pinocytosis and phagocytic activity by the cells to gradually accumulate

sufficient iron [1–6,16,17,21–30]. Many cell types, however, are not amenable to this strategy, and several sophisticated derivitisation strategies were evolved to carry iron oxides intracellularly. One of these was to decorate the dextran coating of iron oxides with HIV–tat peptide, a peptide known to cause translocation across cell membranes [31–33] (Fig. 1). Another approach used transfection agents (cationic lipophilic agents used to carry DNA into cells for transduction work in cell biology) to carry iron oxides into cells, an approach that has proved popular [17,34–42]. Protamine can be used as a transfection agent with already approved iron oxide preparations, an off-label approach with many potential regulatory advantages [43,44]. SPIOs have been conjugated to various complexes to improve cell uptake and biocompatibility [12,16,41,45–57]. Others have tried more physical approaches, and have used electroporesis [40] and magnetoporesis [58] to directly force iron oxides into cells. Some have used kinetic gene gun devices to label cells with iron oxides [59–61].

MR imaging of cell-based therapies also can be accomplished with T1-weighted imaging using appropriate image markers. Gadolinium, the active

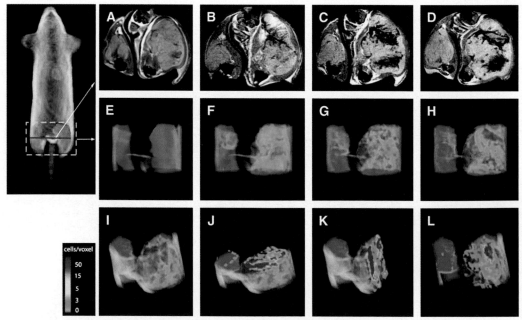

Fig. 1. Cell loading with iron oxides. time-course of CLIO-HD OT-I CD8 + T cell homing to B16-OVA tumor. Serial MR imaging was performed following adoptive transfer into a mouse carrying both B16F0 (*left side*) and B16-OVA (*right side*) melanomas. Axial slices through the mouse thighs (*A*) before adoptive transfer, (*B*) 12 hours, (*C*) 16 hours, (*D*) 36 hours after adoptive transfer of CLIO-HD labeled OT-I CD8 + T cells. Three-dimensional color-scaled reconstructions of B16F0 (*left*) and B16-OVA (*right*) melanomas at (*E*) 0 hours, (*F*) 12 hours, (*G*) 16 hours, (*H, I*) 36 hours following adoptive transfer. Numbers of cells/voxel are color-coded as shown in scale. (*J*) axial, (*K*) sagittal, (*L*) coronal plane slices through the three-dimensional reconstruction shown in *I*. Data are representative of 8 individual animals. (*Adapted from* Kircher MF, Allport JR, Graves EE et al. In vivo high resolution three-dimensional imaging of antigen-specific cytotoxic T-lymphocyte trafficking to tumors. Cancer Res 2003;63: 6838–46; with permission.)

component of the most commonly used clinical MR contrast agent, has been used as part of a polymer [62–66], linked to a peptide [67,68], together with transfection agents [69], in liposomes [16], as part of novel chelators [70], and in porphyrons [71]. In addition, manganese [72] and lanthanides other than gadolinium [73] have been used for labeling.

Nuclear imaging technology is suited for cell tracking, because of the high sensitivity of the imaging modality. Cell labeling with positron emission tomography (PET) has been accomplished with ^{64}Cu-PTSM [74], ^{18}FDG [74], and ^{18}F-FEAU [75], with single photon emission computed tomography (SPECT) using ^{111}Indium-oxine [2,27,76–78] and ^{99m}Tc-HMPAO [77]. Historically, the first cell labeling and tracking studies were done with ^{111}indium–oxine-labeled white blood cells [79,80].

Optical imaging of cell therapies is an emerging field, but several articles have appeared using quantum dots [81] and various fluorophores such s PKH dye [82,83], dil dye [23,84], rhodamine [63,64], and others [7,15,38]. Reviews are available on many aspects of cell labeling technology [39,85–103].

All these approaches have their advocates and detractors, and most likely will find applicability in at least a niche application. Iron oxide labeling technology seems to be the cell-loading technology with the largest number of adherents, and the widest body of literature. Stem cells and immunocytes seem to be the cells most frequently labeled, but bacterial cells and cancer cells also are targeted frequently.

In general, these approaches are safe, but some reports have emerged on potential toxicities of iron oxide labeling [104–106], and also of optical labeling technologies [107] on the cells being imaged. These concerns should be considered as these imaging technologies are developed further in the future.

Cell gene modification

A survey of cell gene modification technologies is presented in Table 3. These are understood most easily by examining the gene that was introduced or modified to render the cells imagable.

Gene modification leads to the production of an intracellular or membrane protein in the cell of interest. This protein product subsequently is probed for with an appropriate imagable chemical or physical agent. An example of an intracellular protein is HSV type 1–thymidine kinase (HSV1-tk). The herpes simplex virus thymidine kinase can be probed for using various radiolabeled markers. Two of

these are FIAU [108–115] and FHBG [116–119]. A modification of the HSV1-tk enzyme has been created, the so-called HSV-1-sr39tk. This variation of the HSV thymidine kinase shows a greater affinity for ganciclovir analogs and is coming into common use in all applications where thymidine kinase is used. It provides improved target–to-background ratios with FIAU [120] and FHBG [121,122].

A genetic modification involving the cell membrane is the dopamine 2 receptor (D2r). This receptor can be probed for with radiotracer agents such as tropane [123] and fluoro-ethyl-spiperone (FESP) [124].

Another genetic modification is to express fluorescent proteins of which a red fluorescent protein (RFP) [116,125] and green fluorescent protein (GFP) [117,126–133] are the most popular.

Cells also can be modified to express the luciferase enzyme. Luciferase catalyzes the breakdown of its substrate, luciferin, with the emission of a photon that can be detected using specialized optical imaging equipment. There are multiple examples of such modifications done in stem cells [116,121, 125–128,134,135] (Fig. 2) immunocytes [129,130, 136–141], bacteria [142–146], cancer cells [114, 133,147–152], and also other cells [114,130,134, 148,153,154].

The transferrin receptor has been used to probe for cells, particularly stem cells [155], and bacteria [156] by means of accumulation of iron and subsequent MR imaging. Ferritin has been used in a similar fashion [132].

An artificial receptor that binds to oxotechnetate [157] has been described as a model system of a receptor that would not be occurring in nature. The enzyme tyrosinase has been used to bind indium [158] and other metals and thus provide imaging contrast for nuclear or MR imaging.

Treatment versus disease modeling in gene modification strategies

A survey of the literature indicates that in multiple cases, cells have genetic modifications applied to them not for the purposes of therapy but for the purposes of studying the disease itself. Confusion can result if clear distinction is not maintained between imaging a disease process and imaging a cell-based therapy. Table 4 lists various studies where cellular gene modification was applied for imaging purposes, sometimes to image a cellular treatment, sometimes to study the disease state, and sometimes to prove technology in basic studies that could be applied either way. There are many examples of each, indicative of the very valuable information that can be gleaned from imaging either a disease model or a treatment model.

Table 3: **Cellular gene Modification technologies**

| | | Material labeled | | | | |
| | | Cells | | | | |
Gene	Probe	Stem cells	Immunocytes	Bacteria	Cancer cells	Other
Labeling method						
HSV1–tk	FIAU		[108,109]	[110,111]	[112–115]	
	FHBG	[116,117]	[118]			[119]
HSV1–sr39tk	FIAU		[120]		[120]	
	FHBG	[121]			[122]	
D2r	Tropane	[123]			[124]	
	FESP					
hSSTr2	99mTc–P2045					
RFP	Exogenous light	[116,125]	[129,130]		[131–133]	[130]
GFP	Exogenous light	[117,126–128]		[268]		
Luciferase	Luciferin	[116,121,125–128, 134,135]	[129,130, 136–141]	[142–146]	[114,133, 147–152]	[114,130,134, 148,153,154]
Transferrin receptor	Exogenous/ Endogenous iron	[155]		[156]		
Ferritin	Endogenous iron				[132]	
Artificial oxotechnetate receptor	99mTc-glucoheptonate				[157]	
Tyrosinase	111Indium				[158]	[158]

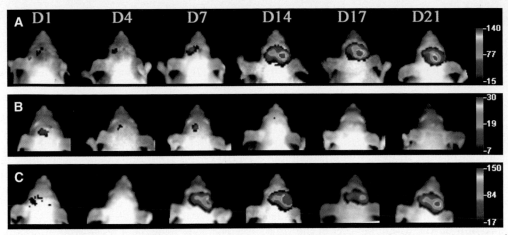

Fig. 2. Genetic modification of cells for bioluminescent imaging. Representative bioluminescent imaging of neu-ral stem cell injections modified to express luciferase (also GFP and LacZ). *(A)* Intraparenchymal injection contra-lateral to a site of superficial MCA infarction. Cells are seen initially at the injection site; they then migrate to the infarct, crossing the midline by day 7 with subsequent increasing photon emissions at the infarct. *(B)* Intrapar-enchymal injection into the left lobe of a control animal with sham infarct surgery. Notice the decline of photon emissions over time, with eventual disappearance of signal. There is no migration to the contralateral hemi-sphere. *(C)* Intraventricular injection contralateral to a site of superficial MCA infarction. Note the initial distrib-uted appearance, consistent with random cell distribution through the cerebrospinal fluid. The infarct is populated by day 7, and shows increasing photon emissions thereafter. *(Adapted from* Kim D, Schellingerhout D, Ishii K, et al. Imaging of stem cell recruitment to ischemic infarcts in a murine model. Stroke 2004;35(4):952–7; with permission.)

Thus, there are imagable treatment models of car-diac disease [116,121], cancer [108–113,117,118, 127,138,141,150], neurodegenerative disease [123], spinal injury [128,155], immune disease [129,136, 140], stroke [126], and transplants [134,135,153]. There are imagable disease models of cancer [114, 122,124,131–133,147,149,151,152,156,157], im-mune disease [129,136,139], transplant disease [130, 137], and infective disease [142–146]. These studies share a common ancestry and often are linked, but they study different entities.

There are also general [119] and basic studies [114,115,120,125,148,154,158] that underlie many of the more specific disease examples.

Many reviews are available dealing with cell gene modifications [93,94,100,159–178]. Some dealing specifically with disease models are also available [179–183].

Table 4: **Treatment versus disease modeling in cell gene modification strategies**

| | What is imaged? | | |
Disease	Treatment	Disease	Basic
Cardiac	[116,121]		
Cancer	[108–113,117,118, 127,138,141,150]	[114,122,124, 131–133,147,149, 151,152,156,157, 269–296]	[297–299]
Neuro–degenerative	[123]		
Spinal injury	[128,155]		
Immune	[129,136,140]	[129,136,139]	
General	[119]		[114,115,120, 125,148,154,158]
Stroke	[126]		
Transplant	[134,135,153]	[130,137]	
Infection		[142–146]	

[129,136] listed twice

Viral loading

Multiple technologies have been used to directly label therapeutic viral vectors for imaging purposes (Table 5). The following section discusses the technologies that have been used.

Nuclear labeling technology has been attempted with [111]indium for HSV [184,185] (Fig. 3) and ^{99m}Tc for the binding motif of adenovirus [186]. MR contrast agents also have been used to mark viral particles or their surrogates with gadolinium viral capsid conglomerates [187], gadolinium polymers [188], and also with SPIOs [189,190]. A unique and interesting way to load viral particles with optical technology has been achieved using the expression of RFP within the coat of the virus [191]. Reviews dealing with viral loading are available [192].

Viral gene modification

The point of viral or viral-based therapies is most often to deliver a gene of interest to a target tissue, and thus the natural way to assess these therapies is to make use of an imagable marker gene. There are various approaches, summarized in Table 6. The easiest way to understand these is to focus on the genetic modifications implemented.

HSV1-tk, the marker gene familiar from its similar use as a cellular marker gene, can be probed with the radiopharmaceuticals such as FIAU in conjunction with HSV vectors [193–195] in adenovirus [196,197] (Fig. 4), in artificial vectors [198–201], and in retrovirus [202]. Radiolabeled ganciclovir [203,204] and penciclovir [205,206] have been used in adenoviral gene therapy. A herpes simplex thymidine kinase variant modified for higher affinity to imaging ligands known as HSV1-sr39tk variety also has been used to be probed with FHBG in the setting of adenoviral applications [207–211].

The D2r has been probed with FESP [209,211–213] in adenoviral gene therapy applications. The human somatostatin receptor type 2 has been probed with ^{99m}Tc-P2045 [196,197,210,214–219], which is a radiolabeled somatostatin analog, and also with ^{99m}Tc-P829 [220], another somatostatin analog, and with [111]indium-DTPA-D-Phe1-octreotide [221,222], all used with adenoviral gene delivery.

Modifications to make viruses and to make viral gene products visible by means of optical imaging have been attempted with RFP [223] in adenovirus and with GFP in HSV [113], adenovirus [224], artificial vectors [189], and canine adenovirus 2 [225]. Luciferase often is used as a marker gene for gene therapy with adenovirus [216,220,226–231], artificial vectors [188], and with adeno-associated virus [232,233].

There are many viral therapeutic approaches in use, but some of the more frequent are the use of the therapeutic gene to induce conversion from a nontoxic prodrug to a cytotoxic drug to kill targeted tissue (typically tumors). An example of this approach is the use of HSV1-tk with pharmacological doses of ganciclovir instead of tracer quantities of radionuclide imaging agent. Thus HSV1-tk can act as a marker and a therapeutic gene. Oncolytic viral therapy is another means of achieving tumor kill. In this approach, replication-deficient virus (that can replicate only in rapidly dividing tissue such as tumors), is injected. The virus proceeds to replicate and lyses tumor cells selectively. These and many other approaches are detailed in reviews available on the use of marker genes with viral-based therapies [94,113,160–162,178,234–257].

Dual/multiple imaging strategies

As image tracking imaging technology matures, there is also an emergence of increasing use of dual or even triple labels in various types of experiments, often blurring the lines between loading and genetic modification, and frequently investigating multiple aspects sequentially or simultaneously. Table 7 lists many of these uses. Surveys of the literature indicate that there are relatively few

---

Table 5: **Viral loading technologies**

			Material labeled			
				Vectors		
			HSV	AV	Artificial vector	Surrogates
Labeling method	Nuclear	[111]Indium–oxine	[184,185]			
		[99m]Tc				[186]
	MR	Gd–viral capsid				[187]
		Gd–polymer			[188]	
		SPIO			[189]	[190]
	Optical	RFP				[191]

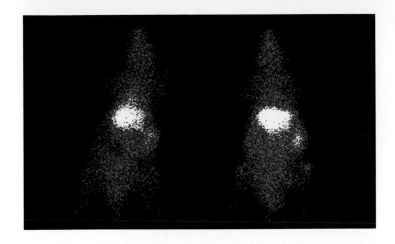

Fig. 3. Viral loading. Planar scintigraphic images of rats immediately after *(left)* and 12 hours after *(right)* intravenous injection of radiolabeled HSV (158 µCi, 5-min acquisitions). Note the predominant distribution to the blood pool or lungs, liver, and spleen on the initial images *(left panel).* Twelve hours later, viral distribution to the blood pool and lung has decreased significantly, with more intense uptake over the liver and spleen *(right panel).* (*Adapted from* Schellingerhout D, Bogdanov A Jr, Marecos E, et al. Mapping the in vivo distribution of Herpes simplex virions. Hum Gene Ther 1998; 9(11):1543–9; with permission.)

comparative studies where more than one label is used for the purpose of weighting the relative advantage of one label with another. One of these is a clinical trial where human dendritic cells are compared in terms of the relative efficacy of [111]indium oxine and ^{99m}Tc-HMPAO as cell-loading agents [77]. A similar study was used to compare ^{64}Cu-PTSM and [18]FDG as PET cell-loading agents in rat C6 glioma cells [74]. As the field matures from invention-driven to clinical-use driven, more comparative studies likely will emerge.

Most studies are not comparative but use multiple technologies to examine different aspects of the biology being investigated. For example, cell-loading strategies that combine MR imaging and optical imaging often are used [7,15,23,63,64,70,71,258]. This makes sense from an experimental point of view, as cell sorting analysis is often very helpful in the experimental setting to purify cell populations, whereas MR imaging can be used to image the intact organism after the cells are injected.

It is possible to use both cell loading technology and cellular gene modification in a single cell-based therapy [38], thus allowing one to image both the initial wave of cells, and the subsequent progeny. Cell loading technology also can be used to combine MR imaging and nuclear imaging [27].

Gene modification technology very frequently combines optical imaging with either nuclear or MR imaging [113,116,117,132]; however, there are also examples of gene modification where various optical markers are combined [126,259] or even nuclear markers are combined [124]. Gene modifications in cells very frequently are done in such a way as to have two optical imaging modalities combined. Frequently this will be a fluorescent

and a bioluminescent marker combined in a single cell [126–129,133]. Again fluorescent markers make it easy to modify and sort purified cell populations, whereas luciferase-based optical imaging is relatively easy to image in the in vivo setting. A triple reporter gene for fluorescent (GFP), bioluminescent (luciferase), and nuclear imaging (HSV1-tk) has been described [260].

Viral-based therapies follow a similar pattern. It is possible to use loading technologies with the viruses and simultaneous gene modification. This is a useful approach as it allows tracking of the administered vector and monitoring of the expression of that vector. This has been achieved using MR loading technology and MR imaging technology [188] or MR loading technology and optical gene expression technology [189].

Virus gene modification has been done using several different nuclear reporters. One approach has been to combine the luciferase marker gene with gene-expressing carcinoembryonic antigen (CEA), allowing correlation between bioluminescent imaging and a serum marker [226]. Another approach has been a dual optical label with the adenoviral capsid expressing RFP, and the reporter gene expressing GFP, a hybrid of loading and genetic modification [223,224]. Fusion genes have been made of HSV1-tk and GFP to allow simultaneous expression assessment with optical and nuclear imaging [113].

In one artificial vector-based gene therapy paradigm administered through catheters to astrocytomas, the delivery of vector was assessed using a surrogate in the form of gadolinium infusion, followed by vector administration and assessment of marker gene expression using HSV1-tk [198]. Similar surrogate imaging approaches have been used

Table 6: Viral gene modification technologies

| Gene | Probe | Material labeled | | | | | |
		HSV	AV	Artificial vector	Canine AV2	STK retrovirus	AAV
HSV1–tk	FIAU	[193–195]	[196,197]	[198,199–201]		[202]	
	FHBG						
	Radiolabeled gancyclovir		[203,204]				
	Radiolabeled pencyclovir		[205,206]				
HSV1–sr39tk	FIAU						
	FHBG		[207–211]				
D2r	Tropane		[209,211–213]				
	FESP		[196,197,210,214–219]				
hSSTr2	^{99m}Tc–P2045		[220]				
	^{99m}Tc–P829		[221,222]				
	^{111}Indium–DTPA-D-Phe1–octreotide		[300]				
	P829		[223]				
RFP							
GFP				[189]			
Luciferase	Luciferin	[113]	[224,301] [216,220, 226–231]	[188]	[225]		[232,233]

Labeling method

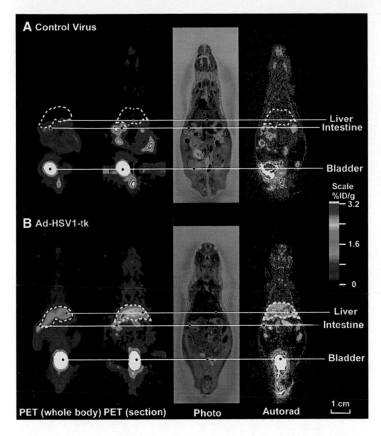

Fig. 4. Viral gene modification with HSV1-tk as marker gene. Images in mice demonstrate differences in thymidine kinase gene expression after tail vein injection of a replication-deficient adenovirus that expresses thymidine kinase (Ad-HSV1-tk) or control virus. %ID/g = percentage injected dose per gram. *(A)* Injection of 1.53 × 109 plaque-forming units of control virus. *(B)* Injection of 1.53 × 109 plaque-forming units of the replication-deficient adenovirus. For each mouse, a whole-body mean coronal projection positron emission tomography (PET) scan *(left)* of the 18F activity distribution was obtained. The location of the liver *(dotted white outline)* was determined from the 8-[18F]-fluoroganciclovir signal and the cryostat slices (second from right). Coronal micro-PET sections *(second from left)* are approximately 2 mm thick. After PET, the mice were sectioned *(second from right)*, and autoradiography (Autorad) was performed *(right)*. Images are displayed on the same quantitative color scale to allow signal intensity comparisons among them. *(Adapted from* Gambhir SS, Barrio JR, Phelps ME, et al. Imaging adenoviral-directed reporter gene expression in living animals with positron emission tomography. Proc Natl Acad Sci U S A 1999;96:2333–8; with permission. © Copyright 1999 National Academy of the Sciences USA.)

where viral particles have proved too difficult to label directly [186,187,190,191]. In others, artificial vectors were easier to label directly with gadolinium–polymer as the loading contrast agent, and transferrin–luciferin as the reporter gene, allowing gene expression monitoring with both MR and bioluminescent imaging [188].

A dual diagnostic–therapeutic approach aimed at the same adenoviral gene expression target, the hSSTr2, uses [111]indium-DTPA-D-Phe1-octreotide as a diagnostic probe to assess gene expression, followed by therapeutic ^{90}Y-SMT487 probe to administer radiotherapy to the cells expressing this receptor.

Of interest in the development of dual and multiple reporter systems is the bicistronic expression system. These expression cassettes are designed to allow the simultaneous, quantitatively equivalent expression of two gene products driven by a single promoter [215]. Bicistronic systems are discussed in multiple reviews [162,196,210,211,215,261–263].

Human applications of cell- and viral-based imaging

There are three different levels of development in a molecular imaging strategy for a cell- or viral-based therapy. Therapies progress from basic chemistry and synthesis to cell testing, animal experiments, and finally to use in people. Table 8 summarizes the level of development of multiple imaging technologies. There is a clear march of development toward clinic use of these emerging technologies. There are relatively few human studies, as one would expect in a nascent field. Only cell loading and viral gene modification studies are represented in clinical trials.

Cell loading in human studies has been performed with iron oxide or nuclear loading. In a landmark comparative study, iron oxide and [111]indium–oxine labeling of dendritic cells were compared in an immunotherapy paradigm of treatment for melanoma [2]. Iron oxide labeling proved superior in this application. A similar study on

Table 7: Dual or triple labeling systems

Type of technology (modalities)	What was labeled?	Use	Reporters used	Reference
Comparative studies				
Cell loading	Rat C6 glioma cells	Animal metastasis model	64Cu-PTSM versus 18FDG	[74]
Cell loading	Human dendritic cells	Human comparative tracer study	111Indium-oxine and 99mTc-HMPAO	[77]
Multi-technology studies				
Cell loading (MR/optical)	Hematopoietic stem cells	Comparative cell labeling study	Gd-HPDO3A an Eu-HPDO3A	[70]
Cell loading (MR/optical)	Human hematopoietic stem cells	Cell tracking	Gadophrin-2	[71]
Cell loading (MR/optical)	Mouse T-cells	Cell tracking	CLIO–Tat peptide–FITC	[258]
Cell loading (MR/optical)	Mesenchymal stem cells	Cell tracking	SPIO and DiI dye	[23]
Cell loading (MR/optical)	Mesenchymal stem cells	Cell tracking	Iron fluorophore particles	[15]
Cell loading (MR/optical)	Hematopoietic and mesenchymal stem cells	Cell labeling	SPIO (large size) with fluorophore	[7]
Cell loading/Cell gene modification (MR/optical)	Embryonic stem cells	Cell tracking	SPIO and GFP	[38]
Cell loading (MR/nuclear)	Mesenchymal stem cells	Cell tracking	SPIO and 111Indium-oxine	[27]
Cell loading (MR/optical)	Neural progenitor cells	Cell tracking	Gd–rhodamine–dextran	[63]
Cell loading (MR/optical)	Neural progenitor cells	Cell tracking	Gd–rhodamine–dextran	[64]
Cell gene modification (optical/nuclear)	Murine embryonic stem cells	Cell tracking	Triple reporter: f-luciferase, RFP, HSV-tk	[116]
Cell gene modification (MR/optical)	Rat C6 Glioma cells	Cell tracking	Ferritin and GFP (Tetracyclin inducible)	[132]
Cell gene modification (nuclear/optical)	Human mesenchymal stem cells	Cell tracking	HSV–tk and GFP	[117]
Cell gene modification (nuclear/optical)	RG2 glioma, 9L gliosarcoma and W256 carcinoma cell lines	Disease model	HSV–tk and GFP	[113]
Cell gene modification (optical/optical)	C17.2 mouse neural progenitor cells	Cell tracking, stroke	Luciferase, GFP and LacZ	[126]
Cell gene modification (optical/optical)	Cell lines and hepatocytes	Two-step transcriptional activation gene therapy	f–luciferase and r–luciferase	[259]
Cell gene modification (nuclear/nuclear)	HeLa transduced tumor cells	Disease model	D2 receptor and HSV1–sr39tk (tetracycline inducible bicistronic system)	[124]
Cell gene modification (optical/optical/nuclear)	U87 glioma cells	Disease model	GFP– luciferase–HSV1–tk fusion gene	[260]
Cell gene modification (Optical/optical)	C17.2 mouse neural progenitor cells	Cell tracking, tumor	Luciferase, GFP and LacZ	[127]
Cell gene modification (optical/optical)	Murine lymphoma cell lines	Disease model	Luciferase-GFP fusion	[133]

Cell gene modification (optical/optical)	Neural progenitor cells	Cell tracking	Luciferase-GFP fusion	[128]
Cell Gene Modification (optical/optical)	Dendritic cells	Cell tracking	Luciferase–GFP fusion	[129]
Virus loading and gene modification (MR/MR)	Artificial vector particle	Vector tracking and expression	PL-DTPA-Gd and Transferrin gene	[188]
Virus loading and gene modification (MR/optical)	Artificial vector particle	Vector tracking and expression	SPIO–polylysine and GFP gene	[189]
Virus gene modification (nuclear/nuclear)	Adenovirus	Vector gene expression	HSV-tk and SSTr2 (bicistronic expression, one marker could be therapeutic)	[215]
Virus gene modification (optical/serum level)	Adenovirus	Vector gene expression	Luciferase and CEA (optical and serum-level reporters)	[226]
Virus gene modification (optical/optical)	Adenovirus	Vector tracking and expression in modified receptor system	Fusion gene for viral capsid RFP and GFP target expression	[224]
Virus gene modification (optical/optical)	Adenovirus	Transfection study in cells	Fusion gene for viral capsid RFP and GFP target expression	[223]
Virus gene modification (optical/optical)	Adenovirus	Transfection study in tumors	Fusion gene for viral capsid RFP and GFP target expression	[223]
Virus gene modification (nuclear/optical)	Adenovirus	Vector expression studies	hSSTr2 and hemagglutinin	[217]
Virus gene modification (nuclear/therapeutic nuclear)	Adenovirus	Vector expression and treatment in tumors	hSSTr2 with both diagnostic ^{111}Indium–DTPA-D-Phe1-octreotide and therapeutic ^{90}Y-SMT487 probes	[222]
Virus gene modification (nuclear/ nuclear)	Adenovirus	Cell transduction studies	hSSTr2 and HSV1-tk (bicistronic expression system)	[196]
Virus gene modification (nuclear/ nuclear)	Adenovirus	Vector expression	D2r and HSV1-sr39tk (bicistronic fusion)	[210]
Virus gene modification (nuclear/ nuclear)	Adenovirus	Vector expression	D2r and HSV1-sr39tk (bicistronic fusion)	[211]
Vector surrogate/vector gene modification (MR/nuclear)	Liposomal artificial vector	Vector surrogate delivery (MR contrast) and vector gene expression during human convection enhanced delivery	MR contrast infusion and HSV1-tk	[198]
Virus gene modification (nuclear/ optical)	HSV	Vector transduction study in cells	HSV1–tk and GFP fusion	[113]
Virus loading/Virus gene modification (MR/MR/ optical)	Artificial vector	Vector delivery and expression in cells	PL-DTPA-Gd loaded in particle with Transferrin-Luciferase gene	[188]

Table 8: Cell- and vector-based therapies: level of development (papers cited by highest level only, or most likely clinical use if dual agent)

		Level of development		
		Humans	*Animals*	*Cells*
Cell loading	Iron oxides and T2 agents	[2,39]	[3,5,6,10–13,15,17, 20,22–31,34,35,38, 40,45,46,49,50, 52,54,56,57,59,60, 258,264,265,302,304] [32,61]	[1,4,7–9,14,16,18,19, 21,33,36,37,41–44, 47,48,51,53,55,58]
	T1 agents		[63,64,70,71]	[62,65–69,72,73,266]
	Nuclear	[2,77]	[27,74–76,267]	[78]
	Optical		[84]	[81–83]
Cell gene modification	HSV–tk		[108–111,114–122]	[112,113]
	D2r		[123,124]	
	hSSTr2		[124]	
	Fluorescence		[131]	
	Bioluminescence		[121,126–129, 133–140,142–151,153,259,305] [141,152,154]	[125]
	Transferrin		[155,156]	
	Ferritin			[132]
	Artificial receptors			[157]
	Tyrosinase			[158]
Viral loading	Nuclear		[184–186]	
	MR		[189,190]	[188]
	Optical		[191]	
Viral gene modification	HSV–tk	[198] [199–201]	[193–195,197, 202–205, 207–211,216]	[196]
	D2r		[209,210,212,213]	
	hSSTr2		[197,214–217, 219–222,300]	[196,218]
	Fluorescence		[189,223,225]	[113,224]
	Bioluminescence		[220,226–233,303]	
	Transferrin			[188]

labeling dendritic cells with two known nuclear labeling technologies, [111]indium–oxine and 99mTc-HMPAO, was done in people [77]. In another landmark study, iron oxide-labeled human neural stem cells were used to treat brain injury in China [39], allowing the tracking of the injected cells by serial MR imaging.

Viral gene modification imaging approaches have been performed in people as part of the treatment of gliomas [198–201]. In this seminal work, the HSV1-tk marker gene was used to image the outcome of gene therapy in human gliomas.

Table 8 lists the vast number of approaches that have been used in animal and cell experiments. A large literature on chemistry and synthesis of labels of interest falls beyond the scope of this article. Many of these will not progress to higher levels, but undoubtedly some will. The relatively high number of comparative studies suggests that there will be a period of consolidation and validation of imaging approaches to find those robust enough to become future clinical standards in humans.

Summary

The molecular imaging literature is increasing in volume and quality, and particularly so in the area of novel therapies. Nonetheless, the basic principles of imaging therapies remain simple, at least until the next innovation wipes away current constructs.

With a large body of literature available, clear trends are emerging, such as the preference for loading technologies in cell-based therapies, and for genetic modification in viral-based therapies. Human use of these technologies is on the horizon, as the logic of therapeutic development inexorably drives clinical trials and molecular imaging together.

Molecular imaging will transform molecular therapeutics, likely be transformed itself, and medicine will become new, and better for patients.

Acknowledgements

Thanks to Lucia G. LeRoux, David Piwnica-Worms and Lee Josephson for helpful discussions and ideas. Thanks to George J. Hunter and colleagues for supporting me during writing.

References

[1] Weissleder R, Cheng HC, Bogdanova A, et al. Magnetically labeled cells can be detected by MR imaging. J Magn Reson Imaging 1997; 7(1):258–63.

[2] De Vries IJM, Lesterhuis WJ, Barentsz JO, et al. Magnetic resonance tracking of dendritic cells in melanoma patients for monitoring of cellular therapy. Nat Biotechnol 2005;23(11):1407–13.

[3] Kleinschnitz C, Bendszus M, Frank M, et al. In vivo monitoring of macrophage infiltration in experimental ischemic brain lesions by magnetic resonance imaging. J Cereb Blood Flow Metab 2003;23(11):1356–61.

[4] Sipe JC, Filippi M, Martino G, et al. Method for intracellular magnetic labeling of human mononuclear cells using approved iron contrast agents. Magn Reson Imaging 1999;17(10): 1521–3.

[5] Yeh T-C, Zhang W, Ildstad ST, et al. In vivo dynamic MRI tracking of rat T-cells labeled with superparamagnetic iron oxide particles. Magn Reson Med 1995;33(2):200–8.

[6] Zelivyanskaya ML, Nelson JA, Poluektova L, et al. Tracking superparamagnetic iron oxide labeled monocytes in brain by high-field magnetic resonance imaging. J Neurosci Res 2003; 73(3):284–95.

[7] Hinds KA, Hill JM, Shapiro EM, et al. Highly efficient endosomal labeling of progenitor and stem cells with large magnetic particles allows magnetic resonance imaging of single cells. Blood 2003;102(3):867–72.

[8] Shapiro EM, Skrtic S, Koretsky AP. Sizing it up: cellular MRI using micron-sized iron oxide particles. Magn Reson Med 2005;53(2):329–38.

[9] Shapiro EM, Skrtic S, Sharer K, et al. MRI detection of single particles for cellular imaging. Proc Natl Acad Sci U S A 2004;101(30):10901–6.

[10] Weber A, Pedrosa I, Kawamoto A, et al. Magnetic resonance mapping of transplanted endothelial progenitor cells for therapeutic neovascularization in ischemic heart disease. Eur J Cardiothorac Surg 2004;26(1):137–43.

[11] Bulte JWM, Douglas T, Witwer B, et al. Magnetodendrimers allow endosomal magnetic labeling and in vivo tracking of stem cells. Nat Biotechnol 2001;19(12):1141–7.

[12] Bulte JWM, Ben-Hur T, Miller BR, et al. MR microscopy of magnetically labeled neurospheres transplanted into the Lewis EAE rat brain. Magn Reson Med 2003;50(1):201–5.

[13] Walter GA, Cahill KS, Huard J, et al. Noninvasive monitoring of stem cell transfer for muscle disorders. Magn Reson Med 2004;51(2): 273–7.

[14] Bulte JWM, Hoekstra Y, Kamman RL, et al. Specific MR imaging of human lymphocytes by monoclonal antibody-guided dextran–magnetite particles. Magn Reson Med 1992;25(1): 148–57.

[15] Hill JM, Dick AJ, Raman VK, et al. Serial cardiac magnetic resonance imaging of injected mesenchymal stem cells. Circulation 2003;108(8): 1009–14.

[16] Daldrup-Link HE, Rudelius M, Oostendorp RA, et al. Targeting of hematopoietic progenitor cells with MR contrast agents. Radiology 2003; 228(3):760–7.

[17] Daldrup-Link HE, Rudelius M, Piontek G, et al. Migration of iron oxide-labeled human hematopoietic progenitor cells in a mouse model: in vivo monitoring with 1.5 T MR imaging equipment. Radiology 2005;234(1):197–205.

[18] van den Bos EJ, Wagner A, Mahrholdt H, et al. Improved efficacy of stem cell labeling for magnetic resonance imaging studies by the use of cationic liposomes. Cell Transplant 2003;12(7): 743–56.

[19] Bulte JWM, Ma LD, Magin RL, et al. Selective MR imaging of labeled human peripheral blood mononuclear cells by liposome mediated incorporation of dextran-magnetite particles. Magn Reson Med 1993;29(1):32–7.

[20] Hawrylak N, Ghosh P, Broadus J, et al. Nuclear magnetic resonance (NMR) imaging of iron oxide-labeled neural transplants. Exp Neurol 1993;121(2):181–92.

[21] Bulte JW, Kraitchman DL, Mackay AM, et al. Chondrogenic differentiation of mesenchymal stem cells is inhibited after magnetic labeling with ferumoxides. Blood 2004;104(10):3410–2.

[22] Garot J, Unterseeh T, Teiger E, et al. Magnetic resonance imaging of targeted catheter-based implantation of myogenic precursor cells into infarcted left ventricular myocardium. J Am Coll Cardiol 2003;41(10):1841–6.

[23] Hauger O, Frost EE, Van Heeswijk R, et al. MR evaluation of the glomerular homing of magnetically labeled mesenchymal stem cells in a rat model of nephropathy. Radiology 2006; 238(1):200–10.

[24] Himes N, Min JY, Lee R, et al. In vivo MRI of embryonic stem cells in a mouse model of myocardial infarction. Magn Reson Med 2004; 52(5):1214–9.

[25] Jendelova P, Herynek V, DeCroos J, et al. Imaging the fate of implanted bone marrow stromal

cells labeled with superparamagnetic nanoparticles. Magn Reson Med 2003;50(4):767–76.

[26] Kraitchman DL, Heldman AW, Atalar E, et al. In vivo magnetic resonance imaging of mesenchymal stem cells in myocardial infarction. Circulation 2003;107(18):2290–3.

[27] Kraitchman DL, Tatsumi M, Gilson WD, et al. Dynamic imaging of allogeneic mesenchymal stem cells trafficking to myocardial infarction. Circulation 2005;112(10):1451–61.

[28] Magnitsky S, Watson DJ, Walton RM, et al. In vivo and ex vivo MRI detection of localized and disseminated neural stem cell grafts in the mouse brain. Neuroimage 2005;26(3):744–54.

[29] Dunning MD, Lakatos A, Loizou L, et al. Superparamagnetic iron oxide-labeled Schwann cells and olfactory ensheathing cells can be traced in vivo by magnetic resonance imaging and retain functional properties after transplantation into the CNS. J Neurosci 2004;24(44):9799–810.

[30] Franklin RJ, Blaschuk KL, Bearchell MC, et al. Magnetic resonance imaging of transplanted oligodendrocyte precursors in the rat brain. Neuroreport 1999;10(18):3961–5.

[31] Lewin M, Carlesso N, Tung C-H, et al. Tat peptide-derivatized magnetic nanoparticles allow in vivo tracking and recovery of progenitor cells. Nat Biotechnol 2000;18(4):410–4.

[32] Zhao M, Kircher MF, Josephson L, et al. Differential conjugation of tat peptide to superparamagnetic nanoparticles and its effect on cellular uptake. Bioconjug Chem 2002;13(4):840–4.

[33] Kaufman CL, Williams M, Ryle LM, et al. Superparamagnetic iron oxide particles transactivator protein–fluorescein isothiocyanate particle labeling for in vivo magnetic resonance imaging detection of cell migration: uptake and durability. Transplantation 2003;76(7):1043–6.

[34] Bos C, Delmas Y, Desmouliere A, et al. In vivo MR imaging of intravascularly injected magnetically labeled mesenchymal stem cells in rat kidney and liver. Radiology 2004;233(3): 781–9.

[35] Cahill KS, Gaidosh G, Huard J, et al. Noninvasive monitoring and tracking of muscle stem cell transplants. Transplantation 2004;78(11): 1626–33.

[36] Frank J, Zywickie H, JOrdan E, et al. Magnetic intracellular labeling of mammalian cells by combining (FDA-approved) superparamagnetic iron oxide MR contrast agents and commonly used transfection agents. Acad Radiol 2002;9: 484–7.

[37] Frank JA, Miller BR, Arbab AS, et al. Clinically applicable labeling of mammalian and stem cells by combining superparamagnetic iron oxides and transfection agents. Radiology 2003; 228(2):480–7.

[38] Hoehn M, Kustermann E, Blunk J, et al. Monitoring of implanted stem cell migration in vivo: a highly resolved in vivo magnetic resonance imaging investigation of experimental stroke in rat. Proc Natl Acad Sci U S A 2002; 99(25):16267–72.

[39] Zhu J, Wu X, Zhang HL. Adult neural stem cell therapy: expansion in vitro, tracking in vivo and clinical transplantation. Curr Drug Targets 2005;6(1):97–110.

[40] Daldrup-Link HE, Meier R, Rudelius M, et al. In vivo tracking of genetically engineered, anti-HER2/neu directed natural killer cells to HER2/neu positive mammary tumors with magnetic resonance imaging. Eur Radiol 2005;15(1):4–13.

[41] Arbab AS, Yocum GT, Wilson LB, et al. Comparison of transfection agents in forming complexes with ferumoxides, cell labeling efficiency, and cellular viability. Mol Imaging 2004;3(1):24–32.

[42] Arbab AS, Wilson LB, Ashari P, et al. A model of lysosomal metabolism of dextran coated superparamagnetic iron oxide (SPIO) nanoparticles: implications for cellular magnetic resonance imaging. NMR Biomed 2005;18(6):383–9.

[43] Arbab AS, Yocum GT, Kalish H, et al. Efficient magnetic cell labeling with protamine sulfate complexed to ferumoxides for cellular MRI. Blood 2004;104(4):1217–23.

[44] Arbab AS, Yocum GT, Rad AM, et al. Labeling of cells with ferumoxides-protamine sulfate complexes does not inhibit function or differentiation capacity of hematopoietic or mesenchymal stem cells. NMR Biomed 2005;18(8):553–9.

[45] Anderson SA, Glod J, Arbab AS, et al. Noninvasive MR imaging of magnetically labeled stem cells to directly identify neovasculature in a glioma model. Blood 2005;105(1):420–5.

[46] Arai T, Kofidis T, Bulte JWM, et al. Dual in vivo magnetic resonance evaluation of magnetically labeled mouse embryonic stem cells and cardiac function at 1.5 T. Magn Reson Med 2006; 55(1):203–9.

[47] Arbab AS, Bashaw LA, Miller BR, et al. Characterization of biophysical and metabolic properties of cells labeled with superparamagnetic iron oxide nanoparticles and transfection agent for cellular MR imaging. Radiology 2003; 229(3):838–46.

[48] Arbab AS, Bashaw LA, Miller BR, et al. Intracytoplasmic tagging of cells with ferumoxides and transfection agent for cellular magnetic resonance imaging after cell transplantation: methods and techniques. Transplantation 2003;76(7):1123–30.

[49] Arbab AS, Jordan EK, Wilson LB, et al. In Vivo trafficking and targeted delivery of magnetically labeled stem cells. Hum Gene Ther 2004;15(4): 351–60.

[50] Yocum GT, Wilson LB, Ashari P, et al. Effect of human stem cells labeled with ferumoxides-poly-L-lysine on hematologic and biochemical measurements in rats. Radiology 2005;235(2): 547–52.

[51] Ahrens ET, Feili-Hariri M, Xu H, et al. Receptor-mediated endocytosis of iron-oxide particles provides efficient labeling of dendritic cells for

in vivo MR imaging. Magn Reson Med 2003; 49(6):1006–13.

[52] Anderson SA, Shukaliak-Quandt J, Jordan EK, et al. Magnetic resonance imaging of labeled T cells in a mouse model of multiple sclerosis. Ann Neurol 2004;55(5):654–9.

[53] Wilhelm C, Billotey C, Roger J, et al. Intracellular uptake of anionic superparamagnetic nanoparticles as a function of their surface coating. Biomaterials 2003;24(6):1001–11.

[54] Yeh TC, Zhang W, Ildstad ST, et al. Intracellular labeling of T cells with superparamagnetic contrast agents. Magn Reson Med 1993;30(5): 617–25.

[55] Berry CC, Charles S, Wells S, et al. The influence of transferrin stabilised magnetic nanoparticles on human dermal fibroblasts in culture. Int J Pharm 2004;269(1):211–25.

[56] Bulte JWM, Zhang S-C, Van Gelderen P, et al. Neurotransplantation of magnetically labeled oligodendrocyte progenitors: Magnetic resonance tracking of cell migration and myelination. Proc Natl Acad Sci U S A 1999;96(26):15256–61.

[57] Bulte JWM, Duncan ID, Frank JA. In vivo magnetic resonance tracking of magnetically labeled cells after transplantation. J Cereb Blood Flow Metab 2002;22(8):899–907.

[58] Walczak P, Kedziorek DA, Gilad AA, et al. Instant MR labeling of stem cells using magneto-electroporation. Magn Reson Med 2005;54(4): 769–74.

[59] Zhang RL, Zhang L, Zhang ZG, et al. Migration and differentiation of adult rat subventricular zone progenitor cells transplanted into the adult rat striatum. Neuroscience 2003;116(2): 373–82.

[60] Zhang Z, Jiang Q, Jiang F, et al. In vivo magnetic resonance imaging tracks adult neural progenitor cell targeting of brain tumor. Neuroimage 2004;23(1):281–7.

[61] Zhang ZG, Jiang Q, Zhang R, et al. Magnetic resonance imaging and neurosphere therapy of stroke in rat. Ann Neurol 2003;53(2): 259–63.

[62] Jacobs RE, Fraser SE. Magnetic resonance microscopy of embryonic cell lineages and movements. Science 1994;263(5147):681–4.

[63] Modo M, Cash D, Mellodew K, et al. Tracking transplanted stem cell migration using bifunctional, contrast agent-enhanced, magnetic resonance imaging. Neuroimage 2002;17(2): 803–11.

[64] Modo M, Mellodew K, Cash D, et al. Mapping transplanted stem cell migration after a stroke: a serial, in vivo magnetic resonance imaging study. Neuroimage 2004;21(1):311–7.

[65] Allen MJ, Meade TJ. Synthesis and visualization of a membrane-permeable MRI contrast agent. J Biol Inorg Chem 2003;8(7):746–50.

[66] Allen MJ, MacRenaris KW, Venkatasubramanian PN, et al. Cellular delivery of MRI contrast agents. Chem Biol 2004;11(3):301–7.

[67] Heckl S, Debus J, Jenne J, et al. CNN-Gd(3+) enables cell nucleus molecular imaging of prostate cancer cells: the last 600 nm. Cancer Res 2002;62(23):7018–24.

[68] Bhorade R, Weissleder R, Nakakoshi T, et al. Macrocyclic chelators with paramagnetic cations are internalized into mammalian cells via an HIV–tat derived membrane translocation peptide. Bioconjug Chem 2000;11(3):301–5.

[69] Rudelius M, Daldrup-Link HE, Heinzmann U, et al. Highly efficient paramagnetic labeling of embryonic and neuronal stem cells. Eur J Nucl Med Mol Imaging 2003;30(7):1038–44.

[70] Crich SG, Biancone L, Cantaluppi V, et al. Improved route for the visualization of stem cells labeled with a Gd-/Eu-chelate as dual (MRI and fluorescence) agent. Magn Reson Med 2004;51(5):938–44.

[71] Daldrup-Link HE, Rudelius M, Metz S, et al. Cell tracking with gadophrin-2: a bifunctional contrast agent for MR imaging, optical imaging, and fluorescence microscopy. Eur J Nucl Med Mol Imaging 2004;31(9):1312–21.

[72] Aoki I, Takahashi Y, Chuang K-H, et al. In vitro cell labeling for manganese enhanced magnetic resonance imaging. Proceedings of the International Society for Magnetic Resonance in Medicine 2004;12:164.

[73] Aime S, Carrera C, Delli Castelli D, et al. Tunable imaging of cells labeled with MRI-PARACEST agents. Angew Chem Int Ed Engl 2005; 44(12):1813–5.

[74] Adonai N, Nguyen KN, Walsh J, et al. Ex vivo cell labeling with 64Cu-pyruvaldehyde-bis(N4-methylthiosemicarbazone) for imaging cell trafficking in mice with positron emission tomography. Proc Natl Acad Sci U S A 2002; 99(5):3030–5.

[75] Balatoni JA, Doubrovin M, Ageyeva L, et al. Imaging herpes viral thymidine kinase-1 reporter gene expression with a new 18F-labeled probe: 2?-fluoro-2?-deoxy-5-[18F]fluoroethyl-1-?-d-arabinofuranosyl uracil. Nucl Med Biol 2005;32(8):811–9.

[76] Chin BB, Nakamoto Y, Bulte JW, et al. 111In oxine labelled mesenchymal stem cell SPECT after intravenous administration in myocardial infarction. Nucl Med Commun 2003;24(11): 1149–54.

[77] Blocklet D, Toungouz M, Kiss R, et al. 111In-oxine and 99mTc-HMPAO labelling of antigen-loaded dendritic cells: In vivo imaging and influence on motility and actin content. Eur J Nucl Med Mol Imaging 2003;30(3):440–7.

[78] Marienhagen J, Hennemann B, Andreesen R, et al. 111In-oxine labeling of tumour-cytotoxic macrophages generated in vitro from circulating blood monocytes: An in vitro evaluation. Nucl Med Commun 1995;16(5):357–61.

[79] Thakur ML, Lavender JP, Arnot RN, et al. Indium-111-labeled autologous leukocytes in man. J Nucl Med 1977;18(10):1014–21.

[80] Thakur ML, Coleman RE, Welch MJ. Indium-111 labeled leukocytes for the localization of abscesses: preparation, analysis, tissue distribution, and comparison with gallium 67 citrate in dogs. J Lab Clin Med 1977;89(1): 217–28.

[81] Dubertret B, Skourides P, Norris DJ, et al. In vivo imaging of quantum dots encapsulated in phospholipid micelles. Science 2002;298(5599): 1759–62.

[82] Askensay N, Farkas D. Optical imaging of PKH-labeled hematopoietic cells in recipient bone marrow in vivo. Stem Cells 2002;20:501–13.

[83] Fox D, Kouris GJ, Blumofe KA, et al. Optimizing fluorescent labeling of endothelial cells for tracking during long-term studies of autologous transplantation. J Surg Res 1999;86(1): 9–16.

[84] Ferrari A, Hannouche D, Oudina K, et al. In vivo tracking of bone marrow fibroblasts with fluorescent carbocyanine dye. J Biomed Mater Res 2001;56(3):361–7.

[85] Aime S, Cabella C, Colombatto S, et al. Insights into the use of paramagnetic Gd(III) complexes in MR-molecular imaging investigations. J Magn Reson Imaging 2002;16(4):394–406.

[86] Bulte JWM, Douglas T, Witwer B, et al. Monitoring stem cell therapy in vivo using magnetodendrimers as a new class of cellular MR contrast agents. Acad Radiol 2002;9(suppl 2): S332–5.

[87] Bulte JWM, Kraitchman DL. Iron oxide MR contrast agents for molecular and cellular imaging. NMR Biomed 2004;17(7):484–99.

[88] Bulte JWM. Magnetic nanoparticles as markers for cellular MR imaging. Journal of Magnetism and Magnetic Materials 2005;289:423–7.

[89] Frank JA, Anderson SA, Kalsih H, et al. Methods for magnetically labeling stem and other cells for detection by in vivo magnetic resonance imaging. Cytotherapy 2004;6(6):621–5.

[90] Jaiswal JK, Simon SM. Potentials and pitfalls of fluorescent quantum dots for biological imaging. Trends Cell Biol 2004;14(9):497–504.

[91] Leroy-Willig A, Fromes Y, Paturneau-Jouas M, et al. Assessing gene and cell therapies applied in striated skeletal and cardiac muscle: is there a role for nuclear magnetic resonance? Neuromuscul Disord 2003;13(5):397–407.

[92] Modo M, Hoehn M, Bulte JWM. Cellular MR imaging. Mol Imaging 2005;4(3):143–64.

[93] Modo M, Roberts TJ, Sandhu JK, et al. In vivo monitoring of cellular transplants by magnetic resonance imaging and positron emission tomography. Expert Opin Biol Ther 2004;4(2): 145–55.

[94] Blasberg RG, Tjuvajev JG. Molecular–genetic imaging: current and future perspectives. J Clin Invest 2003;111(11):1620–9.

[95] Frangioni JV, Hajjar RJ. In vivo tracking of stem cells for clinical trials in cardiovascular disease. Circulation 2004;110(21):3378–83.

[96] Harrower TP, Barker RA. The emerging technologies of neural xenografting and stem cell transplantation for treating neurodegenerative disorders. Drugs Today 2004;40(2):171–89.

[97] Kalish H, Arbab AS, Miller BR, et al. Combination of transfection agents and magnetic resonance contrast agents for cellular imaging: relationship between relaxivities, electrostatic forces, and chemical composition. Magn Reson Med 2003;50(2):275–82.

[98] Lindvall O, Kokaia Z, Martinez-Serrano A. Stem cell therapy for human neurodegenerative disorders— how to make it work. Nat Med 2004; 10:S42–50.

[99] Michalet X, Pinaud FF, Bentolila LA, et al. Quantum dots for live cells, in vivo imaging, and diagnostics. Science 2005;307(5709): 538–44.

[100] Benaron DA, Contag PR, Contag CH. Imaging brain structure and function, infection and gene expression in the body using light. Philos Trans R Soc Lond B Biol Sci 1997;352(1354): 755–61.

[101] Frangioni JV. Self-illuminating quantum dots light the way. Nat Biotechnol 2006;24(3): 326–8.

[102] Frangioni JV. In vivo near-infrared fluorescence imaging. Curr Opin Chem Biol 2003;7(5): 626–34.

[103] Herschman HR. PET reporter genes for noninvasive imaging of gene therapy, cell tracking and transgenic analysis. Crit Rev Oncol Hematol 2004;51(3):191–204.

[104] Emerit J, Beaumont C, Trivin F. Iron metabolism, free radicals, and oxidative injury. Biomed Pharmacother 2001;55(6):333–9.

[105] Kostura L, Kraitchman DL, Mackay AM, et al. Feridex labeling of mesenchymal stem cells inhibits chondrogenesis but not adipogenesis or osteogenesis. NMR Biomed 2004;17(7):513–7.

[106] Krishnan M, Park JM, Cao F, et al. Effects of epigenetic modulation on reporter gene expression: Implications for stem cell imaging. FASEB J 2006;20(1):106–8.

[107] Oh DJ, Lee GM, Francis K, et al. Phototoxicity of the fluorescent membrane dyes PKH2 and PKH26 on the human hematopoietic KG1a progenitor cell line. Cytometry 1999;36(4): 312–8.

[108] Koehne G, Doubrovin M, Doubrovina E, et al. Serial in vivo imaging of the targeted migration of human HSV-TK-transduced antigen-specific lymphocytes. Nat Biotechnol 2003;21(4): 405–13.

[109] Ponomarev V, Doubrovin M, Lyddane C, et al. Imaging TCR-dependent NFAT-mediated T-cell activation with positron emission tomography in vivo. Neoplasia 2001;3(6):480–8.

[110] Soghomonyan SA, Doubrovin M, Pike J, et al. Positron emission tomography (PET) imaging of tumor-localized Salmonella expressing HSV1-TK. Cancer Gene Ther 2005;12(1):101–8.

[111] Tjuvajev J, Blasberg R, Luo X, et al. Salmonella-based tumor-targeted cancer therapy: Tumor amplified protein expression therapy (TAPET?) for diagnostic imaging. J Control Release 2001; 74(1–3):313–5.

[112] Choi SR, Zhuang Z-P, Chacko A-M, et al. SPECT imaging of herpes simplex virus type1 thymidine kinase gene expression by [123I] FIAU. Acad Radiol 2005;12(7):798–805.

[113] Jacobs A, Dubrovin M, Hewett J, et al. Functional coexpression of HSV-1 thymidine kinase and green fluorescent protein: implications for noninvasive imaging of transgene expression. Neoplasia 1999;1(2):154–61.

[114] Ray P, Wu AM, Gambhir SS. Optical bioluminescence and positron emission tomography imaging of a novel fusion reporter gene in tumor xenografts of living mice. Cancer Res 2003;63(6):1160–5.

[115] Blasberg RG, Tjuvajev JG. Herpes simplex virus thymidine kinase as a marker/reporter gene for PET imaging of gene therapy. Q J Nucl Med 1999;43(2):163–9.

[116] Cao F, Lin S, Xie X, et al. In vivo visualization of embryonic stem cell survival, proliferation, and migration after cardiac delivery. Circulation 2006;113(7):1005–14.

[117] Hung S-C, Deng W-P, Yang WK, et al. Mesenchymal stem cell targeting of microscopic tumors and tumor stroma development monitored by noninvasive in vivo positron emission tomography imaging. Clin Cancer Res 2005;11(21): 7749–56.

[118] Dubey P, Su H, Adonai N, et al. Quantitative imaging of the T cell antitumor response by positron emission tomography. Proc Natl Acad Sci U S A 2003;100(3):1232–7.

[119] Green LA, Yap CS, Nguyen K, et al. Indirect monitoring of endogenous gene expression by positron emission tomography (PET) imaging of reporter gene expression in transgenic mice. Mol Imaging Biol 2002;4(1):71–81.

[120] Su H, Forbes A, Gambhir SS, et al. Quantitation of cell number by a positron emission tomography reporter gene strategy. Mol Imaging Biol 2004;6(3):139–48.

[121] Wu JC, Chen IY, Sundaresan G, et al. Molecular imaging of cardiac cell transplantation in living animals using optical bioluminescence and positron emission tomography. Circulation 2003;108(11):1302–5.

[122] Yaghoubi SS, Barrio JR, Namavari M, et al. Imaging progress of herpes simplex virus type 1 thymidine kinase suicide gene therapy in living subjects with positron emission tomography. Cancer Gene Ther 2005;12(3):329–39.

[123] Chen YI, Brownell AL, Galpern W, et al. Detection of dopaminergic cell loss and neural transplantation using pharmacological MRI, PET and behavioral assessment. Neuroreport 1999; 10(14):2881–6.

[124] Sun X, Annala AJ, Yaghoubi SS, et al. Quantitative imaging of gene induction in living animals. Gene Ther 2001;8(20):1572–9.

[125] Tolar J, Osborn M, Bell S, et al. Real-time in vivo imaging of stem cells following transgenesis by transposition. Mol Ther 2005;12(1): 42–8.

[126] Kim DE, Schellingerhout D, Ishii K, et al. Imaging of stem cell recruitment to ischemic infarcts in a murine model. Stroke 2004;35(4):952–7.

[127] Tang Y, Shah K, Messerli SM, et al. In vivo tracking of neural progenitor cell migration to glioblastomas. Hum Gene Ther 2003;14(13): 1247–54.

[128] Okada S, Ishii K, Yamane J, et al. In vivo imaging of engrafted neural stem cells: its application in evaluating the optimal timing of transplantation for spinal cord injury. FASEB J 2005;19(13):1839–41.

[129] Schimmelpfennig CH, Schulz S, Arber C, et al. Ex vivo expanded dendritic cells home to T-cell zones of lymphoid organs and survive in vivo after allogeneic bone marrow transplantation. Am J Pathol 2005;167(5):1321–31.

[130] Tanaka M, Swijnenburg RJ, Gunawan F, et al. In vivo visualization of cardiac allograft rejection and trafficking passenger leukocytes using bioluminescence imaging. Circulation 2005; 112(Suppl 9):I105–10.

[131] Chaudhuri TR, Mountz JM, Rogers BE, et al. Light-based imaging of green fluorescent protein-positive ovarian cancer xenografts during therapy. Gynecol Oncol 2001;82(3):581–9.

[132] Cohen B, Dafni H, Meir G, et al. Ferritin as novel MR-reporter for molecular imaging of gene expression. Proc Int Soc Magn Reson Med 2004;11:1707.

[133] Edinger M, Cao YA, Verneris MR, et al. Revealing lymphoma growth and the efficacy of immune cell therapies using in vivo bioluminescence imaging. Blood 2003;101(2):640–8.

[134] Cao YA, Bachmann MH, Beilhack A, et al. Molecular imaging using labeled donor tissues reveals patterns of engraftment, rejection, and survival in transplantation. Transplantation 2005;80(1):134–9.

[135] Cao YA, Wagers AJ, Beilhack A, et al. Shifting foci of hematopoiesis during reconstitution from single stem cells. Proc Natl Acad Sci U S A 2004;101(1):221–6.

[136] Hardy J, Edinger M, Bachmann MH, et al. Bioluminescence imaging of lymphocyte trafficking in vivo. Exp Hematol 2001;29(12):1353–60.

[137] Beilhack A, Schulz S, Baker J, et al. In vivo analyses of early events in acute graft-versus-host disease reveal sequential infiltration of T cell subsets. Blood 2005;106(3):1113–22.

[138] Chan JK, Hamilton CA, Cheung MK, et al. Enhanced killing of primary ovarian cancer by retargeting autologous cytokine-induced killer cells with bispecific antibodies:

a preclinical study. Clin Cancer Res 2006; 12(6):1859–67.

[139] Costa GL, Sandora MR, Nakajima A, et al. Adoptive immunotherapy of experimental autoimmune encephalomyelitis via T cell delivery of the IL-12 p40 subunit. J Immunol 2001; 167(4):2379–87.

[140] Nakajima A, Seroogy CM, Sandora MR, et al. Antigen-specific T cell-mediated gene therapy in collagen-induced arthritis. J Clin Invest 2001;107(10):1293–301.

[141] Thorne SH, Negrin RS, Contag CH. Synergistic antitumor effects of immune cell-viral biotherapy. Science 2006;311(5768):1780–4.

[142] Burns-Guydish SM, Olomu IN, Zhao H, et al. Monitoring age-related susceptibility of young mice to oral Salmonella enterica serovar Typhimurium infection using an in vivo murine model. Pediatr Res 2005;58(1):153–8.

[143] Chatterjea D, Burns-Guydish SM, Sciuto TE, et al. Adoptive transfer of mast cells does not enhance the impaired survival of Kit(W)/Kit(W-v) mice in a model of low dose intraperitoneal infection with bioluminescent Salmonella typhimurium. Immunol Lett 2005;99(1):122–9.

[144] Contag CH, Contag PR, Mullins JI, et al. Photonic detection of bacterial pathogens in living hosts. Mol Microbiol 1995;18(4):593–603.

[145] Hardy J, Francis KP, DeBoer M, et al. Extracellular replication of Listeria monocytogenes in the murine gall bladder. Science 2004;303(5659): 851–3.

[146] Hardy J, Margolis JJ, Contag CH. Induced biliary excretion of Listeria monocytogenes. Infect Immun 2006;74(3):1819–27.

[147] Craft N, Bruhn KW, Nguyen BD, et al. Bioluminescent imaging of melanoma in live mice. J Invest Dermatol 2005;125(1):159–65.

[148] Contag CH, Spilman SD, Contag PR, et al. Visualizing gene expression in living mammals using a bioluminescent reporter. Photochem Photobiol 1997;66(4):523–31.

[149] Rehemtulla A, Stegman LD, Cardozo SJ, et al. Rapid and quantitative assessment of cancer treatment response using in vivo bioluminescence imaging. Neoplasia 2000;2(6):491–5.

[150] Scheffold C, Kornacker M, Scheffold YC, et al. Visualization of effective tumor targeting by CD8 + natural killer T cells redirected with bispecific antibody F(ab')(2)HER2xCD3. Cancer Res 2002;62(20):5785–91.

[151] Sweeney TJ, Mailander V, Tucker AA, et al. Visualizing the kinetics of tumor cell clearance in living animals. Proc Natl Acad Sci U S A 1999;96(21):12044–9.

[152] Nguyen JT, Machado H, Herschman HR. Repetitive, noninvasive imaging of cyclooxygenase-2 gene expression in living mice. Mol Imaging Biol 2003;5(4):248–56.

[153] Lu Y, Dang H, Middleton B, et al. Bioluminescent monitoring of islet graft survival after transplantation. Mol Ther 2004;9(3):428–35.

[154] Ishikawa TO, Jain NK, Taketo MM, et al. Imaging Cyclooxygenase-2 (Cox-2) Gene Expression in Living Animals with a Luciferase Knock-in Reporter Gene. Mol Imaging Biol 2006;8(3): 171–87.

[155] Ding W, Bai J, Zhang J, et al. In vivo tracking of implanted stem cells using radio-labeled transferrin scintigraphy. Nucl Med Biol 2004;31(6): 719–25.

[156] Moore A, Josephson L, Bhorade RM, et al. Human transferrin receptor gene as a marker gene for MR imaging. Radiology 2001;221(1): 244–50.

[157] Simonova M, Shtanko O, Sergeyev N, et al. Engineering of technetium-99m-binding artificial receptors for imaging gene expression. J Gene Med 2003;5(12):1056–66.

[158] Weissleder R, Simonova M, Bogdanova A, et al. MR imaging and scintigraphy of gene expression through melanin induction. Radiology 1997;204(2):425–9.

[159] Lang P, Yeow K, Nichols A, et al. Cellular imaging in drug discovery. Nat Rev Drug Discov 2006;5(4):343–56.

[160] Blasberg RG, Gelovani J. Molecular-genetic imaging: a nuclear medicine-based perspective. Mol Imaging 2002;1(3):280–300.

[161] Bengel FM, Gambhir SS. Clinical molecular imaging and therapy—moving ahead together. Eur J Nucl Med Mol Imaging 2005;32(Suppl 2): S323.

[162] Tjuvajev JG, Blasberg RG. In vivo imaging of molecular-genetic targets for cancer therapy. Cancer Cell 2003;3(4):327–32.

[163] Weissleder R, Ntziachristos V. Shedding light onto live molecular targets. Nat Med 2003; 9(1):123–8.

[164] Burns SM, Joh D, Francis KP, et al. Revealing the spatiotemporal patterns of bacterial infectious diseases using bioluminescent pathogens and whole body imaging. Contrib Microbiol 2001; 9:71–88.

[165] Contag PR, Olomu IN, Stevenson DK, et al. Bioluminescent indicators in living mammals. Nat Med 1998;4(2):245–7.

[166] Doyle TC, Burns SM, Contag CH. In vivo bioluminescence imaging for integrated studies of infection. Cell Microbiol 2004;6(4):303–17.

[167] Edinger M, Cao YA, Hornig YS, et al. Advancing animal models of neoplasia through in vivo bioluminescence imaging. Eur J Cancer 2002; 38(16):2128–36.

[168] Edinger M, Hoffmann P, Contag CH, et al. Evaluation of effector cell fate and function by in vivo bioluminescence imaging. Methods 2003; 31(2):172–9.

[169] Edinger M, Sweeney TJ, Tucker AA, et al. Noninvasive assessment of tumor cell proliferation in animal models. Neoplasia 1999;1(4):303–10.

[170] Helms MW, Brandt BH, Contag CH. Options for visualizing metastatic disease in the living body. Contrib Microbiol 2006;13:209–31.

[171] McCaffrey A, Kay MA, Contag CH. Advancing molecular therapies through in vivo bioluminescent imaging. Mol Imaging 2003;2(2):75–86.

[172] Negrin RS, Edinger M, Verneris M, et al. Visualization of tumor growth and response to NK-T cell based immunotherapy using bioluminescence. Ann Hematol 2002;81(Suppl 2): S44–5.

[173] Tarner IH, Slavin AJ, McBride J, et al. Treatment of autoimmune disease by adoptive cellular gene therapy. Ann N Y Acad Sci 2003;998: 512–9.

[174] Zhang W, Contag PR, Madan A, et al. Bioluminescence for biological sensing in living mammals. Adv Exp Med Biol 1999;471:775–84.

[175] Chemaly ER, Yoneyama R, Frangioni JV, et al. Tracking stem cells in the cardiovascular system. Trends Cardiovasc Med 2005;15(8): 297–302.

[176] Herschman HR. Micro-PET imaging and small animal models of disease. Curr Opin Immunol 2003;15(4):378–84.

[177] Herschman HR. Molecular imaging: looking at problems, seeing solutions. Science 2003; 302(5645):605–8.

[178] Jacobs AH, Li H, Winkeler A, et al. Pet-based molecular imaging in neuroscience. Eur J Nucl Med Mol Imaging 2003;30(7):1051–65.

[179] Yang M, Luiken G, Baranov E, et al. Facile whole-body imaging of internal fluorescent tumors in mice with an LED flashlight. Biotechniques 2005;39(2):170–2.

[180] Hoffman RM. In vivo cell biology of cancer cells visualized with fluorescent proteins. Curr Top Dev Biol 2005;70:121–44.

[181] Hoffman RM, Yang M. Dual-color, whole-body imaging in mice. Nat Biotechnol 2005;23(7): 790.

[182] Hoffman RM. In vivo imaging with fluorescent proteins: the new cell biology. Acta Histochem 2004;106(2):77–87.

[183] Yamamoto N, Yang M, Jiang P, et al. Color coding cancer cells with fluorescent proteins to visualize in vivo cellular interaction in metastatic colonies. Anticancer Res 2004;24(6): 4067–72.

[184] Schellingerhout D, Bogdanov A Jr, Marecos E, et al. Mapping the in vivo distribution of herpes simplex virions. Hum Gene Ther 1998; 9(11):1543–9.

[185] Schellingerhout D, Rainov NG, Breakefield XO, et al. Quantitation of HSV mass distribution in a rodent brain tumor model. Gene Ther 2000; 7(19):1648–55.

[186] Zinn KR, Douglas JT, Smyth CA, et al. Imaging and tissue biodistribution of 99mTc-labeled adenovirus knob (serotype 5). Gene Ther 1998; 5(6):798–808.

[187] Allen M, Bulte JWM, Liepold L, et al. Paramagnetic viral nanoparticles as potential high-relaxivity magnetic resonance contrast agents. Magn Reson Med 2005;54(4):807–12.

[188] Kayyem JF, Kumar RM, Fraser SE, et al. Receptor-targeted co-transport of DNA and magnetic resonance contrast agents. Chem Biol 1995; 2(9):615–20.

[189] De Marco G, Bogdanov A, Marecos E, et al. MR imaging of gene delivery to the central nervous system with an artificial vector. Radiology 1998; 208(1):65–71.

[190] Rainov NG, Zimmer C, Chase M, et al. Selective uptake of viral and monocrystalline particles delivered intra-arterially to experimental brain neoplasms. Hum Gene Ther 1995;6(12): 1543–52.

[191] Hoshino K, Kimura T, De Grand AM, et al. Three catheter-based strategies for cardiac delivery of therapeutic gelatin microspheres. Gene Ther 2006; May 18.

[192] Schellingerhout D, Bogdanov AA Jr. Viral imaging in gene therapy: Noninvasive demonstration of gene delivery and expression. Neuroimaging Clin N Am 2002;12(4): 571–81.

[193] Jacobs A, Tjuvajev JG, Dubrovin M, et al. Positron emission tomography-based imaging of transgene expression mediated by replication-conditional, oncolytic herpes simplex virus type 1 mutant vectors in vivo. Cancer Res 2001;61(7):2983–95.

[194] Tjuvajev JG, Avril N, Oku T, et al. Imaging herpes virus thymidine kinase gene transfer and expression by positron emission tomography. Cancer Res 1998;58(19):4333–41.

[195] Tjuvajev JG, Finn R, Watanabe K, et al. Noninvasive imaging of herpes virus thymidine kinase gene transfer and expression: a potential method for monitoring clinical gene therapy. Cancer Res 1996;56(18):4087–95.

[196] Zinn KR, Chaudhuri TR, Buchsbaum DJ, et al. Simultaneous evaluation of dual gene transfer to adherent cells by gamma-ray imaging. Nucl Med Biol 2001;28(2):135–44.

[197] Zinn KR, Chaudhuri TR, Krasnykh VN, et al. Gamma camera dual imaging with a somatostatin receptor and thymidine kinase after gene transfer with a bicistronic adenovirus in mice. Radiology 2002;223(2):417–25.

[198] Voges J, Reszka R, Gossmann A, et al. Imaging-guided convection-enhanced delivery and gene therapy of glioblastoma. Ann Neurol 2003; 54(4):479–87.

[199] Jacobs AH, Winkeler A, Dittmar C, et al. Positron-emission tomography monitoring of anti-glioblastoma HSV-1-tk gene therapy. Gene Therapy and Regulation 2003;2(1): 49–57.

[200] Jacobs A, Voges J, Reszka R, et al. Positron-emission tomography of vector-mediated gene expression in gene therapy for gliomas. Lancet 2001;358(9283):727–9.

[201] Reszka RC, Jacobs A, Voges J. Liposome-mediated suicide gene therapy in humans. Methods Enzymol 2005;391:200–8.

[202] Tjuvajev JG, Stockhammer G, Desai R, et al. Imaging the expression of transfected genes in vivo. Cancer Res 1995;55(24):6126–32.

[203] Gambhir SS, Barrio JR, Wu L, et al. Imaging of adenoviral-directed herpes simplex virus type 1 thymidine kinase reporter gene expression in mice with radiolabeled ganciclovir. J Nucl Med 1998;39(11):2003–11.

[204] Gambhir SS, Barrio JR, Phelps ME, et al. Imaging adenoviral-directed reporter gene expression in living animals with positron emission tomography. Proc Natl Acad Sci U S A 1999; 96(5):2333–8.

[205] Gambhir SS, Bauer E, Black ME, et al. A mutant herpes simplex virus type 1 thymidine kinase reporter gene shows improved sensitivity for imaging reporter gene expression with positron emission tomography. Proc Natl Acad Sci U S A 2000;97(6):2785–90.

[206] Penuelas I, Mazzolini G, Boan JF, et al. Positron emission tomography imaging of adenoviral-mediated transgene expression in liver cancer patients. Gastroenterology 2005;128(7):1787–95.

[207] Inubushi M, Wu JC, Gambhir SS, et al. Positron emission tomography reporter gene expression imaging in rat myocardium. Circulation 2003; 107(2):326–32.

[208] Liang Q, Nguyen K, Satyamurthy N, et al. Monitoring adenoviral DNA delivery, using a mutant herpes simplex virus type 1 thymidine kinase gene as a PET reporter gene. Gene Ther 2002; 9(24):1659–66.

[209] Yaghoubi SS, Wu L, Liang Q, et al. Direct correlation between positron emission tomographic images of two reporter genes delivered by two distinct adenoviral vectors. Gene Ther 2001; 8(14):1072–80.

[210] Chen IY, Wu JC, Min JJ, et al. Micropositron emission tomography imaging of cardiac gene expression in rats using bicistronic adenoviral vector-mediated gene delivery. Circulation 2004;109(11):1415–20.

[211] Liang Q, Gotts J, Satyamurthy N, et al. Noninvasive, repetitive, quantitative measurement of gene expression from a bicistronic message by positron emission tomography, following gene transfer with adenovirus. Mol Ther 2002;6(1): 73–82.

[212] MacLaren DC, Gambhir SS, Satyamurthy N, et al. Repetitive, non-invasive imaging of the dopamine D2 receptor as a reporter gene in living animals. Gene Ther 1999;6(5):785–91.

[213] Liang Q, Satyamurthy N, Barrio JR, et al. Noninvasive, quantitative imaging in living animals of a mutant dopamine D2 receptor reporter gene in which ligand binding is uncoupled from signal transduction. Gene Ther 2001; 8(19):1490–8.

[214] Buchsbaum DJ, Chaudhuri TR, Yamamoto M, et al. Gene expression imaging with radiolabeled peptides. Ann Nucl Med 2004;18(4): 275–83.

[215] Hemminki A, Zinn KR, Liu B, et al. In vivo molecular chemotherapy and noninvasive imaging with an infectivity-enhanced adenovirus. J Natl Cancer Inst 2002;94(10):741–9.

[216] Kim M, Zinn KR, Barnett BG, et al. The therapeutic efficacy of adenoviral vectors for cancer gene therapy is limited by a low level of primary adenovirus receptors on tumour cells. Eur J Cancer 2002;38(14):1917–26.

[217] Rogers BE, Chaudhuri TR, Reynolds PN, et al. Noninvasive gamma camera imaging of gene transfer using an adenoviral vector encoding an epitope-tagged receptor as a reporter. Gene Ther 2003;10(2):105–14.

[218] Zinn KR, Chaudhuri TR, Buchsbaum DJ, et al. Detection and measurement of in vitro gene transfer by gamma camera imaging. Gene Ther 2001;8(4):291–9.

[219] Chaudhuri TR, Rogers BE, Buchsbaum DJ, et al. A noninvasive reporter system to image adenoviral-mediated gene transfer to ovarian cancer xenografts. Gynecol Oncol 2001;83(2): 432–8.

[220] Reynolds PN, Zinn KR, Gavrilyuk VD, et al. A targetable, injectable adenoviral vector for selective gene delivery to pulmonary endothelium in vivo. Mol Ther 2000;2(6):562–78.

[221] Rogers BE, McLean SF, Kirkman RL, et al. In vivo localization of [111In]-DTPA-D-Phe1-octreotide to human ovarian tumor xenografts induced to express the somatostatin receptor subtype 2 using an adenoviral vector. Clin Cancer Res 1999;5(2):383–93.

[222] Rogers BE, Zinn KR, Lin C-Y, et al. Targeted radiotherapy with [90Y]-SMT 487 in mice bearing human nonsmall cell lung tumor xenografts induced to express human somatostatin receptor subtype 2 with an adenoviral vector. Cancer 2002;94(Suppl 4):1298–305.

[223] Le LP, Le HN, Dmitriev IP, et al. Dynamic monitoring of oncolytic adenovirus in vivo by genetic capsid labeling. J Natl Cancer Inst 2006; 98(3):203–14.

[224] Le LP, Everts M, Dmitriew IP, et al. Fluorescently labeled adenovirus with pIX-EGFP for vector detection. Mol Imaging 2004;3(2): 105–16.

[225] Le LP, Li J, Ternovoi VV, et al. Fluorescently tagged canine adenovirus via modification with protein IX-enhanced green fluorescent protein. J Gen Virol 2005;86(12):3201–8.

[226] Kanerva A, Zinn KR, Peng K-W, et al. Noninvasive dual modality in vivo monitoring of the persistence and potency of a tumor targeted conditionally replicating adenovirus. Gene Ther 2005;12(1):87–94.

[227] Lee C-T, Lee Y-J, Kwon S-Y, et al. In vivo imaging of adenovirus transduction and enhanced therapeutic efficacy of combination therapy with conditionally replicating adenovirus and adenovirus-p27. Cancer Res 2006;66(1): 372–7.

[228] Liang Q, Dmitriev I, Kashentseva E, et al. Non-invasive of adenovirus tumor retargeting in living subjects by a soluble adenovirus receptor-epidermal growth factor (sCAR-EGF) fusion protein. Mol Imaging Biol 2004;6(6):385–94.

[229] Liang Q, Yamamoto M, Curiel DT, et al. Noninvasive imaging of transcriptionally restricted transgene expression following intratumoral injection of an adenovirus in which the COX-2 promoter drives a reporter gene. Mol Imaging Biol 2004;6(6):395–404.

[230] Rehemtulla A, Hall DE, Stegman LD, et al. Molecular imaging of gene expression and efficacy following adenoviral-mediated brain tumor gene therapy. Mol Imaging 2002;1(1):43–55.

[231] Zinn KR, Szalai AJ, Stargel A, et al. Bioluminescence imaging reveals a significant role for complement in liver transduction following intravenous delivery of adenovirus. Gene Ther 2004;11(19):1482–6.

[232] Lipshutz GS, Gruber CA, Cao Y, et al. In utero delivery of adeno-associated viral vectors: intraperitoneal gene transfer produces long-term expression. Mol Ther 2001;3(3):284–92.

[233] Lipshutz GS, Titre D, Brindle M, et al. Comparison of gene expression after intraperitoneal delivery of AAV2 or AAV5 in utero. Mol Ther 2003;8(1):90–8.

[234] Blasberg RG, Gelovani-Tjuvajev J. In vivo molecular-genetic imaging. J Cell Biochem 2002;(Suppl 39):172–83.

[235] Bogdanov A Jr, Weissleder R. The development of in vivo imaging systems to study gene expression. Trends Biotechnol 1998;16(1):5–10.

[236] Buchsbaum DJ, Chaudhuri TR, Zinn KR. Radiotargeted gene therapy. J Nucl Med 2005;46(Suppl 1):179S–86S.

[237] Contag CH, Bachmann MH. Advances in in vivo bioluminescence imaging of gene expression. Annu Rev Biomed Eng 2002;4:235–60.

[238] Gambhir SS, Barrio JR, Herschman HR, et al. Imaging gene expression: Principles and assays. J Nucl Cardiol 1999;6(2):219–33.

[239] Gambhir SS, Barrio JR, Herschman HR, et al. Assays for noninvasive imaging of reporter gene expression. Nucl Med Biol 1999;26(5):481–90.

[240] Gambhir SS, Herschman HR, Cherry SR, et al. Imaging transgene expression with radionuclide imaging technologies. Neoplasia 2000;2:118–38.

[241] Herschman HR, MacLaren DC, Iyer M, et al. Seeing is believing: noninvasive, quantitative and repetitive imaging of reporter gene expression in living animals, using positron emission tomography. J Neurosci Res 2000;59(6):699–705.

[242] Iyer M, Sato M, Johnson M, et al. Applications of molecular imaging in cancer gene therapy. Curr Gene Ther 2005;5(6):607–18.

[243] Jacobs AH, Voges J, Kracht LW, et al. Imaging in gene therapy of patients with glioma. J Neurooncol 2003;65(3):291–305.

[244] MacLaren DC, Toyokuni T, Cherry SR, et al. PET imaging of transgene expression. Biol Psychiatry 2000;48(5):337–48.

[245] Ray P, Bauer E, Iyer M, et al. Monitoring gene therapy with reporter gene imaging. Semin Nucl Med 2001;31(4):312–20.

[246] Shah K, Jacobs A, Breakefield XO, et al. Molecular imaging of gene therapy for cancer. Gene Ther 2004;11(15):1175–87.

[247] Zinn KR, Chaudhuri TR. The type 2 human somatostatin receptor as a platform for reporter gene imaging. Eur J Nucl Med 2002;29(3):388–99.

[248] Mathis JM, Stoff-Khalili MA, Curiel DT. Oncolytic adenoviruses—selective retargeting to tumor cells. Oncogene 2005;24(52):7775–91.

[249] Min JJ, Gambhir SS. Gene therapy progress and prospects: Noninvasive imaging of gene therapy in living subjects. Gene Ther 2004;11(2):115–25.

[250] Noureddini SC, Curiel DT. Genetic targeting strategies for adenovirus. Molecular Pharmaceutics 2005;2(5):341–7.

[251] Penuelas I, Haberkorn U, Yaghoubi S, et al. Gene therapy imaging in patients for oncological applications. Eur J Nucl Med Mol Imaging 2005;32(Suppl 2):S384–403.

[252] Phelps ME. PET: the merging of biology and imaging into molecular imaging. J Nucl Med 2000;41(4):661–81.

[253] Rots MG, Curiel DT, Gerritsen WR, et al. Targeted cancer gene therapy: The flexibility of adenoviral gene therapy vectors. J Control Release 2003;87(1–3):159–65.

[254] Spear MA, Herrlinger U, Rainov N, et al. Targeting gene therapy vectors to CNS malignancies. J Neurovirol 1998;4(2):133–47.

[255] Yamamoto M, Curiel DT. Cancer gene therapy. Technol Cancer Res Treat 2005;4(4):315–30.

[256] Bornhop DJ, Contag CH, Licha K, et al. Advance in contrast agents, reporters, and detection. J Biomed Opt 2001;6(2):106–10.

[257] Jacobs AH, Dittmar C, Winkeler A, et al. Molecular imaging of gliomas. Mol Imaging 2002;1(4):309–35.

[258] Dodd CH, Hsu HC, Chu WJ, et al. Normal T cell response and in vivo magnetic resonance imaging of T cells loaded with HIV transactivator-peptide-derived superparamagnetic nanoparticles. J Immunol Methods 2001;256(1–2):89–105.

[259] Ray S, Paulmurugan R, Hildebrandt I, et al. Novel bidirectional vector strategy for amplification of therapeutic and reporter gene expression. Hum Gene Ther 2004;15(7):681–90.

[260] Ponomarev V, Doubrovin M, Serganova I, et al. A novel triple-modality reporter gene for whole-body fluorescent, bioluminescent, and nuclear noninvasive imaging. Eur J Nucl Med Mol Imaging 2004;31(5):740–51.

[261] Bogdanov A Jr, Weissleder R. In vivo imaging of gene delivery and expression. Trends Biotechnol 2002;20(8):11–8.

[262] Bogdanov A Jr. In vivo imaging in the development of gene therapy vectors. Curr Opin Mol Ther 2003;5(6):594–602.

[263] Josephson L, Kircher MF, Mahmood U, et al. Near-infrared fluorescent nanoparticles as combined MR/optical imaging probes. Bioconjug Chem 2002;13(3):554–60.

[264] Kircher MF, Allport JR, Graves EE, et al. In vivo high resolution three-dimensional imaging of antigen-specific cytotoxic T lymphocyte trafficking to tumors. Cancer Res 2003;63(20): 6838–46.

[265] Lee I-H, Bulte JWM, Schweinhardt P, et al. In vivo magnetic resonance tracking of olfactory ensheathing glia grafted into the rat spinal cord. Exp Neurol 2004;187(2):509–16.

[266] Alauddin MM, Louie AY, Shahinian A, et al. Receptor mediated uptake of a radiolabeled contrast agent sensitive to beta-galactosidase activity. Nucl Med Biol 2003;30(3):261–5.

[267] Bai J, Ding W, Yu M, et al. Radionuclide imaging of mesenchymal stem cells transplanted into spinal cord. Neuroreport 2004;15(7):1117–20.

[268] Zhao M, Yang M, Li XM, et al. Tumor-targeting bacterial therapy with amino acid auxotrophs of GFP-expressing Salmonella typhimurium. Proc Natl Acad Sci U S A 2005;102(3):755–60.

[269] Yamauchi K, Yang M, Jiang P, et al. Development of real-time subcellular dynamic multicolor imaging of cancer-cell trafficking in live mice with a variable-magnification whole-mouse imaging system. Cancer Res 2006; 66(8):4208–14.

[270] Glinsky GV, Glinskii AB, Berezovskaya O, et al. Dual color-coded imaging of viable circulating prostate carcinoma cells reveals genetic exchange between tumor cells in vivo, contributing to highly metastatic phenotypes. Cell Cycle 2006;5(2):191–7.

[271] Tsuji K, Yamauchi K, Yang M, et al. Dual-color imaging of nuclear-cytoplasmic dynamics, viability, and proliferation of cancer cells in the portal vein area. Cancer Res 2006;66(1):303–6.

[272] Yamauchi K, Yang M, Jiang P, et al. Real-time in vivo dual-color imaging of intracapillary cancer cell and nucleus deformation and migration. Cancer Res 2005;65(10):4246–52.

[273] Yang M, Jiang P, Yamamoto N, et al. Real-time whole-body imaging of an orthotopic metastatic prostate cancer model expressing red fluorescent protein. Prostate 2005;62(4):374–9.

[274] Burton DW, Geller J, Yang M, et al. Monitoring of skeletal progression of prostate cancer by GFP imaging, X-ray, and serum OPG and PTHrP. Prostate 2005;62(3):275–81.

[275] Wang J, Yang M, Hoffman RM. Visualizing portal vein metastatic trafficking to the liver with green fluorescent protein-expressing tumor cells. Anticancer Res 2004;24(6):3699–702.

[276] Yang M, Amoh Y, Li L, et al. Dual-color fluorescence imaging of tumor-host interaction with green and red fluorescent proteins. In:

Proceedings of SPIE—The International Society for Optical Engineering. 2004. p. 54–60.

[277] Katz MH, Takimoto S, Spivack D, et al. An imagable highly metastatic orthotopic red fluorescent protein model of pancreatic cancer. Clin Exp Metastasis 2004;21(1):7–12.

[278] Yamamoto N, Yang M, Jiang P, et al. Determination of Clonality of Metastasis by Cell-Specific Color-Coded Fluorescent-Protein Imaging. Cancer Res 2003;63(22):7785–90.

[279] Goodison S, Kawai K, Hihara J, et al. Prolonged dormancy and site-specific growth potential of cancer cells spontaneously disseminated from nonmetastatic breast tumors as revealed by labeling with green fluorescent protein. Clin Cancer Res 2003;9:3808–14.

[280] Glinskii AB, Smith BA, Jiang P, et al. Viable circulating metastatic cells produced in orthotopic but not ectopic prostate cancer models. Cancer Res 2003;63(14):4239–43.

[281] Katz MH, Takimoto S, Spivack D, et al. A novel red fluorescent protein orthotopic pancreatic cancer model for the preclinical evaluation of chemotherapeutics. J Surg Res 2003;113(1): 151–60.

[282] Yamamoto N, Yang M, Jiang P, et al. Real-time imaging of individual fluorescent-protein color-coded metastatic colonies in vivo. Clin Exp Metastasis 2003;20(7):633–8.

[283] Hoffman RM. Green fluorescent protein imaging of tumour growth, metastasis, and angiogenesis in mouse models. Lancet Oncol 2002; 3(9):546–56.

[284] Hoffman RM. Green fluorescent protein imaging of tumor cells in mice. Lab Anim 2002; 31(4):34–41.

[285] Zhou JH, Rosser CJ, Tanaka M, et al. Visualizing superficial human bladder cancer cell growth in vivo by green fluorescent protein expression. Cancer Gene Ther 2002;9(8):681–6.

[286] Li X, Wang J, An Z, et al. Optically imagable metastatic model of human breast cancer. Clin Exp Metastasis 2002;19(4):347–50.

[287] Hoffman RM. In vivo imaging of metastatic cancer with fluorescent proteins. Cell Death Differ 2002;9(8):786–9.

[288] Rashidi B, Gamagami R, Sasson A, et al. An orthotopic mouse model of remetastasis of human colon cancer liver metastasis. Clin Cancer Res 2000;6(6):2556–61.

[289] Rashidi B, Sun FX, Jiang P, et al. A nude mouse model of massive liver and lymph node metastasis of human colon cancer. Anticancer Res 2000;20:715–22.

[290] Yang M, Jiang P, An Z, et al. Genetically fluorescent melanoma bone and organ metastasis models. Clin Cancer Res 1999;5(11):3549–59.

[291] Yang M, Jiang P, Sun FX, et al. A fluorescent orthotopic bone metastasis model of human prostate cancer. Cancer Res 1999;59(4):781–6.

[292] Yang M, Chishima T, Baranov E, et al. Green fluorescent protein: a new light to visualize

metastasis and angiogenesis in cancer. In: Proceedings of SPIE—the International Society for Optical Engineering. 1999. p. 117–23.

[293] Sun FX, Sasson AR, Jiang P, et al. An ultra-metastatic model of human colon cancer in nude mice. Clin Exp Metastasis 1999;17(1):41–8.

[294] Hoffman RM. Orthotopic transplant mouse models with green fluorescent protein- expressing cancer cells to visualize metastasis and angiogenesis. Cancer Metastasis Rev 1998;17(3): 271–7.

[295] Yang M, Hasegawa S, Jiang P, et al. Widespread skeletal metastatic potential of human lung cancer revealed by green fluorescent protein expression. Cancer Res 1998;58(19):4217–21.

[296] Chishima T, Miyagi Y, Wang X, et al. Metastatic patterns of lung cancer visualized live and in process by green fluorescence protein expression. Clin Exp Metastasis 1997;15(5):547–52.

[297] Yang M, Baranov E, Jiang P, et al. Whole-body optical imaging of green fluorescent protein-expressing tumors and metastases. Proc Natl Acad Sci U S A 2000;97(3):1206–11.

[298] Naumov GN, Wilson SM, MacDonald IC, et al. Cellular expression of green fluorescent protein, coupled with high-resolution in vivo videomicroscopy, to monitor steps in tumor metastasis. J Cell Sci 1999;112(12):1835–42.

[299] Chishima T, Miyagi Y, Wang X, et al. Visualization of the metastatic process by green fluorescent protein expression. Anticancer Res 1997;17:2377–84.

[300] Zinn KR, Buchsbaum DJ, Chaudhuri TR, et al. Noninvasive monitoring of gene transfer using a reporter receptor imaged with a high-affinity peptide radiolabeled with 99mTc or 188Re. J Nucl Med 2000;41(5):887–95.

[301] Katz MH, Spivack DE, Takimoto S, et al. Gene therapy of pancreatic cancer with green fluorescent protein and tumor necrosis factor-related apoptosis-inducing ligand fusion gene expression driven by a human telomerase reverse transcriptase promoter. Ann Surg Oncol 2003; 10(7):762–72.

[302] Rausch M, Baumann D, Neubacher U, et al. In-vivo visualization of phagocytotic cells in rat brains after transient ischemia by USPIO. NMR Biomed 2002;15(4):278–83.

[303] Banerjee P, Reichardt W, Weissleder R, et al. Novel hyperbranched dendron for gene transfer in vitro and in vivo. Bioconjug Chem 2004; 15(5):960–8.

[304] Zhang ZG, Jiang Q, Zhang R, et al. Magnetic resonance imaging and neurosphere therapy of stroke in rat. Ann Neurol 2003;53(2):259–63.

[305] Tanaka M, Swijenburg RJ, Gunawan F, et al. In vivo visualization of cardiac allograft rejection and trafficking passenger leukocytes using bioluminescence imaging. Circulation 2005; 112(Suppl 9):I105–10.

ELSEVIER
SAUNDERS

NEUROIMAGING
CLINICS
OF NORTH AMERICA

Neuroimag Clin N Am 16 (2006) 681–694

Clinical Trials in a Molecular World

Dawid Schellingerhout, MD, Juri Gelovani, MD, PhD*

- The current status of molecular targeted
  therapies in clinic
  Examples of molecular therapies
  Gene therapy of gliomas
  Estrogen receptor
  Androgen receptor
- The problem
  *Problems with current molecular trial
  methodologies*
- Needed for Clinical Trials in a Molecular
  World
  *Improved selection of patient populations
  by imaging (tumor profiling)*

*Improved dose selection
(pharmacodynamic receptor occupancy
studies)*
*Improved monitoring of therapy
(downstream effect assessment)*
Augment biopsies with molecular imaging
- Clinical trials: what is holding molecular
  imaging back?
  *Afflictions of the diagnostic-therapeutic
  duality*
  Afflictions of the imaging marketplace
  Technical limitations
- Summary
- References

Insight into the molecular nature of cancer and other diseases is giving rise to a new generation of therapies aimed at molecular abnormalities. These therapies address specific molecular abnormalities, and thus are generally more efficacious and less toxic than nontargeted therapies.

As experience with these agents grows, however, a gap in knowledge is exposed. The target must be present for a targeted therapy to be effective. Current knowledge is based on biopsy findings at a single point in space and a single instant in time, while targets are known to change dynamically in both space and time. Current technology forces major treatment decisions to be made on the basis of inadequate data.

This gap in knowledge needs to be filled by molecular imaging technology, enabling the noninvasive establishment of the presence of a molecular target, its spatial distribution and heterogeneity, and how this changes over time.

This is a paradigm shift in medical thinking that exposes both a great lack, and a great opportunity in the care of patients. This article discusses the status of molecular imaging in clinical trails today, and looks forward to what physicians would like it to become.

The current status of molecular targeted therapies in clinic

Examples of molecular therapies

Epidermal growth factor receptor

The epidermal growth factor receptor (EGFR) type I growth factor receptor tyrosine kinase family consists of EGFR (also known as HER-1), HER-2, HER-3, and HER-4. All except HER-3 contain a cytoplasmic tyrosine kinase region, and all except HER-2 bind specific ligands at their extracellular domain. Upon ligand binding, receptors dimerize using HER-2 as the preferred binding partner.

M D Anderson Cancer Center, 1515 Holcombe Boulevard, Houston, TX 77030, USA
* Corresponding author.
E-mail address: jgelovani@di.mdacc.tmc.edu (J. Gelovani).

1052-5149/06/$ – see front matter © 2006 Elsevier Inc. All rights reserved.
neuroimaging.theclinics.com

doi:10.1016/j.nic.2006.08.003

Heterodimerization induces tyrosine kinase activity and the downstream MAPK and PI3K signaling pathways [1]. EGFR is a 170-kd cell surface protein with three regions: an extracellular ligand binding domain, a hydrophobic transmembrane domain, and an intracellular domain with tyrosine kinase activity [2,3]. EGFR malregulation is associated with numerous key features of cancer such as autonomous cell growth, inhibition of apoptosis, invasion, angiogenic potential, and development of metastases [2,4–6].

This is of interest, because 40% to 80% of lung cancers overexpress EGFR [7], and lung cancer is the leading cause of cancer-related death in the United States [7a].

HER2 (erbB2/neu), another member of the EGFR family, is overexpressed in 20% to 25% of invasive breast carcinomas [8,9]. HER2 levels correlate strongly with the pathogenesis and prognosis of breast cancer, and HER2 seems to be expressed at much higher levels in cancer than in normal tissues, both at primary and metastatic sites [10]. Many epithelial cancers overexpress EGFR, and clinical trials have suggested that altered EGFR expression or function can influence a patient's response to chemotherapy or radiation [11].

Because of this and other data indicating the importance of EGFR as a driver of cancer, a massive investment has been made by the pharmaceutical industry to develop drugs targeting this pathway. Fig. 1 demonstrates the main features of the EGF receptor, the pathways downstream from it, and the imaging agents and drugs that can inter-react with these.

Gefitinib

Gefitinib is a small molecule that binds to the ATP binding cleft of the EGFR [12]. In so doing, the drug prevents phosporylation of the receptor, and prevents downstream events (eg, activation of AKT, MAPK, and STAT3) that promote tumor growth and survival. Clinical trials have shown that about 10% to 19% of nonsmall cell lung carcinoma (NSCLCA) patients respond favorably to treatment with gefitinib [13,14] even though 40% to 80% of these tumors overexpress EGFR [7]. Lynch and colleagues showed [15] that the subset of NSCLCA patients who respond to gefitinib have mutations in the ATP binding cleft of the receptor. These mutations render the receptor functionally hyperactive with greater and longer phosphorylation activity for equivalent stimuli when compared with normal (wild type) receptor. The receptor mutations are also sensitive to gefitinib inhibition at lower concentration than wild-type receptors, thus explaining the clinical sensitivity of the tumors having these mutations. The remarkable responses induced in

this small group of patients have led to US Food and Drug Administration (FDA) approval for gefitinib in lung cancer [16]. Gefitinib failed to induce clinically significant responses in gliomas [17,18], another type of cancer driven by EGFR. This is likely because the EGFR found in gliomas is not the mutated hyperactive (and gefitinib-sensitive) form of the receptor.

Erlotinib

Erlotinib is an oral EGFR type 1 inhibitor thought to bind to the ATP binding site of HER1/EGFR [19] in a manner similar to gefitinib. It has been approved since 2004 for advanced lung cancer based on a pivotal phase III trial [20]. In this trial, overall response was 8.9% with erlotinib and 0.9% with placebo [20]. The HER1/EGFR status of 325 of 731 patients in the trial was known [20]. Skin rash is being researched as a surrogate marker for drug efficacy [21]. The rationale for this is based on the presence of EGFR in hair follicles and skin, and thus skin toxicity could indicate the presence of pharmacologically significant doses of the agent.

Trastuzumab

The dimerization of HER2/neu with EGFR results in auto- and transphosphorylation and activation of the EGFR complex [15]. Herceptin is a recombinant humanized monoclonal antibody directed at the extracellular domain of the HER2 protein approved for treating metastatic breast carcinoma [10]. Herceptin interferes with the pathophysiology of HER2 by disrupting receptor dimerization and downstream signaling through AKT and other pathways. Other proposed mechanisms include G1 arrest, induction of apoptosis, suppression of angiogenesis, natural killer cell stimulation, and inhibition of DNA repair [10]. The success of Herceptin therapy depends critically on the HER2 overexpressing phenotype and currently is done by immunohistochemistry or *in situ* hybridization of tissue samples. Monitoring serum levels of HER2 extracellular domain is being evaluated as an adjunct or substitute to histology [10]. A pivotal clinical trial demonstrated that combining Herceptin with standard chemotherapy provided higher responses and improved survival than chemotherapy alone [22] in patients who had HER2-overexpressing tumors. Response rates were low, ranging from 12% to 34% for a median duration of 9 months [9], and most Herceptin-responsive tumors acquire resistance by 1 year [22,23]. Proposed mechanisms of resistance are complex but include:

- **Altered receptor–antibody interaction by evolution of a mutated HER2 level or low HER2 level**

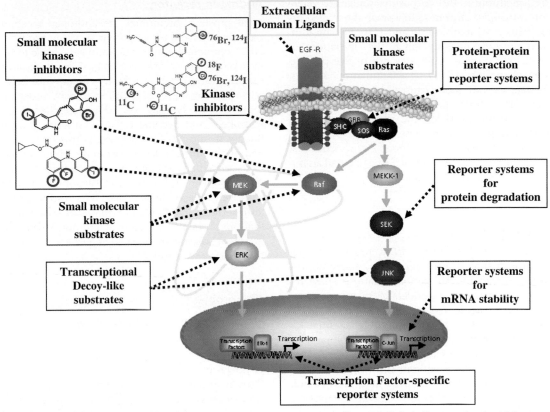

Fig. 1. The EGFR signaling pathway. Notice the many downstream effectors of signaling, each of which represents an opportunity for imaging or therapy.

- Compensatory signaling by other members of the HER family of receptors to downstream effectors
- The activation of other growth-related pathways to circumvent HER2 inhibition [10]

Cetuximab

Cetuximab is a chimeric mouse–human monoclonal antibody that binds competitively and with high affinity to the extracellular portion EGFR. A phase III trial in chemotherapy-refractory metastatic colorectal carcinoma showed a 10.8% response rate for cetuximab as monotherapy (greater when used with chemotherapy) [24]. It is approved for metastatic colorectal carcinoma, but it is undergoing further trials for other malignancies.

Gene therapy of gliomas

Gene therapy is the transduction of therapeutic genes into diseased tissue to induce therapeutic effects. Gene therapy of brain tumors was thought to represent a groundbreaking new therapy, and it was advanced rapidly to clinical trials, reviewed by Jacobs [25]. The first patient was treated in 1994.

Six single-center trials were reported on, along with two multi-center trials using conventional MR imaging and occasionally fluorodeoxyglucose (FDG) or proliferation-based positron emission tomography (PET) imaging as readouts. Results were generally disappointing, with benefit shown only in single patients, most bearing small gliomas.

The first gene marking study was performed by Harsh and colleagues [26]. The authors used stereotactic injection of gene therapy vectors 5 days before tumor resection, with histological examination of the specimens to show thymidine kinase (TK), the transgene thought to be transduced by the gene therapy vector. No tumor transduction was observed in any of five patient samples, with TK expression being limited to vector-producing cells, the carriers of the gene therapy vectors. This study showed limited transduction of tumor tissue to be at the heart of gene therapy's lack of clinical success.

The first gene therapy trial in glioma using imaging as a readout to assess transgene expression was published in 2001 using [124I]FIAU to image TK expression in tumors after catheter-based stereotactic gene therapy of gliomas [27]. This was performed as part of an imaging paradigm that used

[^{11}C]-methionine PET to positively identify viable tumor tissue to target and follow-up the treated tissue with [^{11}C]-methionine and FDG PET in addition to MR imaging after the initiation of ganciclovir therapy. Only one out of five patients showed specific [^{124}I]FIAU accumulation, indicating tracer accumulation caused by transgene expression. The four patients without [^{124}I]FIAU accumulation, however, did show reductions in proliferating cell populations.

Thus there was a gap of about 7 years from first human use, to where molecular imaging had an impact on a molecular therapy.

Estrogen receptor

About two thirds of breast carcinomas are estrogen receptor positive (ER+), identifying those tumors driven in part by estrogen stimulation. These tumors are potential responders to endocrine treatment aimed at depriving the tumor of estrogen. Knowledge of ER status has become essential for managing breast carcinoma [28], and ER+ patients are treated much different from ER- patients, with 30% to 77% of ER+ patients showing a favorable response to endocrine treatments at far less morbidity than alternative chemotherapeutic treatments. In the setting of prior treatment, favorable responses drop to 7% to 21% [29]. ER expression is known to be heterogenous, and knowledge of receptor status at one location does not guarantee that all tumor clones are identical. It is very likely that this heterogeneity in the face of endocrine therapy will select for ER- clones, and a less favorable tumor phenotype. Hence it is of great importance to establish the ER status at all tumor sites as an actual test of ER status, and not to infer this information from a biopsy at a single point in space and time. Fluoroestradiol (FES) is a PET ligand that binds to ER, and it has been shown to predict the response to endocrine therapy in heavily pretreated patients. Standard uptake values (SUV) of greater than 1.5 predicted response in 34% of patients, while no patients with SUV less than 1.5 responded to aromatase inhibitors. In those patients who had HER2/neu-expressing tumors, the response rate was greater, at 46% for SUV greater than 1.5. Estrogen flux measurements of greater than 0.02 mL/min/g had responses of 40% in all patients and 55% in HER2/neu patients [29]. In a given patient, about 15% of sites had FDG avid disease with no FES uptake, indicating some metastatic clones losing their ER+ status [29]. Using FES-PET as a selection tool for patients to undergo endocrine therapy may raise response rates from 23% to 40% by screening out nonresponders predicted by imaging [29].

Androgen receptor

Most prostate carcinomas are androgen receptor (AR) positive, and tumor growth is driven hormonally. Depriving the tumor or androgens leads to tumor cell death or cessation of growth. Medical or surgical castration is an effective therapy for prostate carcinoma [30–32]. Unfortunately, most tumors eventually will lose this dependency on androgens and become resistant to antiandrogen therapy by means of various mechanisms. This process of becoming independent of AR stimulation is likely to be heterogenous, and antiandrogen therapies are likely responsible for selection pressure to androgen-independent clones. Fluoro-dihydroxy-testosterone (FDHT) is a PET analog of testosterone that can probe the AR status of a tumor. This imaging agent is being investigated as a molecular probe in prostate carcinoma [33].

The problem

Problems with current molecular trial methodologies

Heterogeneity between patients and groups of patients

Current thinking in trial design views patients as large homogenous populations to be divided into test and control populations. In the age of targeted therapy, such assumptions are no longer valid. The clear efficacy of EGFR-based drugs in small subgroups of their treatment populations [13,14] and the molecular explanation of why this happens [7] underline the need for targeted therapies to be applied only to those patients who have a valid target.

Heterogeneity within patients: tumor and metastatic heterogeneity

A biopsy samples a small portion of a tumor at a single time point. That small sample then gets processed histologically into 10-μm sections, of which only a few will be examined pathologically for the presence or absence of a molecular target of interest. This is a gross undersampling of the totality of the patient's disease. It ignores the known heterogeneity of tumors and their metastases [34–36], a well-known phenomenon in cancer, and of particular importance in the emergence of resistance to many therapies, particularly molecularly targeted therapies [22,23].

Sampling techniques and tissue processing techniques are heterogeneous between centers

There is little standardization of techniques between centers, particularly for sophisticated tests such as immunohistochemistry and *in situ* hybridization needed to perform molecular targeting studies on tissue samples.

Sampling is ex vivo and teaches nothing of pharmacodynamics
Biopsy is wholly inadequate for studying the interactions of targeted therapies and tumors.

Sampling is usually nonrepetitive, allowing assessment of only a single timepoint
There are hardly any studies that subject patients to repetitive biopsies, implying that most therapeutic decisions are made on a single biopsy at a snapshot in time. It is known that tumor genotype and phenotype are dynamically changing over time.

Current biopsy-based trial methodologies do not translate well to routine clinical practice
Biopsies are complex medical procedures, frequently found only at major centers. Frequently used in clinical trials at major centers, biopsies are used far less frequently once anticancer drugs are administered in the community, and using them as decision makers in the community, where most cancer patients are treated, likely will be difficult to implement.

Needed for clinical trials in a molecular world

Improved selection of patient populations by imaging (tumor profiling)

Epidermal growth factor receptor
An imaging agent is needed that can predict response of a tumor to extracellular (cetuximab) or intracellular (gefitinib, erlotinib) EGFR inhibitors. Such agents are in development [37–59]. An agent that would fit this purpose has been described in animal studies (**Fig. 2**) [60].

HER2/neu
An imaging agent is needed to determine the presence or absence of HER2/neu. Several agents are under development [61–65], with human studies being published [66].

Gliomas
Imaging is needed to delineate and phenotype gliomas. It is becoming possible to gain insight into the major metabolic pathways of brain tumors using imaging (**Fig. 3**) [67,68]. Molecular imaging allows the more precise delineation of glioma borders, thus aiding in better surgical excision [69]. Monitoring glioma therapies is becoming possible [70] and is a key part of the development of experimental therapies for glioma [71–75]. What is needed are predictive imaging tests that can indicate what chemotherapy or gene therapy strategies might be effective for which gliomas. Existing PET tracers need to be advanced to the clinic and subjected to research to determine their benefits in larger patient numbers.

Estrogen receptor
Estrogen receptor status should be an imaging determination primarily, with histologic confirmation. Work with estrogen analog PET agents such as FES is being done to demonstrate how to select patients who have breast cancer for endocrine therapy [29,76–79].

Androgen receptor
PET analogs of testosterone such as FDHT have been synthesized and tested in people, with research into their clinical use underway [33,80,81].

Improved dose selection (pharmacodynamic receptor occupancy studies)
Radiolabeled drug analogs can be used in dynamic competition studies to help determine appropriate dosing regimens for therapeutic agents. This approach is used by the pharmaceutical industry in preclinical drug development [82], but it has yet to make an impact in clinical use. Given the range of interindividual variability between patients and the key importance of knowing if a molecular target has been inhibited/occupied satisfactorily, it seems reasonable to expect this to become a part of the diagnostic armamentarium of the future.

Improved monitoring of therapy (downstream effect assessment)

FDG
FDG is a glucose analog, phosphorylated by hexokinase, the first and rate-limiting enzyme in the glycolytic pathway. Its phosphorylation leads to intracellular entrapment and accumulation in tissues with active glycolysis (such as tumor). Because most tumors have a very active glycolytic pathway, this PET agent is the most universally used of all agents in oncology. Note, however, that there is no molecular specificity in what FDG measures; glycolysis is common to all cells, and is far downstream of any specific interactions. This is both its weakness and its strength; nonspecificity and universal application go hand in hand. As such, the best use of FDG in monitoring therapy is as a far downstream general measure of effect. This was demonstrated in the case of gastrointestinal stromal tumor (GIST) response to imatinib therapy [83–86]. Of significance in these studies is the speed with which a PET response was evident, within

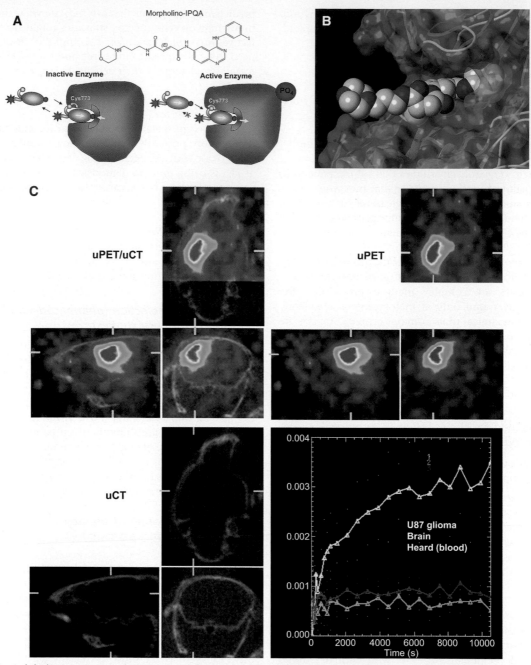

Fig. 2. (*A*) The structure and mechanism of action of Morpholino-IPQA. Note the irreversible binding of the compound to the ATP binding cleft of the EGFR. (*B*) In silico model of 124I-morpholino-IPQA covalently bound to EGFR kinase inside the ATP binding site. (*C*) Noninvasive molecular imaging of EGFR expression activity with 124I-mIPQA PET/CT in orthotopic U87 glioma xenografts in mice.

days of therapy. Feedback that might have taken months, now can be had within a week. This feedback mechanism has vast potential benefits to the patient, as therapy failure potentially could be discovered early, and a rapid change made to more effective therapies (Fig. 4).

¹⁸fluoro-deoxy-L-thymidine (FLT)

FLT is a thymidine analog, phosphorylated by thymidine kinase in the same way that natural thymidine is phosphorylated prior to being used in DNA synthesis. Thus FLT accumulation reflects the activity of the DNA synthetic machinery, and is

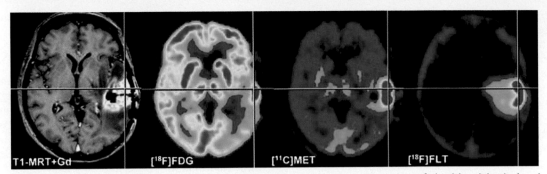

Fig. 3. Mapping the metabolism and pathophysiology of brain tumors. Disruption of the blood–brain barrier and peritumoral edema is shown with gadolinium-enhanced MR imaging. [18F]FDG PET probes glucose uptake and energy metabolism, [11C]MET PET probes amino acid uptake and protein metabolism, while [18F]FLT PET probes DNA synthesis and tumor proliferative activity. *Abbreviations:* FDG, fluoro-deoxy-glucose; FLT, fluoro-L-thymidine; Gd, gadolinium; MET, methionine. (*Reproduced from* Jacobs AH. PET in gliomas. In: Schlegel U, Weller M, Westphal M, editors. Neuroonkologie. Stuttgart: Thieme-Verlag; 2003. p. 72–6; with permission.)

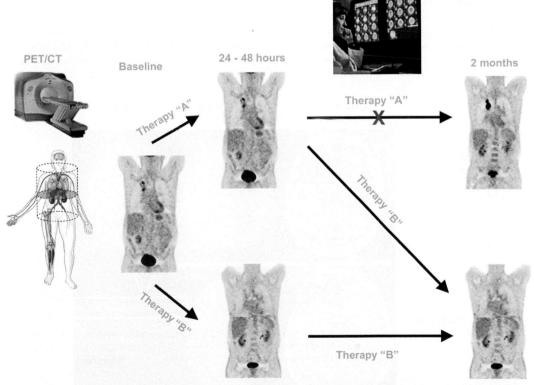

Fig. 4. A future paradigm for diagnostic–therapeutic imaging feedback, allowing the early determination of drug efficacy. Therapy A failed to suppress FDG uptake in this lung carcinoma at 24 to 48 hours, predicting the eventual failure of response at the more usual 2-month follow-up. Therapy B, however, showed an early response, predicting eventual success. Rather than imaging at 2 months or later time points, this early molecular imaging feedback is used to switch the patient from the ineffective therapy to the effective, at the loss of only days, rather than months. This paradigm is likely to be superior to current anatomic measures of effectiveness, as it will allow rapid adjustment of therapy to the individual patient's disease. Feedback can be gained from the specific patient-disease-treatment combination to allow the tailoring of therapies. A paradigm such as this will be necessary for creating and optimizing individualized therapies.

correlated with proliferation of DNA, that is with cell division and growth. Tumors have uncontrolled division and growth as fundamental attributes, thus explaining the success of FLT in imaging cancer. FLT is suited well to measuring the effects of therapy on proliferation, and has a growing body of literature supporting its use [87–90].

Apoptosis/annexin V/caspase

Apoptosis, or programmed cell death, occurs when cells receive a mortal insult and choose to end their own existence. Chemotherapy and radiotherapy very frequently induce apoptosis in cancer cells, and apoptosis is likely a final common pathway for a vast number of anticancer therapies. As an energy-dependent, orderly process, there are predictable changes that occur in cells as they apoptose. Intracellular enzymes, the caspases, control the onset and evolution of the process of apoptosis. One of the predictable changes that cells in apoptosis will undergo is the external display on the cell surface of phosphatidyl serine residues; these residues normally are found only on the cytosolic surface of the cell, and their externalization attracts phagocytes. Annexin V is a protein that binds to exposed phosphatidyl serine residues, and it can be used to label apoptotic cells. Many probes based on this compound have been developed [91–105] and are reviewed elsewhere [106].

Apparent diffusion coefficient

Apparent diffusion coefficient (ADC) measures the water mobility in tissue by means of MR imaging. The use of ADC in diagnosing brain infarctions is established, but ADC also can be used to assess cell death in tumor tissue during therapy [107–110]. The article by Chenevert in this issue has more information.

Hypoxia

[18]F-fluoromisonidazole (FMISO), in combination with ^{15}O-water perfusion imaging, has been used to assess for the presence and severity of intratumoral hypoxia, a major determinant of treatment resistance (Fig. 5) [111]. ^{64}Cu-diacetyl-bis(N4-methylthiosemicarbazone) (ATSM) is another agent being developed to image hypoxia [112–114].

Other agents

There are numerous other agents in development, including agents that target matrix metalloproteinases (MMP) and various disease-related metabolic pathways. As knowledge of the molecular basis of

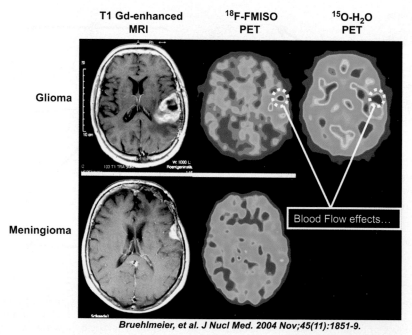

Bruehlmeier, et al. J Nucl Med. 2004 Nov;45(11):1851-9.

Fig. 5. Molecular imaging of hypoxia in brain tumors with 18F-fluoromisonidazole PET and 15O-water. The water scan demonstrates the perfusion to the tumor, while the FMISO scan shows retained tracer in the hypoxic portion of the tumor. Notice the hypoxic (and therefore radioresistant) portion of the glioma, while the meningeoma does not exhibit hypoxia. (*Adapted from* Bruehlmeier M, Roelcke U, Schubiger PA, et al. Assessment of hypoxia and perfusion in human brain tumors using PET with ^{18}F-fluoromisonidazole and 15O-H₂O. J Nucl Med 2004;45:1851–9; with permission.)

disease increases, the scope for molecular imaging will increase with it.

Augment biopsies with molecular imaging

Imaging can demonstrate pertinent molecular features of tumors, confirming biopsy results, but having the benefit of sampling the whole body, not just a single biopsy site. In addition, imaging is repeatable at will and can show dynamic changes in phenotype and disease evolution in ways that biopsy cannot equal. A concerted research effort is needed to correlate biopsy findings to molecular imaging findings. Databases need to be built of spatially tagged biopsies that will allow correlation and study of imaging findings and histological findings, including sophisticated proteomic, genomic and other histological analyses.

Clinical trials: what is holding molecular imaging back?

The question then arises: Why are we not there yet? Many of the technologies are already in place. The questions seem obvious, and the need is great. What follows is a partial, and necessarily subjective, analysis, detailing some of the problems faced by molecular imaging, many of which are common to all emerging fields.

Afflictions of the diagnostic–therapeutic duality

Chicken and egg problem
Therapy and diagnosis evolve as a duality. This is especially true for molecular therapy and imaging. There are many molecular therapies that need imaging support, and will fail without it. There are many molecular imaging tracers that are of vast potential importance in phenotyping disease and assessing the response of therapies that will not get used, because they are not linked to a molecular therapy that would justify the expense and trouble of acquiring this information. The future development of the field requires a far-sighted, balanced approach to allow both therapy and diagnosis to flourish. Without a tight symbiotic relationship between imaging and therapy, coevolution cannot happen.

Conservatism in the therapeutic or imaging community
This translates roughly into: Why do we need this? Why not keep using traditional anatomic imaging and outcomes? Imagers and oncologists are used to using anatomic criteria to judge tumor response. Thinking of imaging as a whole-body biopsy requires a paradigm shift and change in practice that induces short-term discomfort.

Impatience in the therapeutic or imaging community.
CT and MR imaging were adopted by the medical community, because their superiority was obvious. Their usefulness was proven after the fact and validated the common sense notion that this new technology was a good idea. This same common sense (seeing is believing effect) favors the early adoption of molecular imaging, even before efficacy and validation studies, and could theoretically lead to excessively rapid adoption (see Regulation below).

Money
The money available for clinical research is limited, and imaging is expensive. Frequently, it is the major budget item on clinical therapeutic studies. When therapy and diagnosis compete for resources, one or the other will end up with less than requested. Therapists have a bias for therapy, diagnosticians for diagnosis.

Jealousy and meddling
Turf battles can stifle development.

Political inequality (junior partner effect)
Politically, diagnosis is currently subservient to therapy, and resources follow this pattern. Thus, radiology/imaging departments frequently are under-resourced and understaffed. Thus, they often are unable to mount the research effort to move their half of the diagnostic–therapeutic duality forward. As a result, both diagnosis and therapy are held back from their full potential.

Afflictions of the imaging marketplace

Regulation of reimbursement
Because of heavy regulation in the case of PET, there is a large lag between what is possible and desirable clinically, and what is allowed and reimbursed. It took many years and huge amounts of data for regulators and payors to catch up to the well-founded conviction of clinical practitioners that PET imaging is a good and useful thing in the case of FDG (and indications are still strictly limited). The long battle for other tracers still lies ahead. Overzealous regulation can be used as a cost-control tool, with seemingly positive effects on the budgets of payors, but to the long-term detriment of patients.

Regulatory bias against imaging agents
The FDA approval process for drugs of any sort is biased to therapeutics. New imaging drugs have to go through prohibitively expensive tests aimed at screening out toxic therapeutics and proving therapeutic efficacy. These tests often are poorly suited to the evaluation of imaging drugs, and their cost and regulatory burden often unfairly prohibit the

development of useful imaging pharmaceuticals. Regulatory reform is occurring slowly.

Lack of entrepreneurship

There are many imaging advances and drugs, but relatively few translation events. One reason is the shortage of champions to carry these innovations to market.

Lack of industrial interest

The capital and resources of industry, driven by the profit motive, make the therapeutic market thrive. National Institutes of Health (NIH) money is too little and allocated too strongly toward therapy, and at best will supply only a part of the expensive research needed to validate new imaging agents. Once the hope of profit exists, the market will bring its considerable financial and political capital to bear on molecular imaging, and lead to the validation and exploitation of many new imaging agents.

Expense of imaging research

Imaging research is expensive, often comprising the major part of the costs of clinical trials designed to measure therapeutic drug outcomes. Imaging research, by its nature, requires more imaging than most therapeutic trials, and this needs to be paid for by someone. The potential payors are relatively few, commensurate with the current size of the molecular imaging market, and in contrast to the size and activity of the therapeutic market. Companies feel that their payoff is less clear, and hence they have a smaller appetite for risk taking and funding in imaging.

Technical limitations

Lack of clinically suitable radionuclides

Whole families of radionuclides will need to be developed to address such issues as detection, tumor profiling, therapeutic selection, therapeutic dosing, monitoring of early treatment response, monitoring of disease recurrence, and the imaging of imagable therapeutics (theragnostics). This extends far beyond the currently available FDG and a few other tracers, and will require a concerted academic, commercial, and regulatory effort to develop.

Lack of small ^{11}C cyclotrons

There are multiple ^{11}C-based agents available that are suitable only for the research setting, because of the extremely short half-live of the isotope. If ^{11}C could be manufactured reliably and cheaply on site at more centers, the routine use of these agents might become feasible.

Need for more sensitive positron emission tomography systems with longer bores

Current PET systems require the patient to be stepped through the scanner at multiple locations because of the limited length of the PET ring in the Z direction. This multiplies the time needed to perform the examination and puts limits on the area that can be covered. Greater detector sensitivity is needed to reduce the dose of the radiopharmaceutical needed to form a diagnostic quality image yet further.

Positron emission tomography–MR imaging or positron emission tomography–MR imaging–CT systems are needed

Particularly in neurological imaging, where MR imaging is the main clinical diagnostic modality, a combination system with PET would allow significant synergies, similar to that released by CT-PET. Alternatively, flawless automated coregistration technologies that work reliably between differing modalities would need to be developed to allow MR imaging to be wedded to PET.

Summary

The problems described are the problems of a field in its youth or infancy, and is in symmetry with tremendous opportunities. Molecular imaging is destined to be the fulcrum of future clinical trials involving molecular therapies. This future is inevitable, but can it be hastened by improved insight into the complexities faced by the molecular imaging community as it strives to move these technologies forward to the clinic.

References

[1] Graus-Porta D, Beerli RR, Daly JM, et al. ErbB-2, the preferred heterodimerization partner of all ErbB receptors, is a mediator of lateral signaling. EMBO J 1997;16(7):1647–55.

[2] Grunwald V, Hidalgo M. Developing inhibitors of the epidermal growth factor receptor for cancer treatment. J Natl Cancer Inst 2003;95(12): 851–67.

[3] Herbst RS. Review of epidermal growth factor receptor biology. Int J Radiat Oncol Biol Phys 2004;59(Suppl 2):21–6.

[4] Yarden Y. The EGFR family and its ligands in human cancer: signaling mechanisms and therapeutic opportunities. Eur J Cancer 2001; 37(Suppl 4):S3–8.

[5] Schlessinger J. Cell signaling by receptor tyrosine kinases. Cell 2000;103(2):211–25.

[6] Starling N, Cunningham D. Monoclonal antibodies against vascular endothelial growth factor and epidermal growth factor receptor in advanced colorectal cancers: Present and future

directions. Curr Opin Oncol 2004;16(4): 385–90.

[7] Arteaga CL. ErbB-targeted therapeutic approaches in human cancer. Exp Cell Res 2003; 284(1):122–30.

[7a] American Cancer Society. Cancer facts and figures: 2005. Available at: www.cancer.org.

[8] Slamon DJ, Clark GM, Wong SG. Human breast cancer: correlation of relapse and survival with amplification of the HER-2/neu oncogene. Science 1987;235(4785):177–82.

[9] Slamon DJ, Godolphin W, Jones LA, et al. Studies of the HER-2/neu proto-oncogene in human breast and ovarian cancer. Science 1989; 244(4905):707–12.

[10] Nahta R, Esteva FJ. Herceptin: mechanisms of action and resistance. Cancer Lett 2006; 232(2):123–38.

[11] Shin DM, Donato NJ, Perez-Soler R, et al. Epidermal growth factor receptor-targeted therapy with C225 and cisplatin in patients with head and neck cancer. Clin Cancer Res 2001;7(5): 1204–13.

[12] Wakeling AE, Guy SP, Woodburn JR, et al. ZD1839 (Iressa): An orally active inhibitor of epidermal growth factor signaling with potential for cancer therapy. Cancer Res 2002; 62(20):5749–54.

[13] Fukuoka M, Yanso S, Giaccone G, et al. Multi-institutional randomized phase II trial of gefitinib for previously treated patients with advanced nonsmall cell lung cancer. J Clin Oncol 2003;21(12):2237–46.

[14] Kris MG, Natale RB, Herbst RS, et al. Efficacy of gefitinib, an inhibitor of the epidermal growth factor receptor tyrosine kinase, in symptomatic patients with nonsmall cell lung cancer: a randomized trial. JAMA 2003; 290(16):2149–58.

[15] Lynch TJ, Bell DW, Sordella R, et al. Activating mutations in the epidermal growth factor receptor underlying responsiveness of non-small-cell lung cancer to gefitinib. N Engl J Med 2004; 350(21):2129–39.

[16] Cohen MH, Williams GA, Sridhara R, et al. United States Food and Drug Administration Drug approval summary: gefitinib (ZD1839; Iressa) tablets. Clin Cancer Res 2004;10(4):1212–8.

[17] Frederick L, Wang XY, Eley G, et al. Diversity and frequency of epidermal growth factor receptor mutations in human glioblastomas. Cancer Res 2000;60(5):1383–7.

[18] Rich JN, Reardon DA, Peery T, et al. Phase II trial of gefitinib in recurrent glioblastoma. J Clin Oncol 2004;22(1):133–42.

[19] Maslyar DJ, Jahan TM, Jablons DM. Mechanisms of and potential treatment strategies for metastatic disease in nonsmall cell lung cancer. Semin Thorac Cardiovasc Surg 2004;16(1):40–50.

[20] Shepherd FA, Pereira JR, Ciuleanu T, et al. Erlotinib in previously treated nonsmall cell lung cancer. N Engl J Med 2005;353(2):123–32.

[21] Perez-Soler R, Chachoua A, Hammond LA, et al. Determinants of tumor response and survival with erlotinib in patients with nonsmall cell lung cancer. J Clin Oncol 2004;22(16): 3238–47.

[22] Slamon DJ, Leyland-Jones B, Shak S, et al. Use of chemotherapy plus a monoclonal antibody against her2 for metastatic breast cancer that overexpresses HER2. N Engl J Med 2001; 344(11):783–92.

[23] Esteva FJ, Valero V, Booser D, et al. Phase II study of weekly docetaxel and trastuzumab for patients with HER-2-overexpressing metastatic breast cancer. J Clin Oncol 2002;20(7):1800–8.

[24] Cunningham D, Humblet Y, Siena S, et al. Cetuximab monotherapy and cetuximab plus irinotecan in irinotecan- refractory metastatic colorectal cancer. N Engl J Med 2004;351(4): 337–45.

[25] Jacobs AH, Voges J, Kracht LW, et al. Imaging in gene therapy of patients with glioma. J Neurooncol 2003;65(3):291–305.

[26] Harsh GR, Deisboeck TS, Louis DN, et al. Thymidine kinase activation of ganciclovir in recurrent malignant gliomas: A gene-marking and neuropathological study. J Neurosurg 2000; 92(5):804–11.

[27] Jacobs A, Voges J, Reszka R, et al. Positron emission tomography of vector-mediated gene expression in gene therapy for gliomas. Lancet 2001;358(9283):727–9.

[28] Osborne CK. Tamoxifen in the treatment of breast cancer. N Engl J Med 1998;339(22): 1609–18.

[29] Linden HM, Stekhova SA, Link JM, et al. Quantitative fluoroestradiol positron emission tomography imaging predicts response to endocrine treatment in breast cancer. J Clin Oncol 2006;24(18):2793–9.

[30] Huggins C, Hodges CV. Studies on prostatic cancer. I. The effect of castration, of estrogen and of androgen injection on serum phosphatases in metastatic carcinoma of the prostate. Cancer Res 1941;1:293–7.

[31] Buchanan G, Irvine RA, Coetzee GA, et al. Contribution of the androgen receptor to prostate cancer predisposition and progression. Cancer Metastasis Rev 2001;20(3–4):207–23.

[32] Loblaw DA, Mendelson DS, Talcott JA, et al. American Society of Clinical Oncology recommendations for the initial hormonal management of androgen-sensitive metastatic, recurrent, or progressive prostate cancer. J Clin Oncol 2004;22(14):2927–41.

[33] Dehdashti F, Picus J, Michalski JM, et al. Positron tomographic assessment of androgen receptors in prostatic carcinoma. Eur J Nucl Med Mol Imaging 2005;32(3):344–50.

[34] Akabani G, Carlin S, Welsh P, et al. In vitro cytotoxicity of 211At-labeled trastuzumab in human breast cancer cell lines: effect of specific activity and HER2 receptor heterogeneity on

survival fraction. Nucl Med Biol 2006;33(3): 333–47.

[35] Socinski MA, Stinchcombe TE, Hayes DN, et al. The emergence of a unique population in non-small cell lung cancer: systemic or loco-regional relapse following postoperative adjuvant platinum-based chemotherapy. Semin Oncol 2006; 33(Suppl 1):S32–8.

[36] Reardon DA, Wen PY. Therapeutic advances in the treatment of glioblastoma: rationale and potential role of targeted agents. Oncologist 2006;11(2):152–64.

[37] Velikyan I, Sundberg AL, Lindhe O, et al. Preparation and evaluation of (68)Ga-DOTA-hEGF for visualization of EGFR expression in malignant tumors. J Nucl Med 2005;46(11):1881–8.

[38] Babaei MH, Almqvist Y, Orlova A, et al. [99mTc] HYNIC-hEGF, a potential agent for imaging of EGF receptors in vivo: preparation and pre-clinical evaluation. Oncol Rep 2005;13(6): 1169–75.

[39] Calderon Sanchez O, Zayas Crespo F, Leyva Montana R, et al. Direct and indirect labeling with 99mTc of an antireceptor monoclonal antibody of EGF. Rev Esp Med Nucl 2005;24(1): 38–44.

[40] Shaul M, Abourbeh G, Jacobson O, et al. Novel iodine-124 labeled EGFR inhibitors as potential PET agents for molecular imaging in cancer. Bioorg Med Chem 2004;12(13):3421–9.

[41] Mishani E, Abourbeh G, Rozen Y, et al. Novel carbon-11 labeled 4-dimethylamino-but-2-enoic acid [4-(phenylamino)-quinazoline-6-yl]-amides: Potential PET bioprobes for molecular imaging of EGFR-positive tumors. Nucl Med Biol 2004;31(4):469–76.

[42] Wen X, Wu QP, Lu Y, et al. Poly(ethylene glycol)-conjugated anti-EGF receptor antibody C225 with radiometal chelator attached to the termini of polymer chains. Bioconjug Chem 2001;12(4):545–53.

[43] Wen X, Wu QP, Ke S, et al. Conjugation with 111In-DTPA-poly(ethylene glycol) improves imaging of anti-EGF receptor antibody C225. J Nucl Med 2001;42(10):1530–7.

[44] Wang J, Chen P, Su ZF, et al. Amplified delivery of indium-111 to EGFR-positive human breast cancer cells. Nucl Med Biol 2001;28(8):895–902.

[45] Bonasera TA, Ortu G, Rozen Y, et al. Potential 18F-labeled biomarkers for epidermal growth factor receptor tyrosine kinase. Nucl Med Biol 2001;28(4):359–74.

[46] Campa MJ, Kuan CT, O'Connor-Mccourt MD, et al. Design of a novel small peptide targeted against a tumor-specific receptor. Biochem Biophys Res Commun 2000;275(2):631–6.

[47] Reilly RM, Kiarash R, Sandhu J, et al. A comparison of EGF and MAB 528 labeled with 111In for imaging human breast cancer. J Nucl Med 2000;41(5):903–11.

[48] Fredriksson A, Johnstrom P, Thorell JO, et al. In vivo evaluation of the biodistribution of 11C-labeled PD153035 in rats without and with neuroblastoma implants. Life Sci 1999; 65(2):165–74.

[49] Ramos-Suzarte M, Rodriguez N, Oliva JP, et al. 99mTc-labeled antihuman epidermal growth factor receptor antibody in patients with tumors of epithelial origin: Part III. Clinical trials safety and diagnostic efficacy. J Nucl Med 1999; 40(5):768–75.

[50] Kurihara A, Deguchi Y, Pardridge WM. Epidermal growth factor radiopharmaceuticals: 111In chelation, conjugation to a blood-brain barrier delivery vector via a biotin-polyethylene linker, pharmacokinetics, and in vivo imaging of experimental brain tumors. Bioconjug Chem 1999;10(3):502–11.

[51] Deguchi Y, Kurihara A, Pardridge WM. Retention of biologic activity of human epidermal growth factor following conjugation to a blood-brain barrier drug delivery vector via an extended poly(ethylene glycol) linker. Bioconjug Chem 1999;10(1):32–7.

[52] Carlsson J, Blomquist E, Gedda L, et al. Conjugate chemistry and cellular processing of EGF-dextran. Acta Oncol (Madr) 1999;38(3): 313–21.

[53] Iznaga-Escobar N, Arocha LAT, Morales AM, et al. Technetium-99m-antiepidermal growth factor-receptor antibody in patients with tumors of epithelial origin: Part II. Pharmacokinetics and clearances. J Nucl Med 1998; 39(11):1918–27.

[54] Goldenberg A, Masui H, Divgi C, et al. Imaging of human tumor xenografts with an Indium-111-labeled anti-epidermal growth factor receptor monoclonal antibody. J Natl Cancer Inst 1989;81(21):1616–25.

[55] Saga T, Endo K, Akiyama T, et al. Scintigraphic detection of overexpressed c-erbB-2 proto-oncogene products by a class-switched murine anti-c-erbB-2 protein monoclonal antibody. Cancer Res 1991;51(3):990–4.

[56] Cuartero-Plaza A, Martinez-Miralles E, Rosell R, et al. Radiolocalization of squamous lung carcinoma with 131I-labeled epidermal growth factor. Clin Cancer Res 1996;2(1):13–20.

[57] Reist CJ, Garg PK, Alston KL, et al. Radioiodination of internalizing monoclonal antibodies using N- succinimidyl 5-iodo-3-pyridinecarboxylate. Cancer Res 1996;56(21):4970–7.

[58] Rusckowski M, Qu T, Chang F, et al. Technetium-99m labeled epidermal growth factor-tumor imaging in mice. J Pept Res 1997; 50(5):393–401.

[59] Morales AA, Zayas Crespo F, Nunez Gandolff G, et al. Technetium-99m direct radiolabeling of monoclonal antibody ior egf/r3. Nucl Med Biol 1998;25(1):25–30.

[60] Glekas A, Pal A, Doubrovin M, et al. Molecular imaging of EGFR kinase activity in tumors with 124-I-labeled small molecular tracer and PET. Mol Imaging Biol 2006, in press.

[61] Steffen AC, Wikman M, Tolmachev V, et al. In vitro characterization of a bivalent anti-HER-2 affibody with potential for radionuclide-based diagnostics. Cancer Biother Radiopharm 2005; 20(3):239–48.

[62] Olafsen T, Kenanova VE, Sundaresan G, et al. Optimizing radiolabeled engineered anti-p185HER2 antibody fragments for in vivo imaging. Cancer Res 2005;65(13):5907–16.

[63] Tang Y, Scollard D, Chen P, et al. Imaging of HER2/neu expression in BT-474 human breast cancer xenografts in athymic mice using [99mTc]-HYNIC-trastuzumab (Herceptin) Fab fragments. Nucl Med Commun 2005;26(5): 427–32.

[64] Tang Y, Wang J, Scollard DA, et al. Imaging of HER2/neu-positive BT-474 human breast cancer xenografts in athymic mice using 111In-trastuzumab (Herceptin) Fab fragments. Nucl Med Biol 2005;32(1):51–8.

[65] Robinson MK, Doss M, Shaller C, et al. Quantitative immuno-positron emission tomography imaging of HER2-positive tumor xenografts with an iodine-124 labeled anti-HER2 diabody. Cancer Res 2005;65(4):1471–8.

[66] Perik PJ, Lub-De Hooge MN, Gietema JA, et al. Indium-111-labeled trastuzumab scintigraphy in patients with human epidermal growth factor receptor 2-positive metastatic breast cancer. J Clin Oncol 2006;24(15):2276–82.

[67] Jacobs AH, Kracht LW, Gossmann A, et al. Imaging in neurooncology. NeuroRx 2005;2(2): 333–47.

[68] Jacobs AH, Thomas A, Kracht LW, et al. 18F-fluoro-L-thymidine and 11C-methylmethionine as markers of increased transport and proliferation in brain tumors. J Nucl Med 2005; 46(12):1948–58.

[69] Kracht LW, Friese M, Herholz K, et al. Methyl-[11C]-L-methionine uptake as measured by positron emission tomography correlates to microvessel density in patients with glioma. Eur J Nucl Med Mol Imaging 2003;30(6):868–73.

[70] Galldiks N, Kracht LW, Burghaus L, et al. Use of 11C-methionine PET to monitor the effects of temozolomide chemotherapy in malignant gliomas. Eur J Nucl Med Mol Imaging 2006; 33(5):516–24.

[71] Uhl M, Weiler M, Wick W, et al. Migratory neural stem cells for improved thymidine kinase-based gene therapy of malignant gliomas. Biochem Biophys Res Commun 2005; 328(1):125–9.

[72] Reszka RC, Jacobs A, Voges J. Liposome-mediated suicide gene therapy in humans. Methods in Enzymology 2005;391:200–8.

[73] Voges J, Reszka R, Gossmann A, et al. Imaging-guided convection-enhanced delivery and gene therapy of glioblastoma. Ann Neurol 2003; 54(4):479–87.

[74] Jacobs AH, Winkeler A, Dittmar C, et al. Positron emission tomography monitoring of antiglioblastoma HSV-1-tk gene therapy. Gene Therapy and Regulation 2003;2(1):49–57.

[75] Jacobs A, Heiss WD. Towards non-invasive imaging of HSV-1 vector-mediated gene expression by positron emission tomography. Vet Microbiol 2002;86(1–2):27–36.

[76] McGuire AH, Dehdashti F, Siegel BA, et al. Positron tomographic assessment of 16-[18F] fluoro-17-estradiol uptake in metastatic breast carcinoma. J Nucl Med 1991;32(8):1526–31.

[77] Mintun MA, Welch MJ, Siegel BA, et al. Breast cancer: PET imaging of estrogen receptors. Radiology 1988;169(1):45–8.

[78] Dehdashti F, Mortimer JE, Siegel BA, et al. Positron tomographic assessment of estrogen receptors in breast cancer: comparison with FDG-PET and in vitro receptor assays. J Nucl Med 1995;36(10):1766–74.

[79] Mortimer JE, Dehdashti F, Siegel BA, et al. Positron emission tomography with 2-[18F] fluoro-2-deoxy-D-glucose and 16-[18F]fluoro-17-estradiol in breast cancer: correlation with estrogen receptor status and response to systemic therapy. Clin Cancer Res 1996;2(6):933–9.

[80] Bonasera TA, O'Neil JP, Xu M, et al. Preclinical evaluation of fluorine-18-labeled androgen receptor ligands in baboons. J Nucl Med 1996; 37(6):1009–15.

[81] Larson SM, Morris M, Gunther I, et al. Tumor localization of 16beta-18F-fluoro-5alpha-dihydrotestosterone versus 18F-FDG in patients with progressive, metastatic prostate cancer. Journal of nuclear medicine: official publication. Journal of Nuclear Medicine 2004;45(3): 366–73.

[82] Hammond LA, Denis L, Salman U, et al. Positron emission tomography (PET): expanding the horizons of oncology drug development. Invest New Drugs 2003;21(3):309–40.

[83] Stroobants S, Goeminne J, Seegers M, et al. 18FDG-positron emission tomography for the early prediction of response in advanced soft tissue sarcoma treated with imatinib mesylate (Glivec). Eur J Cancer 2003;39(14): 2012–20.

[84] Reddy MP, Reddy P, Lilien DL. F-18 FDG PET imaging in gastrointestinal stromal tumor. Clin Nucl Med 2003;28(8):677–9.

[85] Van den Abbeele AD, Badawi RD. Use of positron emission tomography in oncology and its potential role to assess response to imatinib mesylate therapy in gastrointestinal stromal tumors (GISTs). Eur J Cancer 2002;38(Suppl 5): S60–5.

[86] Joensuu H. Treatment of inoperable gastrointestinal stromal tumor (GIST) with imatinib (Glivec, Gleevec). Med Klin (Munich) 2002; 97(Suppl 1):28–30.

[87] Buck AK, Schirrmeister H, Mattfeldt T, et al. Biological characterisation of breast cancer by means of PET. Eur J Nucl Med Mol Imaging 2004;31(Suppl 1):S80–7.

[88] Buck AK, Halter G, Schirrmeister H, et al. Imaging proliferation in lung tumors with PET: 18F-FLT versus 18F-FDG. J Nucl Med 2003;44(9):1426–31.

[89] Buck AK, Schirrmeister H, Hetzel M, et al. 3-deoxy-3-[(18)F]fluorothymidine-positron emission tomography for noninvasive assessment of proliferation in pulmonary nodules. Cancer Res 2002;62(12):3331–4.

[90] Chen W, Cloughesy T, Kamdar N, et al. Imaging proliferation in brain tumors with 18F-FLT PET: comparison with 18F-FDG. J Nucl Med 2005;46(6):945–52.

[91] Dekker B, Keen H, Lyons S, et al. MBP-annexin V radiolabeled directly with iodine-124 can be used to image apoptosis in vivo using PET. Nucl Med Biol 2005;32(3):241–52.

[92] Dekker B, Keen H, Shaw D, et al. Functional comparison of annexin V analogues labeled indirectly and directly with iodine-124. Nucl Med Biol 2005;32(4):403–13.

[93] Dicker DT, Kim SH, Jin Z, et al. Heterogeneity in non-invasive detection of apoptosis among human tumor cell lines using annexin-V tagged with EGFP or Qdot-705. Cancer Biol Ther 2005;4(9):1014–7.

[94] Haas RLM, De Jong D, Valdes Olmos RA, et al. In vivo imaging of radiation-induced apoptosis in follicular lymphoma patients. Int J Radiat Oncol Biol Phys 2004;59(3):782–7.

[95] Johnson LL, Schofield L, Donahay T, et al. 99mTc-annexin V imaging for in vivo detection of atherosclerotic lesions in porcine coronary arteries. J Nucl Med 2005;46(7):1186–93.

[96] Kartachova M, Haas RLM, Valdes Olmos RA, et al. In vivo imaging of apoptosis by 99mTc-annexin V scintigraphy: visual analysis in relation to treatment response. Radiother Oncol 2004;72(3):333–9.

[97] Keen HG, Dekker BA, Disley L, et al. Imaging apoptosis in vivo using 124I-annexin V and PET. Nucl Med Biol 2005;32(4):395–402.

[98] Lan XL, Zhang YX. Preparation of 99mTc-HYNIC-annexin V. Nuclear Science and Techniques/Hewuli 2005;16(5):299–303.

[99] Sarda-Mantel L, Michel JB, Rouzet F, et al. 99mTc-annexin V and 111In-antimyosin antibody uptake in experimental myocardial infarction in rats. Eur J Nucl Med Mol Imaging 2006;33(3):239–45.

[100] Tait JF, Smith C, Blankenberg FG. Structural requirements for in vivo detection of cell death with 99mTc-annexin V. J Nucl Med 2005;46(5):807–15.

[101] Takei T, Kuge Y, Zhao S, et al. Time course of apoptotic tumor response after a single dose of chemotherapy: comparison with 99mTc-annexin V uptake and histologic findings in an experimental model. J Nucl Med 2004;45(12):2083–7.

[102] Toretsky J, Levenson A, Weinberg IN, et al. Preparation of F-18 labeled annexin V: a potential PET radiopharmaceutical for imaging cell death. Nucl Med Biol 2004;31(6):747–52.

[103] Vanderheyden JL, Liu G, He J, et al. Evaluation of 99mTc-MAG3-annexin V: influence of the chelate on in vitro and in vivo properties in mice. Nucl Med Biol 2006;33(1):135–44.

[104] Watanabe H, Murata Y, Miura M, et al. In vivo visualization of radiation-induced apoptosis using (125)I-annexin V. Nucl Med Commun 2006;27(1):81–9.

[105] Yagle KJ, Eary JF, Tait JF, et al. Evaluation of 18F-annexin V as a PET imaging agent in an animal model of apoptosis. J Nucl Med 2005;46(4):658–66.

[106] Lahorte CMM, Vanderheyden JL, Steinmetz N, et al. Apoptosis-detecting radioligands: current state of the art and future perspectives. Eur J Nucl Med Mol Imaging 2004;31(6):887–919.

[107] Uhl M, Saueressig U, van Buiren M, et al. Osteosarcoma: preliminary results of in vivo assessment of tumor necrosis after chemotherapy with diffusion- and perfusion-weighted magnetic resonance imaging. Invest Radiol 2006;41(8):618–23.

[108] Huang Z, Haider MA, Kraft S, et al. Magnetic resonance imaging correlated with the histopathological effect of Pd-bacteriopheophorbide (Tookad) photodynamic therapy on the normal canine prostate gland. Lasers Surg Med 2006;38(7):672–81.

[109] Tomura N, Narita K, Izumi J, et al. Diffusion changes in a tumor and peritumoral tissue after stereotactic irradiation for brain tumors: possible prediction of treatment response. J Comput Assist Tomogr 2006;30(3):496–500.

[110] Babsky AM, Hekmatyar SK, Zhang H, et al. Predicting and monitoring response to chemotherapy by 1,3-bis(2-chloroethyl)-1-nitrosourea in subcutaneously implanted 9L glioma using the apparent diffusion coefficient of water and (23)Na MRI. J Magn Reson Imaging 2006;24(1):132–9.

[111] Bruehlmeier M, Roelcke U, Schubiger PA, et al. Assessment of hypoxia and perfusion in human brain tumors using PET with 18F-fluoromisonidazole and 15O–H2O. J Nucl Med 2004;45(11):1851–9.

[112] Myerson RJ, Singh AK, Bigott HM, et al. Monitoring the effect of mild hyperthermia on tumour hypoxia by Cu-ATSM PET scanning. Int J Hyperthermia 2006;22(2):93–115.

[113] Yuan H, Schroeder T, Bowsher JE, et al. Intertumoral differences in hypoxia selectivity of the PET imaging agent 64Cu(II)-diacetyl-bis(N4-methylthiosemicarbazone). J Nucl Med 2006;47(6):989–98.

[114] Obata A, Kasamatsu S, Lewis JS, et al. Basic characterization of 64Cu-ATSM as a radiotherapy agent. Nucl Med Biol 2005;32(1):21–8.

NEUROIMAGING CLINICS OF NORTH AMERICA

Neuroimag Clin N Am 16 (2006) 695–699

Index

Note: Page numbers of article titles are in **boldface** type.

doi:10.1016/S1052-5149(06)00112-2

United States Postal Service
Statement of Ownership, Management, and Circulation

1. Publication Title		2. Publication Number								3. Filing Date
Neuroimaging Clinics of North America		0	1	0	-	5	4	8		9/15/06

4. Issue Frequency	5. Number of Issues Published Annually	6. Annual Subscription Price
Feb, May, Aug, Nov	4	$195.00

7. Complete Mailing Address of Known Office of Publication (Not printer) (Street, city, county, state, and ZIP+4)

Elsevier, Inc.
360 Park Avenue South
New York, NY 10010-1710

Contact Person
Sarah Carmichael
Telephone
(215) 239-3681

8. Complete Mailing Address of Headquarters or General Business Office of Publisher (Not printer)

Elsevier, Inc., 360 Park Avenue South, New York, NY 10010-1710

9. Full Names and Complete Mailing Addresses of Publisher, Editor, and Managing Editor (Do not leave blank)

Publisher (Name and complete mailing address)

John Schrefer, Elsevier, Inc., 1600 John F. Kennedy Blvd., Suite 1800, Philadelphia, PA 19103-2899

Editor (Name and complete mailing address)

Barton Dudlick, Elsevier, Inc., 1600 John F. Kennedy Blvd., Suite 1800, Philadelphia, PA 19103-2899

Managing Editor (Name and complete mailing address)

Catherine Bewick, Elsevier, Inc., 1600 John F. Kennedy Blvd., Suite 1800, Philadelphia, PA 19103-2899

10. Owner (Do not leave blank. If the publication is owned by a corporation, give the name and address of the corporation immediately followed by the names and addresses of all stockholders owning or holding 1 percent or more of the total amount of stock. If not owned by a corporation, give the names and addresses of the individual owners. If owned by a partnership or other unincorporated firm, give its name and address as well as those of each individual owner. If the publication is published by a nonprofit organization, give its name and address.)

Full Name	Complete Mailing Address
Wholly owned subsidiary of	4520 East-West Highway
Reed/Elsevier, US holdings	Bethesda, MD 20814

11. Known Bondholders, Mortgagees, and Other Security Holders Owning or Holding 1 Percent or More of Total Amount of Bonds, Mortgages, or Other Securities. If none, check box ► None

Full Name	Complete Mailing Address
N/A	

12. Tax Status (For completion by nonprofit organizations authorized to mail at nonprofit rates) (Check one)
The purpose, function, and nonprofit status of this organization and the exempt status for federal income tax purposes:
☐ Has Not Changed During Preceding 12 Months
☐ Has Changed During Preceding 12 Months (Publisher must submit explanation of change with this statement)

(See Instructions on Reverse)

PS Form 3526, October 1999

13. Publication Title		14. Issue Date for Circulation Data Below
Neuroimaging Clinics of North America		August, 2006

15.	Extent and Nature of Circulation		Average No. Copies Each Issue During Preceding 12 Months	No. Copies of Single Issue Published Nearest to Filing Date
a.	Total Number of Copies (Net press run)		3,125	2,800
b. Paid and/or Requested Circulation	(1)	Paid/Requested Outside-County Mail Subscriptions Stated on Form 3541. (Include advertiser's proof and exchange copies)	1,622	1,549
	(2)	Paid In-County Subscriptions Stated on Form 3541 (Include advertiser's proof and exchange copies)		
	(3)	Sales Through Dealers and Carriers, Street Vendors, Counter Sales, and Other Non-USPS Paid Distribution	529	490
	(4)	Other Classes Mailed Through the USPS		
c.	Total Paid and/or Requested Circulation [Sum of 15b. (1), (2), (3), and (4)]	►	2,151	2,039
d. Free Distribution by Mail (Samples, complimentary, and other free)	(1)	Outside-County as Stated on Form 3541	151	145
	(2)	In-County as Stated on Form 3541		
	(3)	Other Classes Mailed Through the USPS		
e.	Free Distribution Outside the Mail (Carriers or other means)			
f.	Total Free Distribution (Sum of 15d. and 15e.)	►	151	145
g.	Total Distribution (Sum of 15c. and 15f.)	►	2,302	2,184
h.	Copies not Distributed		823	616
i.	Total (Sum of 15g. and h.)	►	3,125	2,800
j.	Percent Paid and/or Requested Circulation (15c. divided by 15g. times 100)		93.44%	93.36%

16. Publication of Statement of Ownership
☐ Publication required. Will be printed in the November 2006 issue of this publication.   ☐ Publication not required

17. Signature and Title of Editor, Publisher, Business Manager, or Owner   Date

[signature] Jan Fanucci – Executive Director of Subscription Services   9/15/06

I certify that all information furnished on this form is true and complete. I understand that anyone who furnishes false or misleading information on this form or who omits material or information requested on the form may be subject to criminal sanctions (including fines and imprisonment) and/or civil sanctions (including civil penalties).

Instructions to Publishers

1. Complete and file one copy of this form with your postmaster annually on or before October 1. Keep a copy of the completed form for your records.
2. In cases where the stockholder or security holder is a trustee, include in items 10 and 11 the name of the person or corporation for whom the trustee is acting. Also include the names and addresses of individuals who are stockholders who own or hold 1 percent or more of the total amount of bonds, mortgages, or other securities of the publishing corporation. In item 11, if none, check the box. Use blank sheets if more space is required.
3. Be sure to furnish all circulation information called for in item 15. Free circulation must be shown in items 15d, e, and f.
4. Item 15h, Copies not Distributed, must include (1) newsstand copies originally stated on Form 3541, and returned to the publisher, (2) estimated returns from news agents, and (3), copies for office use, leftovers, spoiled, and all other copies not distributed.
5. If the publication had Periodicals authorization as a general or requester publication, this Statement of Ownership, Management, and Circulation must be published; it must be printed in any issue in October or, if the publication is not published during October, the first issue printed after October.
6. In item 16, indicate the date of the issue in which this Statement of Ownership will be published.
7. Item 17 must be signed.

Failure to file or publish a statement of ownership may lead to suspension of Periodicals authorization.

PS Form 3526, October 1999 (Reverse)

Moving?

Make sure your subscription moves with you!

To notify us of your new address, find your **Clinics Account Number** (located on your mailing label above your name), and contact customer service at:

E-mail: elspcs@elsevier.com

800-654-2452 (subscribers in the U.S. & Canada)
407-345-4000 (subscribers outside of the U.S. & Canada)

Fax number: 407-363-9661

Elsevier Periodicals Customer Service
6277 Sea Harbor Drive
Orlando, FL 32887-4800

*To ensure uninterrupted delivery of your subscription, please notify us at least 4 weeks in advance of move.

ELSEVIER